To
Scott Burr:

A wonderful man with
greatest courage and
talent.

with Love & Respect.

Omar Bagasra

HIV and Molecular Immunity:

Prospects for the AIDS Vaccine

HIV and Molecular Immunity:

Prospects for the AIDS Vaccine

Omar Bagasra, MD, PhD
Professor of Biology
Center for Transgenic & Recombinant Vaccine Research
Lincoln University
Lincoln University, PA, USA

BioTechniques® Books
(Division of Eaton Publishing)

Omar Bagasra
Center for Transgenic & Recombinant Vaccine Research
P.O. Box 128
Lincoln University
Lincoln University, PA 19352

Library of Congress Cataloging-in-Publication Data

[CATALOGING IN PROGRESS]

ISBN 1-881299-10-4

Printed in the United States of America

9 8 7 6 5 4 3 2 1

Cover graphic depicts the concept of molecular immunity against retroviruses, particularly HIV-1. HIV-1 is entering a CD8+ cell that already expresses a repertoire of mRNAs antisense to an array of retroviral genes. Upon entry, the crucial gene segments of HIV-1 will be blocked and the virus will not be able to enter the nucleus of the host cells.

This book is dedicated to the memory of Dr. Abdus Salam (1926–1996), whose major achievements include a Nobel prize in 1979 for his work on the Standard Model, and the creation of the International Centre for Theoretical Physics, which offered a central forum for scientists of all nationalities to interact. He will forever be remembered as a brilliant scientist and an exceptional spirit.

Foreword

I first became aware of Dr. Omar Bagasra and his work in May of 1992 when he published an article in the *New England Journal of Medicine* (1) presenting the possibility that larger numbers of human blood cells are infected with HIV than was believed at that time. Every scientist now knows that a significant percentage of circulating lymphocytes are infected with HIV, and that control of viral load is one of the major goals of therapy for HIV-infected individuals—but in 1992, his findings were highly controversial.

Dr. Bagasra and his colleagues used a powerful new technique, the in situ polymerase chain reaction. Proper and accurate use of this technique, which allows the detection of specific nucleic acid sequences within single cells at the microscopic level, had the potential to bring many of the hazy issues of HIV retrovirology into clearer focus. But Dr. Bagasra is not only a skillful, innovative laboratory researcher; he is also a discerning scholar who explores novel ideas, many of which he has discussed with me during scientific conferences.

HIV and Molecular Immunity is, I believe, a comprehensive reflection of his provocative theory, which bears on the mechanisms of molecular immunity against retroviruses, as well as on the origin and evolution of the AIDS virus.

HIV research has culminated in several scientific breakthroughs that have allowed us to dream of controlling the AIDS epidemic by treatments and vaccines. However, there are still many unknowns, such as the mechanisms of cell death and the way in which HIV escapes its host's immune responses.

The unraveling of these questions will certainly serve to control the AIDS epidemic, but it may also lead to new developments in the treatment and prevention of other chronic diseases of multifactorial origin in which retroviruses may trigger a cascade of pathologic phenomena.

The reader will find in this book, together with many novel concepts, a wealth of scientific information in the field of HIV research.

Luc Montagnier
Summer 1998

1. **Bagasra, O. et al.** 1992. Detection of human immunodeficiency virus type 1 provirus in mononuclear cells by in situ polymerase chain reaction. N. Engl. J. Med. *326*:1385.

Preface

"The transition from a paradigm in crisis to a new one from which a new tradition of normal science can emerge is far from a cumulative process, one achieved by an articulation or extension of the old paradigm. Rather it is a reconstruction of the field from new fundamentals, a reconstruction that changes some of the field's most elementary theoretical generalizations as well as many of its paradigm methods and applications. During the transition period there will be a large but never complete overlap between the problems that can be solved by the difference in the modes of solution. When the transition is complete, the profession will have changed its view of the field, its methods, and its goals."

Thomas S. Kuhn
The Structure of Scientific Revolutions, 3rd ed.

Over 60% of the world's population is infected with this agent and 8 million individuals develop the resultant disease each year. The majority of those infected live in economically poor nations. Only 20% receive adequate treatment. It accounts for 7% of the deaths in the world and more than 1 in 4 of the preventable diseases. Some of the infected patients live for over 5 decades, with a protracted, indolent illness, while others die in only a few years.

I am not describing AIDS— but tuberculosis. In the next decade, however, this will be the shape of the AIDS epidemic. Tuberculosis has been with us for thousands of years, but when it first gripped our societies, it caused unspeakable devastation. And then this enormously destructive disease receded from Europe and North America. But how? why?

The scientific community has theories and hypotheses, and yet very few facts to explain such occurrences. What sort of immunity was involved in checking the TB epidemic in the Western World? Was it antibodies to tuberculosis bacteria that were protective, or was it the cell-mediated, CD8+ killer T cells that finally conquered the illness?

The development of a system of recognition of foreign invaders, self versus non-self, and pathogenic versus benefactor has been a complex evolutionary process that has taken millions of years to mature. Understanding these defense mechanisms requires clear knowledge of many aspects of biological science as well as immunology. Since the 14th century, man has known that survivors of plague were resistant to subsequent infection. This knowledge of acquired immunity was the basis for the development of modern immunology concepts.

Perhaps the first major attempt to explain a developed resistance to infection came from Ehrlich in 1890, when he presented the side chain theory (1). According to this theory, each cell that is capable of producing an antibody possesses on its surface a repertoire of side chains that can bind many types of antigens. Upon interaction with a specific antigen, these cells stop producing all other types of antibodies and only produce antibodies against the antigen they intercepted. Subsequently, as our understanding of antibody responses to antigens and especially to haptens increased, we realized that the body can produce antibodies to almost any kind of natural or synthetic agent. The side chain theory fell out of favor because we found it difficult to imagine millions of different types of side chains on a single cell.

In 1931, Breinl and Haurowitz (2) forwarded the template theory, which differed radically from the side chain theory. They proposed that antigens actually act as templates and somehow instruct cells to produce a mirror image of the molecules against antigens. However, the basic concepts of molecular biology began to emerge at this time and scientists realized that the shapes of proteins were the result of nucleotide sequences in DNA. After this discovery, it was difficult to imagine an extrinsic protein influencing the formation of nucleotide sequences.

Jerne, Talmage, and Burnet (3) then developed the clonal selection theory, which proposed that antibodies to different types of cells already exist in organisms, each type on a different cell. After an antigen enters the system, it binds its counterpart antibody on the cell surface and this antigen–antibody complex stimulates the cell to proliferate and form many clones, producing large amounts of the same antibody. The molecular mechanisms of this concept are well established and have been confirmed. Currently, the clonal selection theory, with some minor alterations, is considered the accepted paradigm. According to Thomas Kuhn (4), the paradigm is a generally held belief accepted by the mainstream or majority and is therefore very difficult to change, since all experimental designs follow its narrow confines.

Scientists do not always personally arrive at paradigms by critical testing, but rather through education or indoctrination. What we believe to be an absolute truth may have many layers, or may not be as absolute as we once believed. Immunologists do not often study nature directly, but rather observe phenomena and make interpretations that neatly fit into the clonal selection theory paradigm.

In this book, I present a new concept of natural defense that is operational against retroviral infections. I present overwhelming evidence that neither humoral nor cell-mediated immunity can offer adequate protection against retroviral infections. More curiously, the protection against lentiviral infection in the naturally infected nonhuman primates comes about in the absence of humoral or cell-mediated immune responses. What then are the mechanisms and what are the molecules that protect different species from the onslaught of retroviral infection?

This book does not refute the clonal selection theory, which encompasses humoral and cell-mediated immunity, but rather adds another layer to this paradigm. With the addition of this new layer, we will be able to expand our understanding of the defense mechanisms against retroviral infections.

I have been working on this theory for over 15 years and have collected many anomalous findings, which exist mostly as cursory notes. Often they are nothing but a line or two by investigators, who are struggling to explain anecdotal observations they may have made. I have done my best to cite them. On some occasions, I have disagreed with the interpretations of the investigators whose studies I have reported, but I have done my best to be fair and truthful. I have read the original articles cited in this book and all the papers I could find cited in those. Nevertheless, this work is not the unbiased view of a scientist (I don't believe any author could claim that), but it is a specific point of view that I would like to share with the research community and the world. My desire was not to deride others' work or to take on the AIDS research establishment. I want as many readers as possible to see the whole picture as I see it, with all of the critical data, as quickly as possible.

This book is the result of my awareness of the tremendous crisis we are facing regarding AIDS. The majority of treatment efforts are directed towards industrialized nations, while infected persons in poorer countries are ignored. Moreover, many pharmaceutical companies have made a fortune developing anti-HIV-1 agents, knowing full well that these agents will quickly become obsolete and that prices for these agents are higher than many patients can afford. On the other hand, the so-called vaccine trials have failed. Every attempt to develop a vaccine that confers protection in the primate models of AIDS has so far resulted in failure.

So what is the solution? This book offers a new direction for the AIDS research and scientific communities, a new direction towards the development of an HIV-1 vaccine, and it offers the first comprehensive evidence for the existence of a third type of immunity against retroviruses.

This book breaks new ground and reconstructs various old models. It is my hope that it will open new areas of reseach in the race for an HIV-1 vaccine, as well as in many other areas of scientific research. As with many inventors and nonconformists who have brought forth new and radical ideas, I also face the potential negative reaction. But if this work saves a single human life, I know I have done my job as a scientist, a healer, and a human being.

November 1998

REFERENCES

1. **Ehrlich, P.** 1990. The Croonian Lecture on immunity. Proc. R. Soc. Lond. *66*:424.
2. **Breinl, F. and F. Haurowitz.** 1930. Chemical investigation of the precipitate for and anti-hemoglobin serum and remarks on the nature of antibodies [in German]. J. Physiol. Chem. *192*:45.
3. **Burnet, F.M.** 1957. The Clonal Selection Theory of Immunity. Vanderbilt Press, Nashville.
4. **Kuhn, T.S.** 1996. The Structure of Scientific Revolutions, 3rd ed. University of Chicago Press, Chicago.

Acknowledgments

There are many colleagues and friends who deserve my thanks for encouraging me to complete this project and making constructive suggestions. I thank Charles Wood, John Molavi, Robert Marshall Henderson, Mike and John Finney, and Terry Phillips for reviewing the manuscript; my friend and colleague John Hansen whose initial rewrite convinced me to write the rest of the book; my graduate students and post-doctoral fellows, M. Amjad, Matthew Memoli, Maureen Abbey, Lisa Bobroski, Erika Young, and my assistant Saikumari; and my wife Theresa and my children Alex and Anisah, for their support as well as almost daily reading and editing of the manuscript. My thanks to Steve Weaver, Director and Editor-in-Chief of BioTechniques Books, for believing in the project and providing me with encouragement and moral support. And finally, many thanks to Christine McAndrews, Managing Editor of BioTechniques Books, for being so patient and vigilant with this project. English is not my first language, and at times that fact made this book more difficult to edit than to write.

Contents

Chapter 1

Introduction

"It was a radical proposal that ran counter to the generally accepted central dogma of molecular biology: that there is a unidirectional flow of genetic information from DNA to RNA to protein. In this setting, Temin's hypothesis that RSV replicates by transfer of information from RNA to DNA not only failed to win acceptance from the scientific community but was met with general derision."

Geoffrey M. Cooper
The DNA Provirus: Howard Temin's Scientific Legacy

In the course of scientific investigation, data sometimes emerge that cannot be readily reconciled with existing theory. Yet scientists are by their nature reluctant to reach for a new theory when the old concepts are still seemingly viable, albeit in need of revision or update. Usually, the consequence of this scientific reticence is simply enlivened debates at academic conferences or in scholarly journals. However, in the field of human immunodeficiency virus type 1 (HIV-1) pathogenesis, the effect of a decade-long lack of progress in understanding the fundamental biology of retroviral infection can be measured in human terms. Literally 33 million people may be infected with HIV-1 by now, and many will likely die of acquired immunodeficiency syndrome (AIDS) and its complications if rapid progress is not made. Effective treatments must be developed that work at the molecular level, for that is the scale at which retroviruses work, and an effective vaccine for HIV-1 is desperately needed because the epidemic is continuing to expand worldwide.

Clues to effective treatment and the development of a vaccine have long been before us, but conventional wisdom has repeatedly misguided us in the course of scientific investigation. Just 5 years ago, for example, most scientists thought HIV-1 infection included a long latency period in which there was little or no viral activity; we now know this hypothesis may be completely wrong, and the lines of inquiry that resulted were blind alleys (1). Worse still, inconsistencies between anomalous facts and prevailing theory have led to the expenditure of considerable capital in a counterproductive argument over the etiologic agent of AIDS, long after overwhelming data has incontrovertibly shown HIV-1 to be the cause of the disease. The dissenters against the HIV–AIDS hypothesis have made many valid observations, particularly involving the various cofactors that clearly influence the course of HIV-1 pathogenesis (2); however, mainstream scientists have focused more energy upon being appalled at the dissenters than upon trying to examine and accommodate the kernels of truth in their arguments. Of course, existing immunologic theory makes the accommodation of these dissenters' concepts, as well as considerable amounts of enigmatic epidemiological and laboratory data, exceedingly difficult.

The fact is that retroviruses are a unique form of infectious agent and one that has direct access to the genome of the host species (3). The genetic nature of retroviruses is fundamentally different from all other infectious agents—a characteristic that may allow the virus to cause substantial genetic damage to the host (4), even permanent change to the germline of the host species. In fact, some molecular biologists argue that the action of retroviruses has been a critical factor in the course of vertebrate evolution (5–8). Conventional humoral immunity (HI; antibody formation) and cell-mediated immunity [CMI; cytotoxic T cells, natural killer (NK) cells, etc.] seem to be ineffective against most retroviruses (9–22); however, it is almost inconceivable that higher organisms have evolved without some means to control this special sort of pathogen; otherwise retroviruses would have caused massive genetic damage to myriad host species long ago. Furthermore, there is an abundance of data, derived both in vitro and in vivo, that show mammals are indeed quite capable of controlling the actions of retroviruses, but the observed characteristics of the immunologic response do not seem to fit any existing theory of immunology.

Even though the vast majority of humans with high-risk behaviors exposed to significant doses of HIV-1 become infected (in a traditional definition of infectious diseases) and develop antibodies to HIV-1 antigens, many individuals remain uninfected with the virus despite histories of multiple high-risk sexual exposure to the virus (23–26). For example, it has been shown that the CD4+ T cells of some individuals have resisted very high doses of virus (about 1000-fold more virus than what is required to establish infection). Also, in these individuals, the majority of cells have failed to support viral replication (25,26).

While the HIV-1 pandemic has been the central focus for health care providers and has captured the major share of the public's attention, many species of African nonhuman primates infected with various strains of simian immunodeficiency viruses (SIVs) are providing a valuable perspective into our understanding of host–retrovirus interaction (27–37). For example, over 50% of African green monkeys are infected with a substrain of SIV subtype (SIV_{agm}) in the wild, yet no clinical pathology has been associated to date (30,38–46). Similarly, sooty mangabeys have been shown, both in the wild and in breeding colonies, to be infected with another substrain (SIV_{sm}) (31,42,45–46). Like the African green monkey infection, the sooty mangabey infection appears to cause no disease in its native host. These and many African nonhuman primates are the natural hosts of SIVs; they harbor the virus for all of their lives without developing disease (38–46). There is a striking homology between the SIV of sooty mangabeys and human immunodeficiency virus type 2 (HIV-2) (47), but there is a marked difference in the clinical course, with the course of HIV-2 infection being significantly prolonged (47–49).

There is sequence homology between HIV-1 and an SIV isolated from chimpanzees, SIV_{cpz}, which causes no apparent illness in the naturally infected chimpanzees (33–37). Of particular note, chimpanzees experimentally infected with HIV-1 fail to develop overt disease despite establishment of infection as determined by transient viremia, development of HIV-1-specific antibodies, and HIV-1-specific cytotoxic T cells (50–55).

Since 1991, there have been 388 vaccine development trials utilizing various nonhuman primate models of AIDS. Numerous vaccine strategies were utilized, but none except live attenuated virus or genetically related nonpathogenic viruses have resulted in consistently high levels of protection following challenge with pathogenic genetically related virus (56–77). The vaccine efforts utilizing nonhuman primates have shown quite clearly that if the monkeys are first infected with a nonpathogenic lentivirus, then challenged with a genetically closely related pathogenic variety, they do not develop disease (68–77). However, if they are first infected with high doses of a pathogenic variety that is genetically unrelated to any prior lentiviral infection, then the monkeys do develop AIDS-like disease. This complex pattern of clinical expression among lentiviruses is shared by other species of retroviruses that infect humans. For example, the human foamy viruses (HFVs) or spumaviruses (SVs) have yet to be clearly associated with any disease in humans, although a high prevalence of infection exists in certain populations, and infectious virus can be readily cultured in explanted tissues from these individuals (78–83). Human T-cell leukemia/lymphoma virus type II (HTLV-II) has been shown to be endemic in certain Native American populations, but there is no evidence of clinical disease (84,85). Human T-cell leukemia/lymphoma virus type I (HTLV-I) causes disease in a small minority of patients, leading to either adult T-cell leukemia (ATL) if acquired in infancy or to a chronic neuropathic disease if acquired later in life (note the ages of immunoincompetence) (84).

Similarly, although less dramatically, substantial disease variability has been observed in the clinical course of HIV-1 infection. There are reports of long-term survivors, surviving as long as 15 years (86–117), and recent estimates show that at least 1% of HIV-1-exposed individuals may never develop the disease (87,99–106). In contrast, other reports document patients who rapidly progress to immunodeficiency in a matter of a few years (88–90, 92–98).

Pediatric HIV-1 infection is typified by a bimodal pattern of disease progression (91–96). About 20% of perinatally infected infants exhibit a rapid course towards AIDS with immunological deterioration, low CD4+ T-cell count, high viral burden, failure to thrive, delay in development or regression in intellectual capacities, and a very high mortality rate (91–96). About 80%

of children with perinatal HIV-1 infection show a relatively slower development of disease, long-term survival, low viral burden, and limited morbidity (91–98). Some identical, monochorionic, monozygotic twins, born to HIV-1-infected mothers, show discordant results. This means that one is infected with HIV-1, and the other one is uninfected—because in monozygotic, monochorionic fetuses, the blood flow is not equal. One gets more blood than the other. In this situation, the first twin gets exposed to high doses of HIV-1, and the second one gets lower doses; the first one gets infected while the second one is in effect "vaccinated" against HIV-1 (118–120).

The documented exposure of more than 2400 health care workers is a most curious case because only 4 have seroconverted, and none has developed AIDS (99–101). Then there are the cases of spontaneous clearance of HIV-1 (102–105) as well as the low frequency of successful transmission of HIV-1 resulting from a single intercourse with an infected partner, even though HIV-1 is present in 80%–100% of human semen specimens (106–107). Two other anomalous observations are the reported isolation of HIV-1 from individuals who have remained HIV-1 seronegative, and the observation that some men with many different partners with whom they practiced receptive anal sex still remain seronegative (24,26,102–105).

Retrovirus-based vectors have predominated in gene therapy trials, and successful ex vivo transfer of genes has been demonstrated (108–112). However, no human disease has yet been cured utilizing retroviral vectors (109), and even though several studies have demonstrated that therapeutic genes transferred to humans by means of retroviral vectors can be detected in vivo for several years, no long-term biological responses have been documented (110–112). The most publicized therapy, utilizing retroviral vectors containing an adenosine deaminase enzyme expression system, for the treatment of severe combined immunodeficiency, has resulted in failure (110–112). In every case, the retroviral vectors appear to have shut down a few days to a few months after the infusion of vector-containing cells. It is hypothesized that this phenomenon is the result of natural intracellular defenses against retroviruses, and until these intracellular mechanisms have been well defined and are better understood, gene therapy protocols that use retroviral vectors will prove useless.

In mice, the presence of 2 different endogenous proviruses have been identified as protective against infection with certain exogenous retroviruses (113). A similar phenomenon has been noted in chickens in which the presence of certain endogenous retroviruses seems to protect against exogenous viruses, most probably through intracellular molecular immunity (114). *Fv1*, an endogenous *gag*-related gene, has been described recently in certain strains of mice, which makes them resistant to murine leukemia virus (MuLV) (115–117). The *Fv1* gene product is able to block virus in the early phase of the viral life cycle. The course of infection is blocked after reverse transcription (RT) but before the establishment of the integrated provirus in the host genome.

Most of the research efforts on retroviruses over the past 10–15 years have focused on the mechanisms of disease production by these pathogens. Now it is time to explore the mechanisms by which infected hosts defend themselves. The main postulate of this book is that evolution has created some sort of intracellular protective mechanism to specifically battle retroviruses. Many of the previously anomalous phenomena reported by various investigators can be explained on the basis of the hypothesis presented here. For example, it is possible to explain why SIV_{agm}, which has the same overall genomic organization as other lentiviruses, causes no known disease in its native host, the African green monkey. Similarly, it is possible to explain why the SIV_{sm} causes no significant disease in its natural host, the sooty mangabey, and yet causes an AIDS-like illness in experimentally infected, naive rhesus macaques; the same is true for cynomolgus monkeys experimentally exposed to SIV_{agm} (27–46). Extensive analyses of the immune responses of African green monkeys and sooty mangabeys against their respective SIVs show no unusual activity against the virus. They exhibit weak, if any, neutralizing antibodies and no cell-mediated immune response; viral loads in their system are completely independent from their immune responses to the viruses (9–14,16–30,45,46,55,56,60–69,121–125).

I hypothesize both on the basis of much experimental data and on the unintentional experiments of nature that the final disease potential of retroviruses depends on the host–retrovirus interaction, which is primarily governed by the size of the initial dose of virus, the replication capacity of the virus, and the immunocompetence of the host (61,64–77,121). The survival of the host primarily depends on the rapid development of an intracellular molecular immunity that is altogether independent of humoral or cell-mediated immune responses. Molecular immunity can prime the majority of target cells that lack the appropriate defenses, outracing the pathogenic effects of the retroviruses. In humans and nonhuman primates, retroviral-specific molecular immunity could be enhanced under the following circumstances:

(*i*) The host is exposed to very low doses of the pathogenic virus. Low seroconversion in health care workers, clearance of HIV-1 virus from certain individuals, and long-term nonprogressors (LTNPs) with *nef*-defective HIV-1 strains are examples of this situation (68–79,121).

(*ii*) The host is exposed to a nonpathogenic strain of the retrovirus before any exposure to a genetically related pathogenic strain of the virus. Reports of natural immunity in various monkey species against relatively pathogenic SIVs could be explained on the basis of this hypothesis. Since the African primates are exposed to various types of lentiviruses in the wild, they may be protected against a wide range of lentiviruses. On the other hand, the Asian primates who are evolutionarily naive for certain lentivirus strains would be susceptible to even relatively mild types of lentiviral infection. Similarly, neonates and young humans or primates exposed to even relatively mild pathogenic strains of lentiviruses would develop immunodeficiency, due to the late maturation of this molecular immunity system. For example, Ho et al. (122) reported a case in which a woman delivered a baby infected with HIV-1; 12 years later she was without symptoms, although her child had died of AIDS. Baba et al. (70) reported that an attenuated SIV, designated SIVΔ3 (a mutant of SIV deleted in the *nef* and *vpr* genes), induced a lethal AIDS-like disease in 2 of the 4 macaque neonates infected orally, but the infection remained attenuated in the adult after intravenous infection (70). Deacon et al. (123) reported that the 6 recipients of blood or blood products from a single HIV-1-infected donor have remained free of HIV-1-related disease after 10–14 years. The HIV-1 isolated from this donor was found to be defective at the *nef* gene, similar to SIVΔ3 described above (70).

Recently it has been shown that 3 chemokines, MIP-1α, MIP-1β, and RANTES, suppress the ability of HIV-1 to infect CD4+ T cells (126) and, more recently, that the cellular receptors through which these chemicals exert their effect, the coreceptors CCR5 and CXCR4, can also play a role (127,128). Intense genetic analyses of the CCR5 coreceptors have revealed that certain individuals (about 1%) have a 32 base pair (bp) deletion allele, $CCR5\Delta^{32}$. The individuals who possess the homozygous defect in CCR5 are resistant to monocyte-tropic strains of HIV-1 (129,130). It has also been documented that about 11%–17% of Caucasians and up to 1.7% of African-Americans are heterozygous for this $CCR5\Delta^{32}$. However, it appears that only possessing a deleted CCR5 coreceptor does not protect individuals from HIV-1 infection (126,129,130), but there is an indication that it may slow down the progression of AIDS (129,130). Regardless, the excitement over these new discoveries is premature. There is mounting evidence to show that the affinity antibodies generated against the chemokine receptors (i.e., CXCR4 and CCR5) have shown no protection against the primary strains isolated from HIV-1 patients. The findings regarding chemokines explain why different isolates of HIV-1 enter different cell types, but I believe that these chemokine-associated viral tropisms are oversimplified and do not accurately reflect the cellular tropism of the virus (reviewed in Reference 131). They do not explain the fact that the majority of health care workers who have been exposed to HIV-1 have not become infected with the virus nor why several investigators have reported isolation of HIV-1 from individuals who remained HIV-1 seronegative and free of disease (26,102–105).

The central role of CD8+ T cells and their anti-retroviral factor(s) has been well documented (132–139). CD8+ T cells and their anti-retroviral factor(s) from healthy HIV-1-infected or uninfected individuals can suppress HIV-1 replication without killing the infected cells. These are noncytotoxic T cells, noncytolytic, non–major histocompatability complex (MHC) restricted CD8+ T cells, characterized by their ability to reduce HIV-1 replication. I wish to present an abundance of published data, including our own, and new evidence from our laboratory, to support the hypothesis that CD8+ T cells and their anti-retroviral factors belong to a unique form of immunity, distinct from cell-mediated and humoral arms of immunity. I also wish to show how several substances of abuse may adversely affect the anti-retroviral effects of CD8+ T cells.

In the subsequent chapters I will explain many of the relevant aspects of this still relatively unknown molecular immunity and describe how we may utilize our present knowledge to develop vaccines against the AIDS virus.

Chapter 2

Retroviruses and AIDS: Birth of a New Pandemic

"Live poliovirus vaccines were licensed in the United States in 1961, although they had been used extensively in other parts of the world for several years before. Initially, both types of poliovirus vaccines were grown in monkey kidney cells and safety tested in monkeys. The enormous demand for monkeys for these purposes in Europe and North America could initially be met only by importing wild-caught animals, and this was done on a very large scale—mostly from countries in Asia but also from Africa, especially western Africa.

At that time there was no active 'Animal Welfare' movement, nor were large monkey breeding facilities available in Europe or the United States. There was great pressure to get enough animals to satisfy the demand. Holding conditions in both the exporting and importing countries were poor, species of animals were often intermingled at shipping interchanges and stopover points, and handling of animals in the importing countries was such as to facilitate cross-infection between animals of the same and different species. It is not surprising, therefore, that imported primates were often infected with a variety of parasites, not only those common to particular species, but with viruses and other pathogens derived from a variety of other species, including man."

Z. Jezek and F. Fenner
Human Monkeypox

INTEGRATION INTO THE HOST GENOME

Retroviruses are a unique form of infectious agent—one that has direct access to the genome of the host species. The genetic nature of retroviruses is fundamentally different from all other pathogens known; they possess a characteristic that allows the virus to cause substantial genetic damage to the host and even permanent change to the germline of the host species (in fact, some molecular biologists argue that the action of retroviruses has been a critical factor in vertebrate evolution—it is estimated that about 5%–10% of the mammalian genome has been manipulated by reverse transcriptase of retroviral origin during evolution). Yet the 2 well-characterized forms of immunologic response, HI and CMI, do not seem to be effective against retroviruses. What are retroviruses, where do they come from, and how old are they?

Life forms containing reverse transcriptase are not new. It is hypothesized that the first self-replicating molecules in the prebiotic era were RNAs. This concept is based on the assumption that a primitive ribozyme might have served as a template for self-replication (3–8,140–170). Examples of such prebiotic evolutionary index molecules are apparent in bacterial retrons, in mammalian telomerases, in mobile introns of fungal mitrochondria, and in the retroplasmids of fungi (reviewed in References 171 and 172).

It is estimated that over one-third to one-half of the human genome consists of or is the result of reverse transcriptase enzymes found in retroviruses. These include highly repetitive *Alu* sequences, retroviruses, pseudogenes, retrotransposons, and retroelements. The human genome consists of about 3 billion nucleotide base pairs and contains approximately 100 000 genes. If one estimates the total contents of an actual human genome, one may start from the number of expressed mRNAs, which on average contain about 2000 bp per gene. By analyzing the total number of mRNA types, from every cell type in the human system, the total structural genes represent less than 10% of the 3 billion bp of the human genomic DNA. The rest of the genome is made up of regulatory genes, introns, various promoters, many repetitive elements, and many fossilized DNAs of retroelements.

It is estimated that the human genome contains at least 1000 different types of endogenous proviruses (about 0.3%), 4000 long terminal repeats (LTRs: about 0.05%), 40 000 mammalian LTR-transposones (MaLRs: about 5.3%), 90 000 *Alu* sequences (about 6.3%) and about 5×10^8 bp (about 15.2%) of long interspersed repeat sequences (LINES). In addition, about 10% of the human genome consists of pseudogenes, bringing the total to about 37% of the total human genome arising from reverse transcriptase enzyme activity (3,4–8,84,140–175). This information on reverse transcriptase-generated insertions into the host genome indicates that more than one-third of the human genome is composed of already defined retroelements, and as the database on the retroelements increases, it is possible we will discover that a significantly larger portion of the human genome originated from, or is the result of, RT (140–172).

INTERVENING SEQUENCES OR INTRONS

In 1977 the startling discovery was made that eukaryotic genes contained extra segments of DNA which did not appear in the mRNA. These sequences have been named intervening sequences or introns, and the sequences that make up the mRNA are called exons. In many situations, the total length of the introns is significantly greater than the exons (144,164–165). Based upon structural consideration, introns are divided into 4 types (types I–IV). Type I and II are found in many bacteriophages and mitochondria and have endogenous splicing functions in vitro. In vivo, they require additional enzymes called maturases, which are encoded within these introns and have significant sequence homology to reverse transcriptases. These data indicate that the fossilized introns were, at one time, capable of self replication (172). It has been hypothesized that introns were originally self-replicating retroelements that had an independent capacity to enter into and exit out of host genes with ease and without causing any damage to their hosts' genomes (140,144,164–165, 172). Phylogenetic analyses have shown a close relationship between introns and mitochondrial reverse transcriptases. However, at some point during evolution, perhaps the host developed molecular mechanisms to eliminate their reverse transcriptase activities and also devised a method to splice them out during their gene expression phase (146,166). This molecular-based removal of molecular parasites must have been an important evolutionary step in controlling the retroelements that had been assimilated into their genes. In fact, limiting the insertion of retroelements and retroviruses appears to be a major evolutionary step, which probably started several hundred million years ago. By analyzing the *Alu* elements found in humans, Wu et al. estimated that most of the *Alu* insertions occurred before 30 million years ago (168).

The signs of anti-retroelement defense mechanisms have been reported in plants and insects (reviewed in References 6 and 108). For example, both plants and insects can splice the retroelements at the RNA level. In addition, a transcription inhibitory mechanism has been reported in plants (108).

Retroelements are the origin of reverse transcriptase-based life forms. They originated from RNA-based infectious life forms that used reverse transcriptase to weave DNA from the RNA and integrate it into the host DNA. They are abundant among prokaryotes and eukaryotes and include retrotransposons (found in fungi, plants, insects, and other lower life forms), retroviruses (endogenous and exogenous; see below), retrotranscripts (which include *Alu* sequences and pseudogenes) and bacterial retrons. The retroelements have many forms and shapes. Many of them have the ability to integrate into and out of their specific host DNA and are therefore considered mobile genes. However, not all retroelements integrate into the host genome, and certain types have very unique life cycles. For example, pararetroviruses do not integrate but use an RNA intermediate to replicate in the cytoplasm of the host. A very unusual form of retroelements called Mauriceville and Varkud plasmids inhabit the cellular organelles (i.e., mitochondria; 108).

Non-LTR retroposons are found in many species of prokaryotes and eukaryotes. Some exhibit integration site and orientation specificity, and others appear to be random, as far as integration sites are concerned (140,149). Some of these retroelements are up to 9 kb long and encode *gag*- and *pol*-like products (149,167).

A significant portion of the moderately repetitive DNA of mammalian genomes comes from retroposons, which contain LTRs. These include a number of distinct retroposons, such as LINES, SINES (short interspersed sequences, including *Alu* repeats in humans), pseudogenes (cDNA copies of processed mRNA), and tRNA transposons, which resemble tRNA but are completely nonfunctional (169). LINES are derived from transcripts of RNA polymerase II, while SINES are derived from transcripts of RNA polymerase III.

LINES are about 6500 bp long and very abundant in mammalian genomes, about 20 000–50 000 copies of L1 LINES (a subtype of LINES) per genome. They have sequence homologies with reverse transcriptase and an open reading frame, indicating that the LINES originated from active mobile elements.

SINES are usually 75–500 bp in length and contain an adenine-rich 3′ tail similar to the polyadenine tail of mRNA. The best known abundant retroelement family in *Homo sapiens* is *Alu* repeats (because they contain the recognition sequence AGCT for the restriction enzyme AluI), which make up over 5% of the human genome. There are over one million copies of *Alu* repeats in the human genome. The human *Alu* family has a dimerized structure, meaning that the left side is similar to the right side but without the active promoter boxes. The AluI repeats contain a polyadenine tail at the 3′ end, indicating that they have integrated at a new genomic position through an RNA intermediate of the AluI (see Figure 1). A particular SINE from 2 people (except identical twins) would show 80% homology, whereas from 2 different species it would show only 50% homology. The individual members of the *Alu* family are not identical but are related. Therefore, *Alu* repeats and other

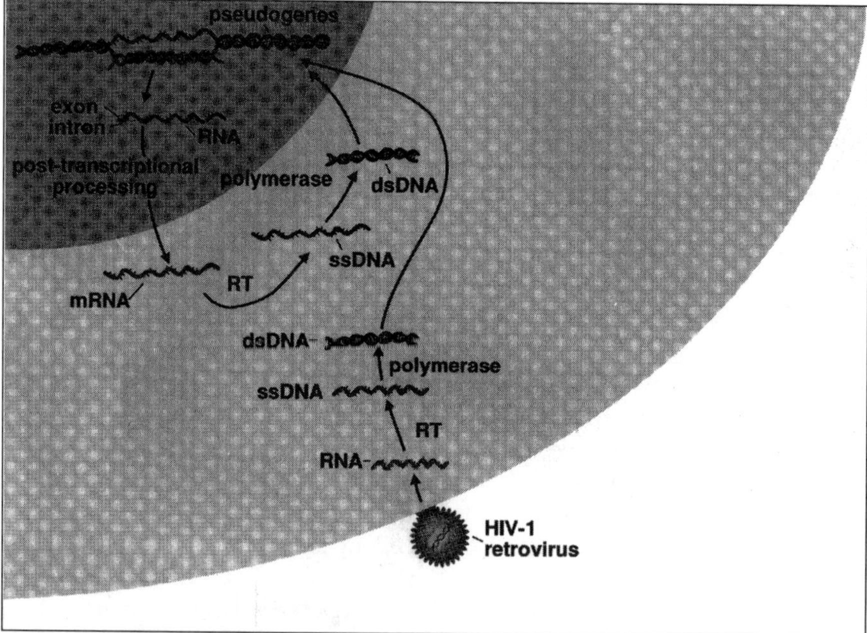

Figure 1. Concept of pseudogene formation. Pseudogenes are formed when cellular mRNAs are exposed to retroviral reverse transcriptase, which results in formation of cDNA copies of mRNA(s). These cellular cDNAs of mRNA subsequently form double-stranded copies of cDNA and then integrate into cellular genomic DNA. The copies of mRNA lack intron sequences and have poly(A) tails. Pseudogenes are inactive genes and may interfere with the normal functions of cellular DNA expression and regulation.

SINES are useful in mapping molecular phylogenetic analyses. For example, comparison of *Alu* repeats in the α-globulin genes of humans and chimpanzees indicates that *Alu* repeats in α-globulin remain in the same position in both species. The analyses of these *Alu* genetic sequences indicate that since the divergence of these 2 species, *Alu* genes mutated at a normal rate: 0.25%–0.5% per million years (168,170–175).

VL30 elements are LTR retrotransposons found in various rodents as well as in humans. These elements are expressed in abundant copies because the mRNA in most cells has the potential to be transmitted. In addition, VL30 elements have been known to transmit host genes and probably play a role in evolution (114,176,177). In the murine genome where VL30 is most studied, they are about 5 kb in length and over 100 VL30 elements are found in the mouse genome with divergent LTR promoters. Other rodents, like rats, also contain numerous VL30 elements but with different gene sequences. In humans there are several retroelements, such as THE1 and MaLR-like elements, which bear close resemblance to VL30 (114,176,177).

PSEUDOGENES AND ANTI-RETROVIRAL IMMUNITY

Many molecular biologists believe that eukaryotic pseudogenes are the result of retroviral reverse transcriptase activity [since they lack promoter and intron sequences and contain stretches of adenine at the 3′ end of the gene, reminiscent of the host's poly (A) tail]. Thus, one of the adverse effects of retroviruses may be the development of pseudogenes, which result from incorporation of mRNA into the host genome (153,178–181). Several recent studies indicate that the numbers of pseudogene copies are about the same in humans, chimpanzees, gorillas, orangutans, and baboons (Figure 1), indicating that appropriate defense mechanisms are in place against retroviruses and that such natural defenses are apparently the result of millions of years of evolution. I believe that higher organisms, including primates and humans, have developed retroviral-directed natural defenses. For example, endogenous retroviral as well as HIV-1 sequences have been detected by various investigators in HIV-1-seronegative individuals (178–181). The high immunogenicity of HIV-1 and the large numbers of circulating HIV-1-specific cytotoxic T cells in humans reported might explain why humans develop a strong immune reaction to HIV-1 upon initial infection (182). Several reports indicate that cytotoxic T-cell clones capable of recognizing HIV-1 gp120, associated with the MHC class II antigens, can be generated from HIV-1-seronegative donors (15,25,26,132,135).

The above information about the abundance of retrovirus and retroviral elements in the mammalian genomes makes 2 points very clear: (*i*) that very few autonomous retroviruses are detected in the mammalian populations, and (*ii*) that these reverse transcriptase-containing elements are rarely pathogenic. The evidence provided here shows that the traditional arms of the immune system, HI and CMI, play an insignificant role in combatting retroviruses. Instead, I believe that higher organisms control retroviruses through much more sophisticated intracellular molecular mechanisms. Furthermore, I will provide an abundance of data, derived both in vitro and in vivo, which show that mammals are indeed quite capable of controlling the actions of retroviruses.

By observing the evolution of retroelements and multicellular organisms, one can conclude that these microparasites coevolved with more complex life forms and reached a symbiotic relationship with higher organisms millions of years before the appearance of mammals, even though we became aware of the harmonious relationship only very recently. For example, in the early 1950s, McClintock et al. (reviewed in Reference 141), observed an unusual phenomenon in maize plants. These investigators noticed the existence of movable genes that inserted themselves randomly into the plant genes and later excised themselves. These genes, which McClintock called “controlling elements”, inhibited the expression of maize genes, but the host functions returned when they were excised. Many microorganisms have developed symbiotic relationships with retroelements. For example, yeast symbiotically utilize an infectious retroviral agent for the creation of a Mating Type locus (140,171–172). Drosophila seem to use a Gypsy-like retrovirus for the same purpose. The yeast and drosophila retroelements are phylogenetically conserved. Similarly, endogenous retroviruses and their derivatives, like medium interspersed sequences (MIRS), LINES, and SINES, are highly abundant in rodents and mammals, and are highly conserved, clearly indicating a symbiotic and harmonious relationship between mammals and their related retroviruses (3,5,6–8,140–176). There appears to be more than one reason why higher organisms harbor such a large number of retroviruses and retroelements. In fact, the survival of both types of life forms may depend on this symbiotic relationship. I will discuss this in a later chapter where I will show that the existence of mammals may be dependent on the expression of certain endogenous retroviruses, and protection against newly emerging retroviruses may lie in the expression of certain repeating retroviral elements. However, one example of this expression can be easily seen in telomerases.

Telomerases are the extreme ends of chromosomes that consist of TTAGGG repeats, about 10 kb long in humans (173–176). During normal somatic cell division, telomeric ends are progressively shortened with each round of replication, which presumably limits the proliferative capacity of normal cells. This is due to the inability of DNA polymerases to fully replicate the 5′ end of the chromosome; since DNA polymerases require a primer and polymerize DNA in only the 5′ to 3′ direction, it is not possible for DNA polymerases to copy the termini of linear chromosomes without an additional mechanism (161–162,173–175). Primordial cells, pluripotent cells, germline cells, several types of tumor cells, and immortalized cell lines can compensate for this telomeric shortening by utilizing an enzyme called telomerase, a ribonucleoprotein that adds new repeats to the 3′ ends of chromosomes, compensating for the shortening that occurs on the opposite strand with each round of replication (161–162,173–175). As primordial cells begin to differentiate during ontogeny, telomerases are inactivated, which results in the shortening of telomeric lengths with each somatic cell division, resulting in limited life span for each cell type. For example, cross-sectional studies have revealed a loss of 30–50 bp per year for human lymphocytes, in vivo (173–175). Telomerases are essentially retrovirus-derived reverse transcriptases. Thus, telomerases are very old enzymes in evolutionary terms and have played a pivotal role in the evolution of higher life forms. Many scientists believe that telomerases evolved a few billion years after bacterial retrons and before the retroplasmids and mobile introns (type II introns) of lower eukaryotic life forms (144,161–162,164–165,173–175). Recently, Linger et al. (140) isolated and characterized the RT motifs in the catalytic subunit of telomerase, which showed a 123-kDa protein with RT activity.

We are at the point where we have a better picture of retroviruses and know more about how rampant they are in our own genome. It is now time to explore how and why a new form of retrovirus, HIV-1, has done so much damage in the human population, as well as where it came from, why it is so pathogenic, and what can be done to stop it from harming us. It is my goal to explore the mechanisms by which higher organisms could disable an invading retrovirus and then explain the causes and events that can lead to the pathogenic manifestations of a retroviral infection. I will also explain how we can make these newly arrived rebellious life forms (i.e., HIV-1 and HIV-2) surrender.

HISTORY, ORIGIN, AND EVOLUTION OF HIV-1

The first report of AIDS dates from June 1981, when the Centers for Disease Control and Prevention (CDC) reported 5 cases of Kaposi's sarcoma (KS) among young homosexual men in Los Angeles (183). Different causes for this cluster of rare skin cancers and the associated *Pneumocystis carinii* pneumonia were considered, including infectious agents, drug abuse (e.g., use of amyl nitrite), and lifestyle factors. Over the next several months, similar cases were described elsewhere, as well as apparent outbreaks of other immunodeficiency-associated conditions. Within the next 12 months after the initial 1981 report, 800 additional cases were reported, and the patients infected included Haitian immigrants, hemophiliacs, transfusion recipients, sex partners of risk group members, and children born to mothers at risk (reviewed in References 1,2,5 and 184). By 1983, an etiologic virus for the disease was discovered by a group led by Luc Montagnier of the Pasteur Institute in Paris (reviewed in Reference 184) through the use of standard virological methods available at that time (tissue culture and electron microscopy techniques). Montagnier and his colleagues had identified one of the first retroviruses to infect humans ever discovered (HTLV-I was the first retrovirus discovered by Robert Gallo's group, but at the time of this new discovery, the real pathogenic nature of HTLV-I was still controversial), which was first dubbed lymphadenopathy-associated virus (LAV) by its discoverers and HTLV-III by Robert Gallo, but its name was later changed to human immunodeficiency virus type 1. The morphology and genome sequences of LAV and HTLV-III were similar to members of the lentivirus genus of the family *Retroviridae*. Soon, a lentivirus causing an AIDS-like disease was discovered in Asian macaques, labeled simian T-lymphotropic virus type III (STLV-III) (38). Finally, in 1986 the designations human immunodeficiency virus and simian immunodeficiency virus were adopted for the lentiviruses of humans and nonhuman primates, respectively (5). HIV-1, described in this study, includes the related viruses worldwide. HIV-2 is the virus prevalent in West African countries (32,47–49, 70).

Serologic detection assays for the virus were soon developed, and scientists across the globe embarked on the quest to better understand the pathogenesis of this novel virus (184). For over a decade, there was little progress. With the benefit of hindsight, we now know many mistakes were made in discerning the proper lines of inquiry, and I believe there are 2 primary reasons for these failures. First, the malady itself was highly unusual: AIDS was a totally new disease with no historical precedent; there was no convenient animal model for in vivo experimentation [and there still is no real animal model that exactly mimics human conditions (185–187)]; and the etiologic agent was a human retrovirus, a poorly understood class of viruses at the time. Second, early investigators did not have any reliable laboratory techniques with sufficient sensitivity to accurately detect the virus intracellularly or quantitatively. Thus scientists had great difficulty gleaning vital pathologic data regarding the activities of HIV-1 inside cells, such as the degree of expression, the nature of this so-called latency, the viral load in lymphoid tissues and other organ systems, etc.

Unfortunately, the inadequate sensitivity of the existing detection methodologies, such as in situ hybridization without amplification, led to false negatives in assays of infected tissues, and these red herrings led most scientists to believe that HIV-1 infected only a very small number of cells, about 1 in 10 000–100 000 peripheral blood mononuclear cells (PBMCs) (188). In response to this rather unusual hypothesis of viral pathology, and other anomalous data, some investigators, whose ideas would later be deemed insupportable, began arguing that this low level of infection showed that HIV-1 was not the cause of AIDS (2). Instead, alternative hypotheses were proposed to explain the CD4+ T-cell destruction that is characteristic of AIDS, such as autoimmunity, antibody-dependent cytotoxic cells, and many other possibilities (88–90). However, as more sensitive techniques to detect the virus developed over time, an abundance of data was produced showing that indeed HIV-1 is the cause of AIDS and the viral burden is at least a thousand times greater than had previously been assumed (189–195).

Now we find ourselves in a situation where over 33 million humans are exposed to HIV-1 worldwide, yet no vaccine is in sight (19–21). Rather, every attempt thus far has failed to produce a vaccine that is even partially effective, and in my opinion, most current lines of inquiry are doomed to failure. The reasons for this are simple—we are either relying upon tried-and-true vaccination techniques that are ineffective against a retrovirus which is rapidly mutating and capable of hiding within the genome of the host before CMI or HI has enough time to intercept them, or we are using synthetic devices to stab in the dark at immunologic phenomena that we simply do not understand.

ENDOGENOUS AND EXOGENOUS RETROVIRUSES

The *Retroviridae* family has been divided into several genera (Figure 2), some of which (HTLV-I-like viruses, the SVs, and the lentiviruses) have not been shown to enter the germline of mammalian species. Therefore, these viruses are regarded as true exogenous retroviruses. On the other hand, the eukaryotic genome contains a wide variety of endogenous retroviruses and retrovirus-like elements that are transmitted as heritable mendelian elements yet exhibit genomic organizational and sequence homologies to infectious exogenous retroviruses (196–201). The majority of these endogenous retroviruses are defective and do not independently replicate. As a result of the symbiotic relationship with their host genome over a great span of time, their survival and duplication is guaranteed and, in return, they no longer have the potential to cause harm to the host. However, one should look at this division between endogenous and exogenous viruses with caution, since pseudotyping can take place, meaning that an exogenous virus can exchange genes with the dormant genes of the endogenous viruses and form a new virus (202–208). Similarly, not all endogenous viruses are completely dead and certain endogenous viruses have been known to express themselves and form particles in various hosts (179–181,200,202–208)—for example, endogenous MuLV in mice (171); avian endogenous retrovirus (113,208–211); feline endogenous virus (212–214); type D endogenous viruses from simian, baboon, and gelada (215–227); type C viruses of macaques (181,220,228–239); and human endogenous retrovirus type K and VL30 (202–208,234–238). Why do these endogenous viruses still replicate and form particles? Do they perform some sort of function for their respective hosts? Are they still active because of their relatively short history of insertion into the host genome, and because of this, are they not completely inactivated? There are many in the field of retrovirology who believe that retroviruses have played a pivotal role in the evolution of mammals (3,5), and there are some who believe that they play an essential role in survival of the viviparous fetus (3,5–6). Recently, Villarreal (6) proposed that the survival of the placental mammalian embryo is totally dependent on the ability of these types of mammals to express certain types of endogenous retroviruses during pregnancy. They suggest that since the embryo is like a foreign allogenic graft and requires specific means to suppress a maternal immune response against it, the activation of endogenous retroviruses in the placental cells provides sufficient immunosuppression (229,234–236). Boyd et al. (236) proposed that the replication of human endogenous retrovirus-like elements (HERV-K and HERV-H) is involved in preventing immune recognition of an embryo by the mother's immune system (45,237). Several families of HERVs have been identified and partly characterized in humans (237–239). HERV-L-related sequences are found at a low copy number in all mammalian species, except in primates and in the murine rodent where they have been amplified up to 100–200 copies. In contrast to HERV-L, amplification of murine endogenous retrovirus-L sequences (MuERV-L) appears to be a recent evolutionary event, as suggested by the uninterrupted open reading frames of the *gag* and *pol* genes in the cloned elements and almost fully identical LTRs, as well as the conservation among all the genomic copies of a series of restriction sites that can be tested by Southern blot analysis (239). Rat genomes do not contain these sequences (239). Interestingly, Benit et al. (239) recently showed a homology between *gag* MuERV-L, *gag* HERV-L, and *Fv1*, the gene that appears to render certain strains of mice resistant to Freund's leukemia virus (FLV)-infection. HERV

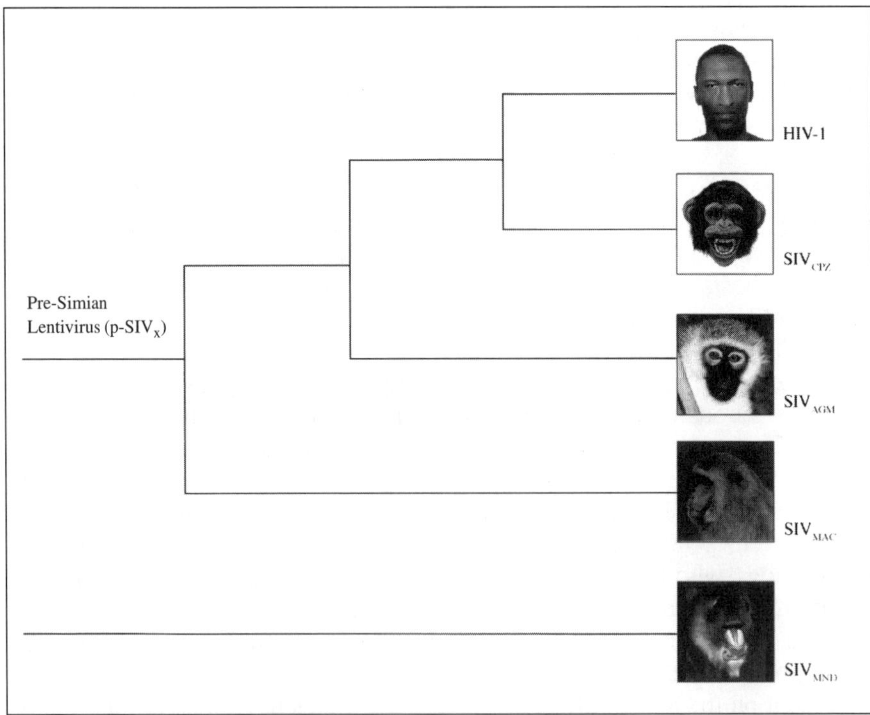

Figure 2. A family tree of lentiviruses: relationship of some selected lentiviruses to their natural hosts. This relationship tree is based on amino acid sequence homologies in the reverse transcriptase protein of the lentiviruses shown.

sequences are estimated to constitute at least 0.6% of human genome. One of the HERV families, HERV-H, constitutes one of the most abundant retroelements, consisting of about 1000 full-length elements and a similar number of solitary LTRs (240). However, the most interesting among the HERV family is HERV-K. HERV-K-derived transcripts have been reported in numerous cell types, including several cell lines like testicular, teratocarcinoma, and lung (241–244). Curiously, normal placental tissue expresses high levels of HERV-K genes, including *pol* and *env* genes (233–238). The human genome contains about 50 copies of HERV-K (108), and it is the only known HERV with open reading frames for all structural and enzymatic proteins (108). It is estimated that HERV-K entered the human genome over 30 million years ago (108), and its sequences are absent in the New World primates. It is the only known HERV that encodes virus-like particles, and similar particles have been repeatedly reported in human placentas (108). I believe that expression of HERV-K in the trophoblasts and in the microvascular endothelial cells, which form a barrier between the maternal and fetal immune systems, creates focal immunosuppression, protecting the fetus from rejection (239–241). The potential role of endogenous retrovirus-like elements in the survival of embryos of viviparous mammals comes from studies of the mouse. All wild mouse embryos have been known to produce very high levels (>10^5 particles/cell) of mouse intracisternal A-type particles (IAP) (207). In addition, human and rhesus monkey syncytiotrophoblasts have been shown to express HERV-K-related reverse transcriptase enzyme, *gag* and *env* gene products (233–239). As a matter of fact, all viviparous mammalian embryos examined so far have demonstrated high levels of expression of endogenous viruses, indicating a symbiotic relationship between the endogenous retroviruses and their respective hosts (43,181,241–246). This symbiosis guarantees the survival of both species. It is not difficult to reach the conclusion that both viviparous mammals and their nondefective endogenous retroviruses have reached harmony in their reproductive cycles. Therefore, during early embryonic implantation and subsequent development of the hosts' new progenies, they require a high expression of these viruses for the survival of their species (239–255) and in return, these hosts provide their endogenous viruses with ample opportunity to propagate and enter into their germlines.

Recently, my laboratory evaluated over 30 placentas and found HERV-K sequences in all of them (Figure 3A; 235–237). This explains why viviparous mammals, as compared to other vertebrates, have accumulated so many proviral variants (like MIRS, LINES, etc.) and why viviparous species possess their unique varieties of proviral genetic elements (5). Based on preliminary observations made in my laboratory, I believe that this system also serves an additional purpose: if a host's differentiation is abnormal, defective due to genetic errors, or is infected early on with some other infectious agents [e.g., syphilis, cytomegalovirus (CMV), rubella virus, toxoplasmosis], the endogenous retroviruses are able to spread beyond the evolutionary boundaries of the placenta (i.e., microvascular endothelial cells and syncytiotrophoblasts), to infect and destroy the host's embryo (235–245,250–261). Currently, my laboratory is evaluating placentas obtained from women who chronically abort after conceiving. It is possible that somehow the expression of HERV is shut down in these women, and the immune system of the mother actually destroys the fetus. These studies are under way. My laboratory has recently evaluated 68 placentas from HIV-1-infected mothers in a blinded fashion and has observed expression of HIV-1 in the syncytiotrophoblasts and microvascular cells of a significant percentage of placental tissues from HIV-1-infected individuals cells (Figure 3B). However, a relatively low percentage of babies born to HIV-1-infected mothers are infected with HIV-1 in utero. We have also observed that if other cell types, besides the microvascular endothelial cells, are infected, then the babies are either stillborn or born with HIV-1 infection. In our studies, we have observed that many cell types are infected with HIV-1 in aborted and stillborn tissues, whereas such infections are limited only to microvascular endothelial cells and syncytiotrophoblasts in babies who appear to be healthy at birth (Figure 3B; unpublished preliminary data). Interestingly, a certain species of wasp has been known to utilize a similar adaptive mechanism to that proposed for viviparous mammals (6,247). The wasp deposits its fertilized eggs with a high concentration of the wasp-encoded polydnavirus into parasitized host larvae. The virus causes immunosuppression of the host larva's immune system, which then is unable to recognize and destroy the wasp eggs (247). Sequence analyses of endogenous proviruses in inbred mice show considerable variation of endogenous retroviruses among different inbred mice. Of over 150 mice proviruses analyzed, only one was common to all strains (248). In almost all cases, about 50% of the proviruses in any one strain shared sequences with some other strains, and each inbred strain also possessed its own

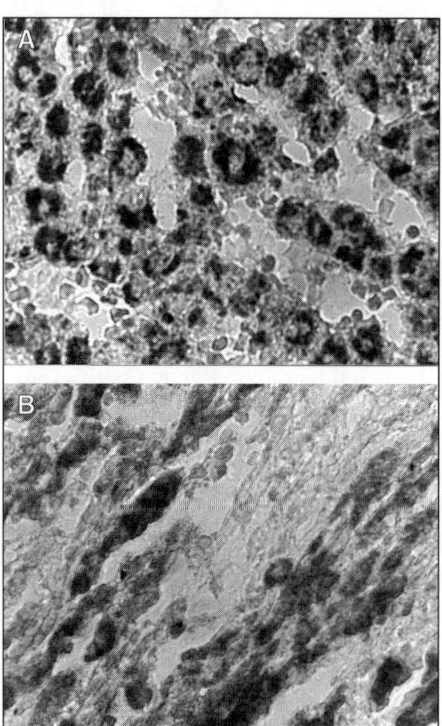

Figure 3. Expression of HERV-K and mammalian survival. (A) Expression of human endogenous retrovirus (HERV-K) mRNA in various cell types of human placenta. Notice the proposed defense lines of immunosuppression at the microvascular endothelial cells. (B) Very similar pattern of viral expression is seen in HIV-1-infected placenta.

unique brand of endogenous proviral sequences. From the detailed sequence analyses, it has been suggested that the different species of inbred mice were invaded by a closely related but different endogenous retrovirus (5,7,140,248, 261–269). These viruses spread clonally within the germline of each species and only recognize each other during cross-mating. This mating may not be without pathogenic consequences. The expression of 3 types of viruses (one from each inbred strain and one as recombinant), can give rise to pathogenic viruses that can lead to a fatal outcome in the form of lymphoma (7,140,248, 249). I will describe below the way I believe the AIDS virus came into existence, possibly by a recombinant event between various simian retroviruses, which were completely nonpathogenic to their native host, but developed into a new recombinant variant(s) when grown in vitro while the polio vaccine was being prepared.

More is known about the evolution of exogenous nonhuman primate lentiviruses than about their endogenous counterparts. Simian lentiviruses, similar to HIVs, have been identified in many genera of nonhuman primates including *Macacus* (rhesus monkeys, pig-tailed macaques, cynomolgus monkeys, and stump-tailed monkeys), African green monkeys or *Cercopithecus* (grivets, green, skyes, tantalus, and vervets), sooty mangabeys, white-crowned mangabeys, mandrills, and chimpanzees (270). These SIVs are related to HIVs in their overall physical structure, genetic makeup, and replication cycle; they induce no clinical symptoms or disease in their native hosts (38–46,271–314). Currently, there are 233 species in the mammalian order of primates, including 77 species of monkeys and 13 species of great apes (including gorillas, chimpanzees, orangutans, and gibbons; the fourteenth species is *Homo sapiens*), which evolved about 60 million years ago from 41 prosimian species (315). The nonhuman primates are divided into 2 distinct groups: the monkeys of the Eastern Hemisphere are called Old World monkeys, and those of the tropical areas of Western Hemisphere are called New World monkeys. SIVs are mainly found in Old World monkeys; they are prevalent in African green monkeys of the genera *Cercopithecus*, and *Cercocebus* (sooty mangabey). Over 30 distinct strains of SIV have been isolated just from African green monkeys captured in the wild (27–49,215,221,223, 286,288,293,316–334) and many more strains of SIVs are found in other wild primates. SIVs are very common among African nonhuman primates and are absent in Asian monkeys. On the other hand, endogenous type D retroviruses are common in Asian monkeys and absent in African green monkeys (44,30,215–230,335,336). Sera isolated from many other primates and apes do not cross-react with SIV or HIV, but this does not mean that they do not harbor lentiviruses, since they may express entirely different antigen dominant epitopes, and hence may not induce the cross-reacting antibodies. A similar situation has been reported in human sera: many humans are infected with certain HIV-1 subtypes but do not show antibodies reacting with screening antigens (337–340). In addition, a significant percentage (up to

70%) of African monkey species held in captivity in various zoos and 19 primate centers in the United States have been demonstrated to have antibodies to SIVs (23,30,37,43–45). In addition, a large percentage (>40%) of animals caught in the wild also have antibodies to SIVs (341–348). In all cases, various strains of SIVs are carried by their natural hosts as a harmless infection in their natural conditions (27–46). The species specificity of SIV for each of their respective monkey species strongly suggests the coevolution of these retroviruses and their natural hosts (27–46). This harmonious coevolution of microparasites and complex hosts is not novel; it exists among many microorganisms and higher animals.

Coevolution between microparasites and macroorganisms has occurred for eons. A virus, bacterium, fungus, or parasite that kills off its host rapidly creates a crisis for itself, since it has to find a new live host quickly and often enough to keep itself alive. Therefore, the ideal condition for the microparasite and the host would be to coexist in a fashion that allows both to survive and creates no harmful side effects for the other. Many examples of such harmonious coevolution exist. Humans carry a huge number of *Bacteroides* in our lower gastrointestinal system as normal flora. We also carry in our mouth and on our skin various species of bacteria and fungi; in return, these microorganisms protect us from the harmful effects of certain more aggressive microorganisms. However, there are other microparasites that have failed to reach a balance with their mammalian hosts (e.g., salmonella, shigella, cholera, malaria, African trypanosomiasis, schistosomiasis, and several others); there are others that are still pathogenic but seem to be less so as time passes (e.g., tuberculosis and influenza). There are also other microorganisms to which the host develops lifelong immunity; if the host survives the early phase of infection it develops a permanent protection (e.g., measles, mumps, smallpox, chickenpox, whooping cough, diphtheria, tetanus, polio, etc.). However, in biological life forms, host–microparasite interactions are not always so simple. Protection against microparasites is not always dependent upon developing antibodies or CMI. Even in the presence of these antibodies and CMI, infections with certain microparasites linger on throughout the life of the host. For example, herpesviruses [i.e., herpes simplex type 1 and 2, CMV, Epstein-Barr virus (EBV), and other related viruses] will keep recurring even in the presence of antibodies and T-cell responses. Shingles will recur after the pathogenic effects of the chickenpox virus have disappeared. The newly discovered human herpesvirus type 8 (HHV-8), appears to be ubiquitous, and apparently most healthy individuals have antibodies to it; however, in immunosuppressed individuals it can cause KS (349–357) or even encephalitis (357).

In the case of humans and nonhuman primates, the process of coevolution is very long, and host–parasite interaction is gradual before a harmonious, stable, and balanced biological relationship is achieved for both life forms. In addition, as the parasites learn to find new ways to exploit the host defenses, the host also develops new weapons and new ways to counter the effects of the parasite, including accommodating the parasite, if necessary. For example, the role of antibody production in mammalian survival is pivotal and hence has gone through many layers of evolutionary change, including immunoglobulin gene rearrangement, various classes of immunoglobulins, isotype switching, T-helper cell dependent and independent antibody formation, and B-cell development. Similarly, the evolutionary importance of the various functions that T cells perform clearly provides a strong impetus for the evolution of these cells (i.e., there are at least 20 subtypes of T cells with apparently different functions). Similarly, I believe that evolution of what I call molecular immunity against genetic parasites like retroviruses had to be of paramount importance for the survival of the genes of any host invaded by these unusual germs. Retroviruses can directly invade the host's DNA; they enter the host cells, reverse transcribe, and integrate into the host's genomic DNA before CMI or antibodies have a chance to develop (both of which take days to weeks to develop). Therefore, there has to be a different mechanism of defense. It appears that hosts and parasitic retroviral RNAs have reached an understanding; the presence of retrovirus-like elements, introns, and retrovirus-related genes in over one-third of human DNA speaks loudly about this understanding. Retroviruses are genetic parasites, and their presence can literally consume and replace hosts' reproductive capabilities. The mere presence of the reverse transcriptase enzyme can create pseudogenes (utilizing the host's own mRNA as a target: see Figure 1) (358,359).

I believe that while various hosts were being invaded by these genetic parasites, some hosts were also developing new means to counter the actions of these parasites by developing a genetic (molecular) immunity, which can block the entry of these agents at every level: at the cellular surface, at the viral uncoating step, at the reverse transcriptase step, and, most importantly, at the entry steps of proviruses into the nuclear membrane (integration step). I believe that the most successful of these evolutionary developments was blocking the entry of a preintegration complex (PIC) of retroviruses into the nucleus of the host (see below for the molecular details). The success of this evolutionary strategy had an advantage over blocking the attachment of the retrovirus onto the cell membrane. Since blocking integration into the nucleus only requires a few molecular mechanisms to counter the parasite, the host may take control of the situation with the least cost to itself, rather than trying to prevent the parasite from bypassing the attachment receptors, perhaps by developing the capability to enter by utilizing the cell-surface molecules that may be essential for the host survival (85,87,127,131,220,289, 340,361–364). Also, by blocking the entry of retroviral proviruses into the nucleus, the host counters the integration of retroviral genes as well as its own pseudogenes. The host has also taken advantage of the preexisting retroviral genes, since their presence reduces the chance of lethal mutations (since all mutations are spread out throughout the whole genome and because retroelements make up one-half to one-third of the total genome, their presence reduces the chance of any lethal damage to the actual host genome). In the event of an encounter with a new, more advanced retroviral pathogen, the integration would also be more likely to take place in the host's retroviral area (due to the sequence homology to common LTR, *gag*, *pol,* or *env* genes. Kantor and Herzenberg (365) have suggested that the existence of distinct B-cell and T-cell lineages that develop successively during ontogeny may mirror the evolutionary stages of the immune system, i.e., lymphocytes capable of more advanced functions were acquired in layers as mammals evolved from more primitive organisms to advanced primates.

I believe (and my laboratory has recently found experimental evidence for this notion) that the existence of multiple copies of various retroelements, SINES and LINES, may indicate an additional function. The millions of copies of small RNAs of endogenous retroviruses containing thousands of different types of RNA may be present in certain subsets of T cells (i.e., CD8+ T cells or NK+ cells) and serve as a repertoire of RNA, with all possible sequences found in all the retroviruses present in nature (similar to immunoglobulin and T-cell receptor repertoires that can bind any possible antigen found in nature). These RNA repertoires would, upon exposure to a new type of retrovirus, bind the critical portion(s) of the invading retrovirus, inhibiting its entry into the cellular nucleus and stopping it at the PIC (347,348; see Figure 4). Therefore, these multiple endogenous retroviruses serve as a first defense line against retroviruses. It is possible that a few weeks after exposure to retroviruses the other types of immune defenses might become activated (i.e., antibodies and cytotoxic T cells) but the real defense exists at the molecular level, and other arms of the immune system play an accessory role, if any. I also believe that once certain sequences of RNAs firmly bind the specific segments of the invading retrovirus, the same inhibitory RNA sequence(s) is synthesized in large numbers by the CD8+ T cells, which initially encountered the invading retrovirus. These newly synthesized RNAs enter many cell types throughout the body and serve as antisense–antiretroviral agents (Figure 4). Some experimental evidence for the existent of protective endogenous retroviral gene sequences is found in mice resistant to FLV. The *Fv1* gene has been known to control the replication of murine leukemia retroviruses and prevent disease in mice infected with FLV (212–214). I will discuss *Fv1* further in a later section.

Now, let us look at what happens when a population of humans is exposed to a entirely new kind of virus. The transfer of a new microparasite into a population from a group of hosts who have no evolutionary history or coevolution with that parasite can create havoc in the new and evolutionarily naive host. One of the most remarkable examples of such an introduction in modern history is the conquest of the Aztec Empire, estimated at 13 million people, by the few thousand in the army of Cortez. A paralyzing epidemic of smallpox killed half of the Aztec population, while the Cortez army had become immune to this virus before their arrival. Black Death, introduced by the Mongol army into fourteenth century Europe, killed over 30 million; cholera epidemics of the nineteenth century killed an estimated 32 million; and the flu epidemic in 1918 killed 21 million people. These are some examples of the devastating outcome of such encounters. Moreover, the introduction of a new parasite that devastates a naive population is not limited to humans; introduc-

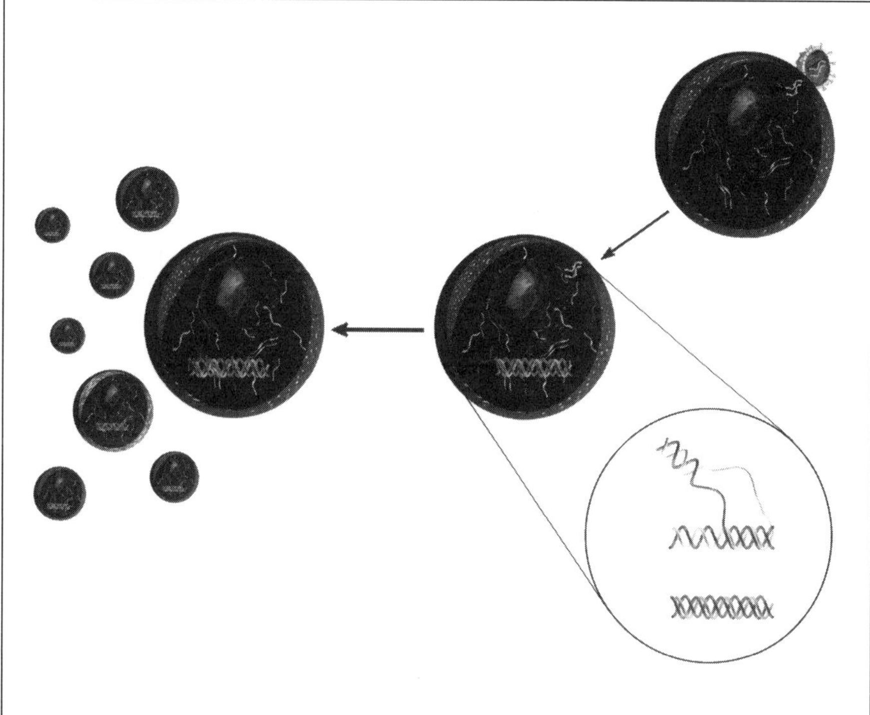

Figure 4. Molecular immunity concept. Top right: HIV-1 or any retrovirus enters the target cells and CD8+/NK+ cells. Upon entrance, they encounter millions of small RNA repertoires. Some of these small RNAs exactly match the gene sequences of the invading target retroviruses. Figure 8 suggests that the most effective step of the defense lies at the preintegration step, where they block the further processing of the retrovirus and its integration step. **Middle center:** The small RNAs that are complementary to the invading provirus form "triple helices" with the retrovirus and block its integration. **Left:** Meanwhile, by utilizing the reverse transcriptase enzyme of the invading retrovirus, millions of additional copies of the "protective" RNAs are replicated at the site of triple helices by the CD8+/NK+ cells, in which the protective RNAs themselves serve as primers for reverse transcriptase. These small protective RNAs are sent off all over the body (like immunoglobulins or cytotoxic T cells), where they enter many different cell types and protect them from the invading retrovirus. This molecular immunity is effective only against the type of the invading retrovirus or against genetically related viruses. The only time this protective barrier is broken is when any of the cells that received the protective RNAs are stimulated. Since in the human body a small number of cells are always stimulated, these cells, if they were infected with retrovirus in question, would produce a low viral load. These virions will enter other target cells but will be stopped at the PIC levels. According to this hypothesis, a low viral burden will always be present but an immunocompetent host will not develop immunodeficiency. However, if initial inoculation viral load is very high or if the host is immunocompromised at the time of inoculation (very young, old, or transiently immunosuppressed), then an overwhelmingly high number of the target cells would be infected, preventing the protective CD8+/NK+ cells from performing optimally.

tion of rinderpest in Africa in 1891 by the Europeans resulted in the destruction of over 90% of domesticated cattle and wild antelope (366). Tuberculosis has been called the number one scourge of native American populations, including those who are natives of Alaska (367). Prehistoric evidence clearly shows that this disease did not exist in the native American peoples before the arrival of Europeans, who had coevolved with the disease for over 3000 years [evidence of tuberculosis exists at least back to 2000 BC (367–369)].

Infections of various monkey species with SIVs, the lentiviruses most closely related to HIV, cause no harmful effects in their natural hosts (27–46, 349–360). However, if one type of monkey gets infected with SIV from another monkey species, variable outcomes can occur, depending on the degree of genetic relatedness of the infecting SIV and the initial inoculating dose. Cross-species transmission of primate lentiviruses has caused several outbreaks in the captive primates (231,306,370–373). For example, accidental or experimental introduction of SIV_{mac} and SIV_{stm} has caused immunodeficiency indistinguishable from human AIDS in rhesus and stump-tailed macaques (56,196–197,272–276,297,310,374–383). Therefore, the lentiviruses that infect various primates in the wild are not necessarily nonpathogenic under all circumstances. They are nonpathogenic in certain species only because of their coevolution with their respective hosts or because of exposure of specific primates to low doses of certain lentiviruses, either during gestation or in the early neonatal period. Similarly, the host species is not intrinsically immune to SIV-induced disease but is only resistant if it has coevolved with that particular strain of lentiviruses or has been exposed to low doses of these viruses early in life. What makes these nonhuman primates resistant to the pathologic consequences of these lentiviruses, which intrinsically are not nonpathogenic? I believe that monkeys get their initial exposure to very low doses of certain strains of SIVs, which are predominant in their particular colony, during fetal life or during delivery or the early neonatal period through breast feeding (58,222,321,335,355,371,378,384–391). Breast milk has been reported to contain lentiviruses as well as other retroviruses and horizontal transmission of such viruses is well documented (392–394). This initial exposure of very low doses of SIVs primes neonates with specific molecular immunity against that particular type of SIV (72,121,395,396). This is similar to human immunization against various vaccines, including diphtheria, smallpox, and polio, except that the mechanisms of defense are entirely different.

THE POSSIBLE ORIGIN OF HIV

The origin of HIV-1 is still an enigma (397). The analyses of an evolutionary tree, based on nucleotide variation in the *gag* and *env* regions of various SIVs, HIV-1, and HIV-2, suggest that HIV-1 diverged from the SIV_{agm}/ SIV_{cpz} group as recently as 50 years ago (reviewed in Reference 19). By similar analyses, it is suggested that SIV_{sm} and HIV-2 could have diverged as recently as 40 years ago (32,47–48). Lentiviruses related to HIV-1 and HIV-2 have been isolated from various nonhuman primate species. Based on their genetic sequences and their antigenic and biological characteristics, these retroviruses are very closely related to HIVs (281,325–330, 398–403). Based on DNA sequence analyses, SIVs fall into 3 subtypes. The HIV-2-related subtype is related to the SIV from macaques and sooty mangabeys (SIV_{mac} and SIV_{sm}; 32,47–49). SIVs from African green monkeys and mandrills (SIV_{agm} and SIV_{mnd}) are distinct and more or less equidistant from HIV-1 and HIV-2 (22–25). HIV-1-related subtypes are related to SIVs isolated from wild-captured, naturally infected chimpanzees from Gabon in West Equatorial Africa and raised in captivity in Belgium and Cote D'Ivoire (28–31). None of the animals naturally infected with these 3 subtypes show any sign of lentivirus-induced pathology (27–50,404–406).

The evolutionary analyses still leave us in the dark regarding the origin of HIV-1. It could have come from SIVs. However, as we concluded from the above examples and discussion, low-dose exposure (through animal bites) of SIV to an immunologically naive person has not caused symptoms of infection (407–411), indicating that perhaps humans who have been accidentally infected with low doses of SIVs through monkey bites do not develop any significant illness because they already have some form of protection against these viruses, or, due to the low dose of the exposure, they have developed resistance instead of illness (407–411). Therefore, it is possible that initial human exposure to pre-HIV-1 lentiviruses was in the form of some mass inoculation with a man-made vaccine containing a high inoculum of pre-HIV-1 or a mixture of various SIV viruses, which subsequently developed into HIVs. Many vaccine trials took place in Central Africa in the 1950s and 1960s (411). Some of the attenuated viral vaccines were produced in monkey kidneys, which might have been contaminated with cells infected with various strains of SIVs and cultured for an extended period of time with different nonhuman cells (like African green monkey kidneys, Asian monkey kidneys, and even chimpanzee kidneys), which could have resulted in more than one recombinant virus. I am offering all of these scenarios in order to explore the possibility that these manipulations might have provided the optimal environment to create new forms of recombinant lentiviruses, like pre-HIV-1 and pre-HIV-2, and also to provide reasons why African monkeys and chimpanzees do not get AIDS from HIV-1 infection. Both types of SIVs, from monkeys and chimpanzees, are known to infect human T cells (412–423). SIV-infected monkeys are numerous in many regions of Central and East Africa, but there is little or no evidence of any human epidemic spreading from monkey bites (407–411) or from ingestion, since monkeys are a frequent source of dietary protein in Africa. Therefore the introduction of recombinant SIVs, developed during the culture of different SIV strains or pre-HIVs, into humans could potentially have formed HIVs. The experimental insight into these mechanisms comes from several laboratories. For example, Horwitz et al. (424) showed that the normal human genome, as well as the normal genomes of primates and apes, contain endogenous retrovirus-related sequences that are closely related to HIV-1. They cloned 2 genes, *EHS-1* and *EHS-2*, from normal human DNA. *EHS-1* showed sequence homologies to certain portions of HIV-1 *env*, while *EHS-2* had sequence homologies to portions of HIV-1 *rev* and *gp41*, as well as certain genes in the rhesus monkey and chimpanzee. It is possible that cocultures and cross-contaminations of various SIVs with human cells and human endogenous viruses could have created new recombinant viruses. In addition, an African SIV_{sm} isolated from African sooty mangabeys has been shown to posses homology to HIV-1 (425). As stated above, many SIVs exhibit >90% homology to HIV-2 (15,18,19,21,23), and SIV_{cpz} isolated from chimpanzees has >90% homology to HIV-1 (33–36). So, is it possible that various types of SIVs present in vaccine-producing cultures might have recombined and formed new types of viruses? The answer to this question is probably affirmative. Harvey and Kirsten MuLVs resulted from recombination of exogenous MuLV with endogenous VL30 elements (108,114, 176–177). These recombinant viruses have been known to form new viruses with new tropism and pathology (178). For example, in a study reported by Vanin et al. (178), a replication-defective MuLV vector was used to transduce bone marrow cells from macaques with a marker gene. Instead, recombination took place, and a replication-competent virus arose and lymphomas developed in 3 out of 10 monkeys within a year. Another example is feline leukemia viruses that acquired altered tropism and pathogenesis from recombination with their endogenous counterparts (214). The acquisition of endogenous genes by exogenous retroviruses demonstrates that a cellular sequence merely needs to provide desirable characteristics to bring about a selectable recombination event.

Recently, a group of investigators from Wright State University, Harvard Medical School, and the New England Primate Research Center have provided direct proof of SIV's recombination in evolutionarily native rhesus macaques. As you may recall, like humans, rhesuses are also naive to SIVs. Recombination of 2 different strains of lentivirus can occur when their RNA genomes are brought together into the same virus particle to create a heterozygous virion. An RT reaction of heterozygous RNA genomes by a copy choice mechanism will produce genetic recombinants (214). (Copy choice mechanism occurs when, in the presence of more than 2 types of RNA, the growing DNA chain switches from one RNA template to another during minus-strand DNA synthesis.) A heterozygous virion is the result of packaging of 2 different types of RNA molecules replicated in a cell infected with 2 types of retroviruses. Another mechanism of recombination could be intracellular recombination of 2 or more different types of retroviruses. In order to directly demonstrate retroviral recombination events in vivo, these investigators infected rhesus macaques with 2 different molecularly cloned strains of SIVs.

One strain of virus had a deletion in *vpx* and *vpr*, and the other strain had a deletion in *nef* (nonpathogenic clones of SIV). When injected into rhesus alone, each strain induced low viral loads and manifested no pathogenic effect in the monkeys. However, when injected simultaneously into separate legs of the same primate, persistent high viral load and depletion of CD4+ cells were noted. Analysis of proviral DNA isolated directly from PBMCs revealed that full-length, nondeleted SIV_{mac} (214) predominated by 2 weeks after infection. These observations provide direct proof of genetic recombination between 2 different, nonpathogenic strains in an infected host. These results also clearly illustrate how easily and quickly an intravirion or intracellular recombination can take place in a host infected with different nonpathogenic SIV strains and result in a pathogenic form.

If an evolutionarily naive human population were exposed to such newly created viruses through some other viral vaccine, these viruses initially could have caused flu-like symptoms (which would have gone unnoticed because it would have been a typical side effect of the vaccine); but years later, this newly formed virus (HIV-1) would cause havoc within the immune system and ultimately devastation for humans (426). In Africa, unfortunately, the most common cause of death due to AIDS is wasting syndrome, in which individuals suffer from various gastrointestinal (GI) diseases, usually diarrhea, and die from malnutrition (as compared to AIDS patients in the Western World, who usually exhibit generalized lymphadenopathy and pulmonary symptoms; 427–433). Therefore, in Africa, if early symptoms of AIDS (i.e., GI malfunctions) appeared, they would have gone unnoticed (434–443). However, there is one AIDS manifestation which is common in both: dermatological symptoms, or KS (349–353,442).

Exposure to new types of HIVs would be like a slow motion version of the exposure of Aztec and Inca peoples to smallpox; millions of people from these populations succumbed to death, whereas the European armies were already immune to this virus and remained completely healthy (426). One can argue that introduction of SIVs from a single individual (i.e., by a bite from a monkey) might have caused the HIV-1 epidemic, but it is highly improbable. In the last several years many laboratory workers dealing with SIVs have become seropositive. Some of them were bitten by macaques infected with SIVs, but none have shown signs of serious illness (407–411).

In the late 1960s and early 1970s, a large number of KS cases and other immunodeficiency-related diseases began to appear in Zaire and several other parts of Central Africa (349–353,442,444). Initiation of an epidemic of such proportions from a virus that spreads by heterosexual intercourse is difficult to reconcile unless significant numbers of individuals were initially inoculated with mixtures of multiple lentiviruses (421,439,444). My reasons for reaching this conclusion are many: (*i*) Spread of HIV-1 through heterosexual intercourse is not very efficient (23–26, 102–104, 338–340, 385–386) and a single index case (a person who is primarily infected with pre-HIVs by an accidental bite from a monkey) would have had to have had sex with several hundred individuals within a few months of initial viremia, and each of the contact persons would have had to do the same for the epidemic to be effectively spread to such a large number in the Central African population [current estimates shows that 14 million individuals are infected with HIV-1 on the African continent, most in Central Africa (427)]. (*ii*) In the Central African population where HIV-1 first appeared, there was no such group of very highly promiscuous individuals who could have spread the epidemic in such a manner (428). (*iii*) On the other hand, in San Francisco and other areas of the US where a large gay population existed, initial exposure to actual HIV-1 from an African source could have spread the HIV-1 epidemic, since the spread of HIV-1 through homosexual intercourse is very efficient and many of the infected persons had been known to have had sex with several hundred individuals (429–431). Also, the human GI tract contains large numbers of CD4+ T cells that are prime targets for HIV-1 infection, making the GI track an efficient source of viral transmission. (*iv*) There are many accidental cases of monkey bites in Africa and elsewhere in the world, but they have not led to HIV-1-like illness or epidemics (407–410). I also believe that both pre-HIV-1 and pre-HIV-2 were introduced at the same time and were part of several recombination events, resulting in several types of new retroviruses. It is also possible that the various SIVs from different species of monkeys, as well as from chimpanzees, were cross-contaminated by utilizing culture supernatants when kidney cells from many different primates were used to prepare vaccine. It is possible that pre-HIVs were recombination events from these animal cells' exogenous retroviruses and endogenous viruses. Almost all major infectious diseases of civilization have been transferred to human populations from animals. Smallpox is related to cowpox, measles is related to rinderpest, influenza is found in pigs and birds, bubonic plague and Lassa viruses in rodents, and yellow fever in monkeys. Almost all the major epidemics in human history are the result of human interference with the balance of nature. For example, the plague, or Black Death, was introduced to the European community as the result of Tamerlane's invasion of Eastern Europe (426). Therefore, it is not unlikely that new lentiviruses introduced into human populations could be the result of new recombinant viruses, originating from SIVs from the cultured monkey kidneys (421). The new forms of lentiviruses created a new epidemic. Recently, the poliovirus has become the domain of public scrutiny and subject of various mass media articles and books (reviewed in References 354,421,433,437,439).

THE GROWTH OF THE AIDS EPIDEMIC

The question still remaining is why did the AIDS epidemic not start in the 1960s, since the HIV-1 incubation period is usually 3–10 years (88–98)? Why did it take 15–22 years before a full-blown AIDS epidemic in Central

Africa became evident? This question could possibly be answered by several experimental observations and calculations, made independently. I propose that the pre-HIVs which existed in vaccines were not exactly the HIV-1 virus we see today. It took time for the viruses to form new recombinant viruses, by combining with each other and perhaps by combining with human endogenous retroviruses, and for them to adapt and weed out the competing viruses from the population. It can be further clarified by this example: suppose pre-HIVs were introduced with the mass polio vaccination from 1957 to 1958, as has been hypothesized (354,421,439); then, depending on the dose of retrovirus inoculated, the route of the inoculations, and the immune status of individuals who received the vaccine, the outcome scenarios would be different. If we take the polio vaccine example (and it is just an example because many books and articles have been written on this subject; a partial list has been reviewed in Reference 421), the route was oral (343). The most vulnerable groups would be those who received relatively high doses of pre-HIVs, including young infants with immature immune systems (97–98; also see Chapter 6), individuals who were ill, and those who had oral sores or bleeding gums (including children between the ages of 4 and 10, who were losing baby teeth and getting permanent ones). These individuals might not have been able to muster an appropriate response to these new forms of recombinant retroviruses. If one assumes that only an estimated 3%–8% of individuals who accidentally received pre-HIVs with the polio vaccine were infected with the pre-HIVs (meaning that pre-HIVs successfully entered into their system without being destroyed by the gastric acids), even within this population, the majority probably did not get exposed to high enough doses of pre-HIVs, since the GI tract could have destroyed the majority of these viruses. However, suppose 0.05%–0.01% of the individuals actually were infected with relatively high doses of pre-HIVs, which allowed the development and propagation of intrahost pre-HIVs of the present-day HIV-1-like viruses thus serving as the launching pad for the present-day AIDS pandemic. Since (if we take the polio vaccine scenario as an example) there were >310 000 individuals who were inoculated with this vaccine, there would be an estimated 3100 to 15 500 individuals who actually carried HIV-like viruses in their bodies [if one takes the estimated example of 0.05%–0.01% of 310 000 individuals who were inoculated with the polio vaccine CHAT 1 strain (354,421, 439)]. If, out of this group, a small percentage developed a real AIDS-causing virus and spread HIV-1, it could have started the epidemic.

It could be argued that the oral route of SIV (or HIV) transmission is exceedingly rare and requires rather high doses of HIV-1 to infect humans (very few cases of HIV-1 transmission have been documented through kissing; reviewed in Reference 438). Such is not the case, however; experimental evidence has shown that it takes a 6000 times lower viral dose to achieve systemic infection with SIV in macaques by oral route than to achieve infection by the rectal route (438). In addition, the oral route of HIV-1 infection is well documented in neonates, who can acquire the virus by breast feeding (reviewed in References 392–394). Recently a group of researchers at the Harvard University, Tufts University, and Tulane University primate centers have evaluated the risk of systemic infection with cell-free SIV by oral route in adult macaques. They concluded that the risk of systemic infection by oral route, in the absence of mucosal lesions, was much higher than the rectal route and required much lower viral doses. In addition, this group had previously reported that neonate macaques were much more susceptible to SIV infection than adult macaques (72). Therefore, it would not be surprising to conclude that neonates and young children who were inoculated with 1 mL of liquid solution containing polio virus (and possibly other contaminants) were susceptible to infection by SIVs/HIVs (421,438,439).

Intrahost evolution of HIV-1 has been described by Lukashov et al. (440). They obtained the genomic RNA sequences from 44 individuals both at seroconversion and 5 years later. They found that the mean number of nonsynonymous nucleotide substitutions in the V3 region of the viruses circulating in 31 nonprogressors (the HIV-1 infected individuals who managed to avoid adverse effects of HIV-1 infection, even temporarily) was significantly higher ($P<0.001$) than the corresponding value for 13 progressors. From this they concluded that antigenic sites of HIV-1 (or in the case of this hypothesis it would be pre-HIVs) evolve more rapidly during the symptom-free period. Therefore, it might have taken much longer for pre-HIV subtypes or clades to develop and subsequently reach a threshold from which they could cause an epidemic. Moreover, in areas where the initial exposure might have taken place, the early signs of an epidemic might have existed, but because of enormous poverty, lack of medical care, the almost nonexistent data collection system, civil wars (which are still going on), and the total absence of an infrastructure for clinical follow-ups, such cases probably went unnoticed. There have been numerous case reports documented in the literature providing evidence for the existence of AIDS-like illness in Africa since the 1960s and in other parts of the globe as well (441–444). I also believe that AIDS was present in Central Africa much earlier than the early 1980s because thousands of cases of KS, which is strongly associated with AIDS, were being reported in the mid-1960s (Figure 5; 286, 349–356,441–444). If one looks at the map of Central Africa and the number of KS cases, it is not difficult to reach the conclusion that AIDS probably existed in that same area where hundreds of thousands of individuals, including young infants, were vaccinated in what was then the Belgian Congo (now Democratic Republic of Congo, until recently Zaire; Figure 5; 349–356). The epidemiological map illustrates a ripple effect, as if a major germ-bomb had exploded in the Belgian Congo and then radiated across the rest of Africa. The farther one gets from the epicenter of the explosion, the weaker the effect is of this figurative radiation (see Figure 6).

Direct evidence for the existence of AIDS before 1972, and as early as 1962, has been provided in 2 reports; one published in *Science* and the other in *The*

Lancet. Both were published in 1985 (442,443). One of these groups of investigators had previously collected 75 serum specimens from clinically healthy children as controls for their studies on Burkitt's lymphoma. After the discovery of HIV-1 and the availability of the enzyme-linked immunosorbent assay (ELISA) test to detect HIV-1, these investigators tested the sera for the presence of HIV-1 (in 1985 it was still called HTLV-III). The HIV-1 ELISA test showed that 66% of the samples were positive for HIV-1 (2 standard deviations above the background). The results of the ELISA test were further confirmed by Western blot, which exhibited a strong reaction to several of the HIV-1 antigens. Since the subjects for collection of specimens were chosen as representative of Burkitt's lymphoma patients by age, sex, and community, and the mean ages of the subjects were low (6.3 years), it was rather surprising that such a

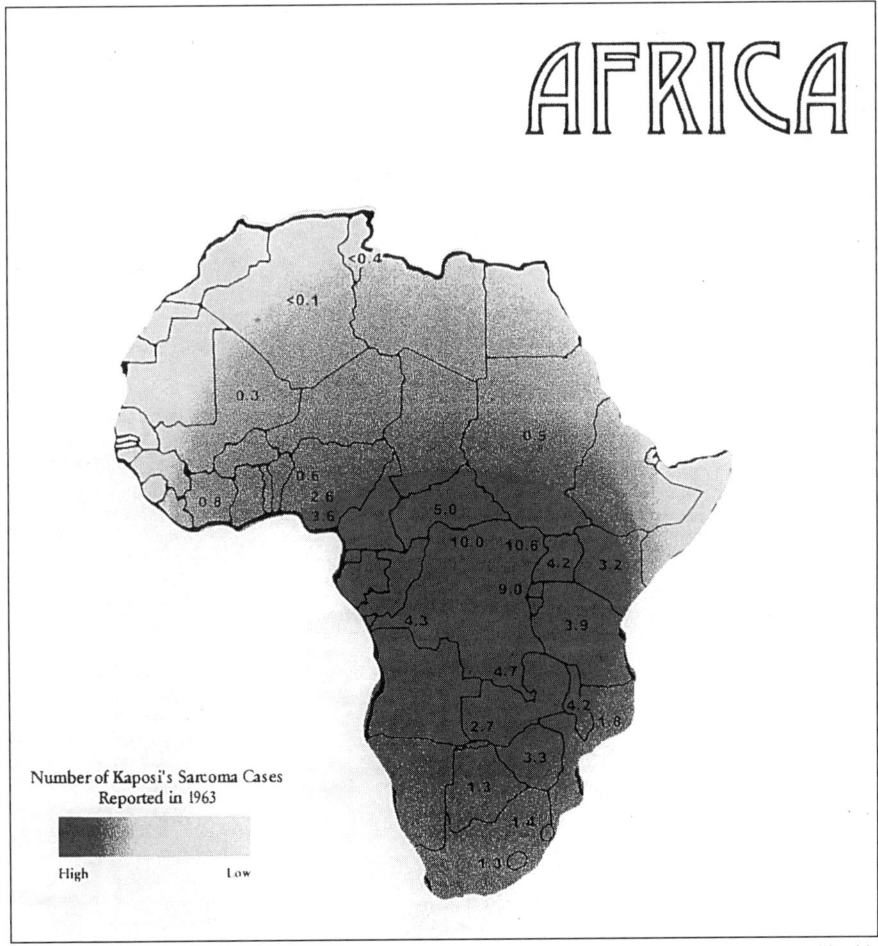

Figure 5. Distribution of incidence of Kaposi's sarcoma in Africa in 1963. The data illustrated in this map was generated from Figure 1 of Hutt et al. (351).

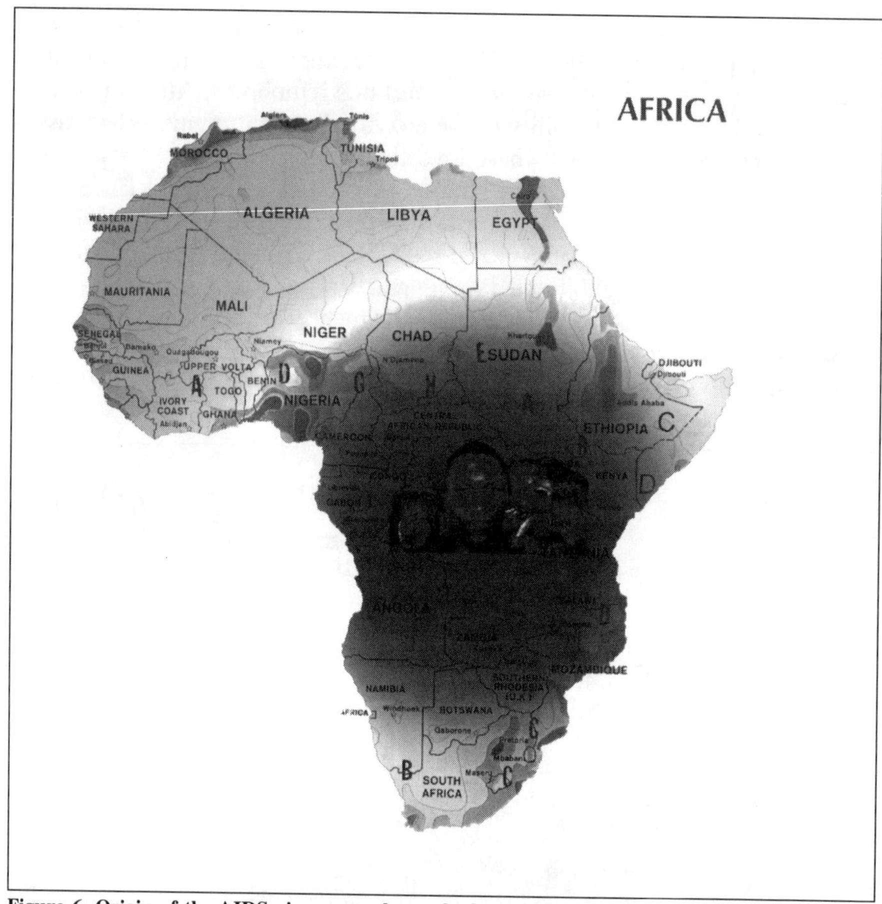

Figure 6. Origin of the AIDS virus map shows the hypothetical point of impact, near lake Tanganyika. It is assumed that over 214 000 individuals were inoculated accidentally with several pre-HIVs, which were contaminants from African green monkey kidney cells or perhaps chimpanzee kidney cells. Both of these nonhuman primates have been known to carry SIVs, which have over 90% sequence homology to current HIV substrains. It is postulated that there would be a ripple effect from the epicenter of infection, and AIDS-related diseases would spread in an almost circular fashion from the epicenter. The map shows the number of individuals infected with HIV-1 diverging from the original point of impact. Number of AIDS cases by territory:

Kenya	56 573	Togo	5609	Guinea	1548	Cape Verde	92
Tanzania	53 247	Cameroon	5375	Eritrea	1539	Equatorial Guinea	74
Uganda	46 120	Namibia	5101	Senegal	1297	Mauritania	59
Zimbabwe	41 298	Central African Republic	4463	Gabon	990	Mauritius	27
Malawi	39 989	South Africa	3849	Angola	895	Madagascar	18
Zambia	32 492	Burkina Faso	3722	Benin	856	Seychelles	6
Zaire	26 131	Chad	3457	Guinea-Bissau	707	Comoros	5
Ivory Coast	25 236	Botswana	3110	Lesotho	515		
Ethiopia	19 493	Mali	2594	Swaziland	413		
Ghana	15 890	Mozambique	1815	Gambia	340		
Rwanda	10 706	Niger	1691	Algeria	217		
Congo	7773	Nigeria	1591	Liberia	191		
Burundi	7024			Sierra Leone	155		

high percentage of individuals tested positive. I believe that these individuals were infected with a milder variant of HIV-1, as I have described above.

Another study reported cases of "slim disease." This is a well-known manifestation of AIDS, especially in Africa; individuals suffer severe weight loss and diarrhea, and a strong association with HIV-1 infection is well established (427,443). This manifestation of HIV-1 infection is also mimicked by nonhuman primates who are experimentally infected with SIV_{mac} (432). This disease had been reported to be very common in Zaire. In addition to weight loss, the majority of the patients who tested positive for HIV-1 by ELISA showed generalized immunosuppression and lymphadenopathy, and some showed KS lesions. The old medical records in Uganda showed the existence of slim diseases as early as 1962, but not before (medical records in Uganda go back to 1944; 443). This information again points to an infectious agent that started spreading a few years before 1962. The most amazing part of the report indicates that the source of the infectious agent might have come from or near the Ruzizi Valley and Lake Victoria. The report states: "The first recognized cases [of slim disease] came from a small village on Lake Victoria, just north of the Tanzanian border." This village was one of many from which goods were traded across the border to Tanzania. The notion that the disease may have been transmitted sexually from Tanzania is interesting since it fits historically with the movements of the Tanzanian army in 1980, and subsequent regular visits by Tanzanian traders. Of the 15 traders tested for evidence of HTLV-III (HIV-1) antibodies, 10 were positive. These traders admitted to both heterosexual and homosexual casual contacts. Tanzanian soldiers entering Uganda since 1980 have had frequent heterosexual contact with the local population. The only Tanzanian army soldier tested also had serological and clinical evidence of HTLV-III (HIV-1) infection. If a virus indeed came from Tanzania, then where did Tanzania get it? It appears that the disease might have started from the area neighboring Lake Tanganyika, only a few miles from Lake Victoria.

Recently, David Ho's group from the Aaron Diamond AIDS Research Center, New York, has reported analyses of an African plasma sample obtained in 1959 (356). This sample was obtained from a Bantu male with a sickle cell trait and glucose-6-phosphate-dehydrogenase deficiency, residing in Leopoldville, Belgian Congo (now Kinshasa, Democratic Republic of Congo). Multiple phylogenetic analyses not only authenticated this case as the oldest reported HIV-1 case, but viral sequence analyses indicate that they are genetically close to subtype B and D. Also, the authors claim that this ancestral virus, evolutionarily, is very close to the original theoretical HIV-1 subtype, which was probably introduced a few years before 1959. As stated earlier, there were reportedly over 300 000 individuals inoculated with live polio vaccine between 1957 and 1959, around the same areas where this sample was obtained (354,421,439). Interestingly, out of 1213 samples they examined, 21 were HIV-1 seropositive, but could not be confirmed by Western blot or radioimmunoprecipitation methods; this finding indicates that there were more forms of HIV-1-like viruses present at that time, as would be predicted from the hypothesis I forwarded earlier, based on recombinant events which might have taken place due to multiple co-infection of monkey kidney cells with various subtypes of SIVs and other lentiviruses (354,421).

Let us get back to this adaptive evolution of pre-HIVs into full-scale pathogenic HIV-1 (445,446). Of course, no one can go back in time and evaluate these situations, but many investigators have worked on this question in patients infected with HIV-1. For example, Wolinsky's group has explored this adaptive evolution of HIV-1 during the natural course of infection in 6 HIV-1-infected individuals (446). They have tracked the evolution of HIV-1 from the blood samples, obtained semiannually by analyzing V3 and V5 proviral sequences. They have demonstrated that the patients who are rapid progressors have less diversified quasispecies of HIV-1, whereas slow progressors exhibit more diverse genetic evolution of HIV-1 quasispecies (446,447). The same group has also analyzed the viral evolution in 6 perinatally infected children. Greater HIV-1 genetic diversity has been found in children with a low viral burden whereas the reverse has been found in children with a high HIV-1 burden (445,446). This also confirms the hypothesis that new, diverse, and possibly pathogenic strains of HIV-1 could have emerged from multiple pre-HIVs/SIVs potentially present in the polio vaccine or other vaccines given during this period to the population in this part of the Belgian Congo (355,421,439).

Two other points should be kept in mind. First, at the time the polio vaccine was being developed, several investigators were competing in this endeavor. When they were ready to begin human trials, their primary concern may not have been where the monkey kidneys used to produce the vaccine came from. Therefore, the millions of doses of polio vaccine used in the Belgian Congo from 1957 to 1960 by one of the investigators (354,439) must have taken several hundred liters of brew (if one assumes that 1 liter is enough to vaccinate 1000 individuals, it would have required at least several hundred liters of fluid to vaccinate over 300 000 people). In addition, in order to grow poliovirus to manufacture the vaccine, it would have required several hundred monkey kidneys from many nonhuman primates, and would have required an enormous effort to collect monkey kidneys from various available sources. Therefore, it would have been very difficult to determine where all of those kidneys came from. Second, during the recombinant events, the resultant new viruses could have formed 3 different types of viruses: (*i*) nonpathogenic variants, (*ii*) low pathogenic, causing immunosuppression in a few years, and (*iii*) a highly pathogenic strain, causing acute fatal immunosuppression, killing the recipient in a few weeks to months. I believe that the highly pathogenic strain would have killed the host without spreading the illness to many other people. The second type of virus, however, probably is the new lentivirus with which we are all familiar—the slow immunosuppression-inducing agent we call the AIDS virus.

THE PATHOGENICITY OF HIV-1

If we accept the hypothesis that HIV-1 was the result of recombinant events between multiple strains of SIVs, some genetically closer to SIV_{cpz} (resulting in HIV-1) and others genetically closer to SIV_{sm} (resulting in HIV-2), then we can expect multiple substrains and significant diversity within HIV-1. We know that genetic diversity is a hallmark of HIV-1; by the same token, HIV-2 should also possess several subtypes. HIV-2 within West African humans can actually be classified into 5 subtypes: A–E (32,42,48). Phylogenetic analyses have shown 2 distinct groups of HIV-1 viruses: M and O. On the basis of *env* and *gag* sequences, at least 10 genetically unique clades have been identified in group M alone (A–J). All 10 clades are found in the sub-Sahara African regions. If HIV-1 is the result of multiple SIVs' recombination events, then one should expect that multiple clades of HIV-1 would be present at the center of its putative origin (Africa). However as one moves farther away from the epicenter, one should find fewer clades (but in certain cases, newer forms of HIV, due to new recombinant events with the lentiviruses indigenous to that particular part of the world may develop.) Currently there are unique clades that predominate in different parts of the world. On the bases of genetic databases for HIV-1 (which now contain over 40 full-length sequences, over 250 *env* sequences, about 100 *gag* sequences and numerous bits and pieces of HIV-1 gene sequences), subtype E may have spread from sub-Sahara Africa to Thailand, and then more widely to the Western Hemisphere (427). Subtype G recombinant HIV-1 spread across Africa and to several European countries. Subtype B is predominant in the American, European, and South African subtype; subtype C predominates in Brazil and D in Zaire. Phylogenetic tree analyses of the *env* gene have shown that all 9 major subtypes (A–G) have an average nucleotide distance of 10%–13% (427). Recombinations between various clades also take place and have been reported extensively (7,427). The mosaic nature of HIV-1 genomes, particularly showing the existence of various SIVs within them, clearly indicate that numerous clades of HIV-1 and HIV-2 have emerged from recombinant events from an accidental inoculation of multiple SIVs, from different strains of primates into humans (see Figure 7).

Since genetic recombinations between several SIVs can produce a large number of possible lentiviruses, many capable of causing various degrees of immunodeficiency, it is expected that with more sophisticated sequencing tools and computer programs, we will undoubtedly find numerous variants of HIV. Some may be more closely related to SIV_{sm} (like HIV-2) and some more closely related to SIV_{cpz} (like HIV-1); the products of recombinant events with various SIV strains will not fit into any group or clade.

HIV-1 is divided into 2 groups: M for major and O for outlier. O indicates that we already have so many genetically divergent strains that do not fit into the accepted parameters of HIV-1 gene sequences and we do not know where to put them.

More recently, a divergent HIV-1 isolate designated YBF30 was isolated from a Cameroonian woman with AIDS (428). A team of French investigators, in collaboration with investigators from Cameroon and Gabon, analyzed the genetic sequences of this HIV-1 isolate. The structural genes and *tat*, *vpr*, and *nef* of YBF30 were found to be almost equidistant from those of HIV-1 group M and $SIV_{cpz\text{-}gab}$, originally isolated from 2 chimpanzees from Gabon. On the other hand, *vif* and *rev* of YBF30 were closely related to HIV-1 M, and HIV-1 *vpu* was totally divergent from HIV-1 and SIV_{cpz}. They also utilized a special ELISA test based on YBF30 envelope V3 protein. Out of 700 sera they collected in Cameroon, 3 tested positive.

Once again, molecular data point toward a catastrophic genetic recombinant event that took place after humans were inadvertently infected with multiple strains of SIVs; after multiple cycles of recombinations, these strains resulted in an array of new lentiviruses, some pathogenic and others completely innocuous. However, the most pathogenic new lentiviruses quickly killed off their hosts,whereas the least pathogenic ones would have outlived their hosts, spreading through sexual/parenteral/vertical transmission routes, radiating their influence slowly from the epicenter (349–356,428,435–439,441–443). This also explains why only 1 or 2 subtypes are predominant in lands far

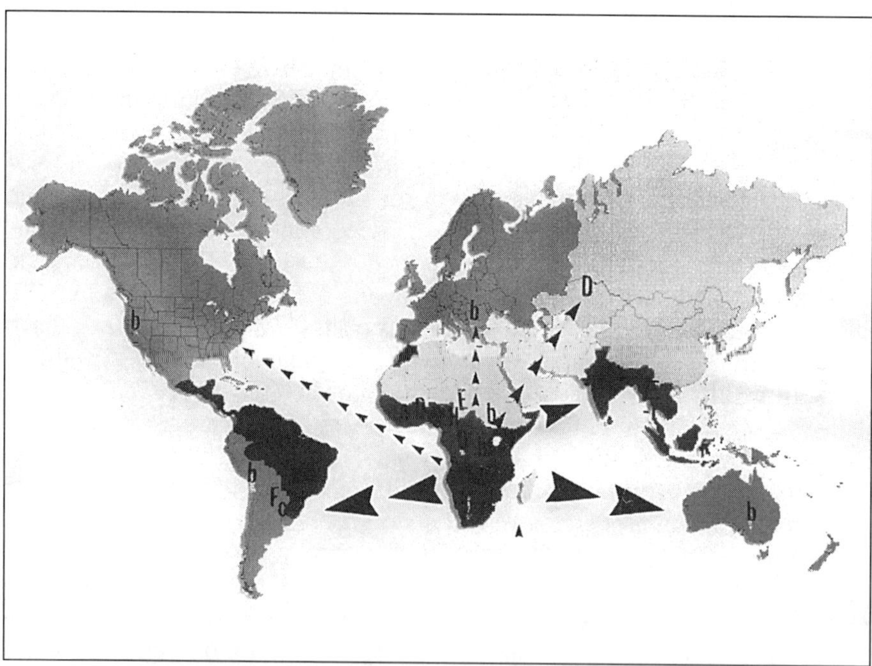

Figure 7. Global prevalence of various HIV-1 subtypes. The map shows the prevalence of all known subtypes in and around the Ruzizi Valley in the Republic of Congo, the original site of one of the polio vaccine trials in the 1950s. Only 1 or 2 subtypes of HIV-1 are prevalent in various parts of the globe and all appear to have spread from its hypothetical point of origin—the Ruzizi Valley.

from sub-Sahara Africa, because the original index host probably only carried 1 or 2 subtypes upon immigration (Figure 7).

The question remaining to be answered is why HIV-1 is so pathogenic to humans when it is not pathogenic to primates or great apes. HIV-1 might have been the result of the recombinant events from SIV_{cpz} (which has >90% homology to HIV; 15,18–19,21–23,33–36) and other African SIVs, including African sooty mangabey SIVs (which have >90% homology to HIV-2; 33–50) or type D viruses from rhesus macaques (4,224–238,321–336). In these cases, the retroviruses from many nonhuman primates share significant portions of their genetic structures with HIV-1. All these species of lentiviruses have coevolved with these nonhuman primates, and several types of viruses share >60%–90% of their genes. Therefore, by simple logic, HIV-1 or HIV-2 should not be terribly pathogenic to chimpanzees or African green monkeys in normal circumstances (when the immune system is competent). However, humans are naive hosts for these lentiviruses and would be vulnerable unless exposed to very low doses.

Finally, we need to consider whether we have any evidence of AIDS in the area of Africa that was vaccinated between 1957 and 1958. Even if less than 0.05% of the individuals got high enough doses of pre-HIVs, there should be some evidence to support this assumption. The incidence of KS in the region serves as a valuable guage.

Until the advent of AIDS, KS was exceedingly rare and was regarded as a relatively benign disorder of elderly males in the Mediterranean area. Only a little over 1200 cases were reported from 1872 to 1956 (reviewed in References 349–356). It was known that the risk of KS was increased in immunosuppressed transplant recipients. We have now discovered that KS is about 300 times more common in HIV-1-infected persons than in other immunosuppressed groups, and it is 20 000 times more common than in the general population.

If one assumes that the 1957–1958 polio vaccine was contaminated with pre-HIVs, then infants who received 1 mL of oral polio vaccine could have gotten sick and developed KS-like skin lesions (which is rare in infants with AIDS) or could have shown the lymph node variety of KS (common in children with AIDS–KS). In late 1957, Thijs reported 8 cases of KS in the Belgian Congo, in the same area where the vaccination took place (reviewed in References 349–356). In 1972, Taylor et al. (349,350) published the largest series of data collected from 339 cases of KS in the Northeast Congo and in Rwanda and Burundi from 1957 to 1970. They provided a detailed map of the area where the incidence of KS was highest (Figure 5). The largest number of individuals with KS was near the same area where polio vaccinations took place, particularly the area near Lake Victoria and Tanganyika (within a 40-mile radius of Ruzizi Valley, where >214 000 children and adults were given oral polio vaccines). One may wonder whether KS was already endemic to this area before 1957 (before vaccination), but Dorn and Culter reported in 1955 that the crude incidence rate of KS in Caucasians was the same as it was in blacks: 0.08/100 000 (reviewed in Reference 350). Earlier, Dorfell conducted a worldwide survey of KS that included 356 cases of KS, and none from Africa (reviewed in Reference 351). However, Oettle published a report in 1962 stating that KS was significantly higher in the Bantu population (352). Amazingly, the majority of cases occurred in men and women under 16 years of age. Hutt published a comprehensive study in 1984 comprising 500 malignant cases in Africa before 1950; only 10 cases out of 500 were KS (0.02%) (351). However, from 1957 to 1961, Lothe had accumulated 211 KS cases, the majority from Eastern Zaire, where >10% of all malignancies were KS, an apparent 500% jump from 1956 to 1961, 2 to 3 years after the mass polio vaccination. Again the epicenter of the incidence was the same area where the polio vaccine trials were conducted (reviewed in Reference 351). Numerous reports have documented that before the discovery of HIV-1 (1983), the highest incidence of KS was found in essentially the same area where >214 000 people were given oral polio vaccines (351). In this area, KS accounted for >10% of registered cancers. As one of the investigators commented, it was rather surprising that blacks in the US, England, and the Caribbean did not have an increased incidence (351). Oettle, in 1962, reported that >12% of all malignant tumors in Zaire were KS (340), and Hutt in 1984 reported that KS accounted for 12.8% of cancers in Zaire, 5% in Equatorial Africa, 4.5% in Tanzania, 4.2% in Uganda, and 2.9% in Kenya (351). Again, if one looks closely at this map, it is clear that the epicenter of the KS epidemic is around the Ruzizi Valley (Figures 5 and 6). Also, from the 1960s onward when endemic KS exploded from the epicenter of Lake Tanganyika, it was not the result of some environmental problem, rainfall, or altitude, since there was no such incidence of KS in similar areas of equatorial India or Brazil.

LIFE CYCLE OF HIV-1

In order to understand the connection between HIV-1 and AIDS, we must first understand the life cycle of HIV-1. Details of our current understanding of the HIV-1 life cycle have been reviewed by several investigators (5, 448–450). An overview of the HIV-1 life cycle is illustrated in Figure 8. Briefly, HIV-1 (as well as SIVs) has a selective tropism for CD4 molecules (found on T-helper cells, monocyte/macrophage cells, and several other cell types; 451–454). Once the virus binds to the CD4 molecules, it requires coreceptors to be internalized (87,127–131,361–364, 415,451). It is currently believed that various HIV-1 subtypes may have tropisms for different cell types (i.e., monocytes, CD4+ T cells; 361-364). Since many cell types carry a low density of CD4 molecules on their cell surfaces, it is the presence of coreceptors that appears to determine the susceptibility of a particular cell type to a specific variant of HIV-1 (87,127–131,361–364,415,451). There are 5 coreceptors, of which only 2 have been described in detail (361–364). One of these is called Fusin (recently renamed CXCR4), an α-chemokine that has tropism for CD4+ T cells (determined in T-cell line adapted strains of HIV-1). A second is β-chemokine, CCR5, which appears to serve as a coreceptor for primary HIV-1 strains, including those that infect macrophages (87,127–131,361–364,415). After internalization, the virus is uncoated, and the viral genome (which is RNA in nature) is transcribed into DNA by reverse transcriptase, an enzyme present in the viral core and necessary for synthesis of proviral DNA. After RT, the proviral DNA may integrate into the host chromosomal DNA or remain unintegrated for an undetermined length of time (451, 455–461). After integration, the proviral HIV-1 may enter a latent phase in certain cell types until the infected cells are activated. The host also enters into a clinically latent state in which HIV-1 is being produced constantly by the HIV-1-infected CD4+ T cells, but being replaced by the new ones (462), thus creating a so-called "steady-state" phase. This latent phase may last from a few months to several years before the clinical symptoms of

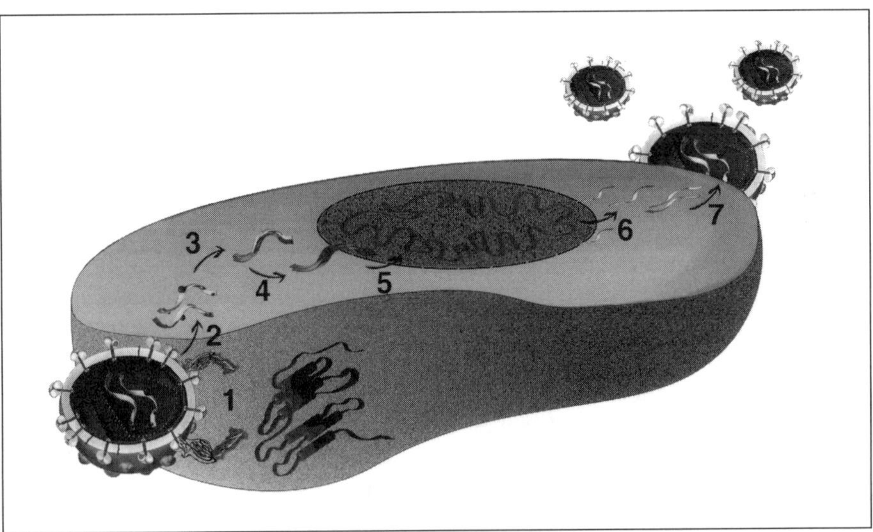

Figure 8. An overview of the HIV-1 life cycle. Step 1: Attachment. HIV-1 consists of 2 strands of RNA and several enzymes necessary for its replication. Viral coat proteins gp120/gp41 interact with CD4+ T cells and bind to CD4+ molecules, which serve as receptors and 7-domain transmembrane proteins called chemokines, which serve as coreceptors. **Step 2:** Entry. The virus then enters the cellular cytoplasm, the viral core opens up, and viral RNAs move into the cell. **Step 3:** Reverse Transcription. With the enzymatic activity of reverse transcriptase, which the virus carries inside the cell, viral RNAs convert into cDNA. **Step 4:** Provirus. With the help of an another viral enzyme, RNase H, the viral cDNA makes a complementary copy of the viral cDNA. This double-stranded HIV-1, now called provirus, enters the nucleus of the cell. **Step 5:** Integration. The genetic parasite integrates with the help of an another viral enzyme, integrase, and the provirus integrates into the host genome. At this step, the only way to detect the virus in the individual cells is by in situ PCR. **Steps 6 and 7:** Viral Replication and Budding. Proviral genes get transactivated if viral envelope proteins (gp120/gp41) accumulate at the hosts' cytoplasmic membranes, whereas the viral core is assembled in the cellular cytoplasm, which subsequently migrates towards the cellular plasma membrane—subsequently budding out from it and forming a viral envelope or coat.

AIDS appear. We will discuss the significance of low versus high HIV-1 viral load during the course of HIV-1 infection in a later section, but for now I would like to emphasize that it is probably one of the most important factors in the battle for survival against HIV-1 infection.

MOLECULAR EVENTS DURING HIV-1 REPLICATION

HIV-1, like many lentiviruses, has a very complex viral life cycle (448–462). Since the discovery in 1970 of the retroviral enzyme reverse transcriptase by Howard Temin (463), this virus-encoded protein has been demonstrated to be critically important to the fuller understanding of retroviral pathogenesis. The infectious virion of HIV-1 contains 2 identical copies of single-stranded positive RNA approximately 9.2 kb long (5). Once inside the cell the RNA is converted into double-stranded linear DNA and integrated into the host cell genome to produce the provirus (5). Figure 9 shows the genomic organization of the linear viral DNA of HIV-1. HIV-1 encodes precursor polypeptides for virion proteins as well as several additional open reading frames. Full-length HIV serves 3 roles: (*i*) as genomic RNA, which gets incorporated into the viral core of the progeny virions, assembled at the plasma membrane; (*ii*) as mRNA for translation of Gag and Gag-Pol polyprotein in the cytoplasm; and (*iii*) as precursors for over 30 alternatively spliced mRNAs that are also translated in the cytoplasm to produce envelope glycoprotein and accessory and regulatory proteins (5). The *gag* gene encodes the precursor for virion capsid proteins; the *pol* gene encodes the precursors for several virion enzymes including protease, reverse transcriptase, and integrase; the *env* gene encodes the precursors for envelope glycoprotein (gp); *tat* is the transcriptional transactivator; and *rev* is the regulator of viral expression (more below). *vif*, *vpr*, *vpu*, and *nef* are the accessory genes, and under certain conditions appear not to be essential for viral replication in vitro (5).

The capsid core proteins package genomic viral RNA into virions and participate in uncoating the virus as well as in efficient viral RT and in viral replication after its entry into the cell (5). The mature capsid proteins, capsid, nucleocapsid, and matrix protein, are produced by cleavage of the Gag polyprotein by the viral-coded protease (5). The capsid protein forms the capsid shell and is 240 amino acids long (5). While the exact functions of the capsid protein remain unknown, it is thought that it may be involved in nucleocapsid assembly, uncoating of virions upon entry into the cell cytoplasm, and stabilization of reverse transcriptase enzymes during the cDNA syntheses (5). The matrix protein is 130 amino acids long and is located between the nucleocapsid and the virion envelope (5). The matrix protein targets membranes for the Gag polyprotein to membranes and helps incorporate the envelope glycoprotein into virions (5). The nucleocapsid protein is 70 amino acids long, and its function may be to condense the viral RNA genome for packaging into capsids and help virion uncoating during entry into the cell (5).

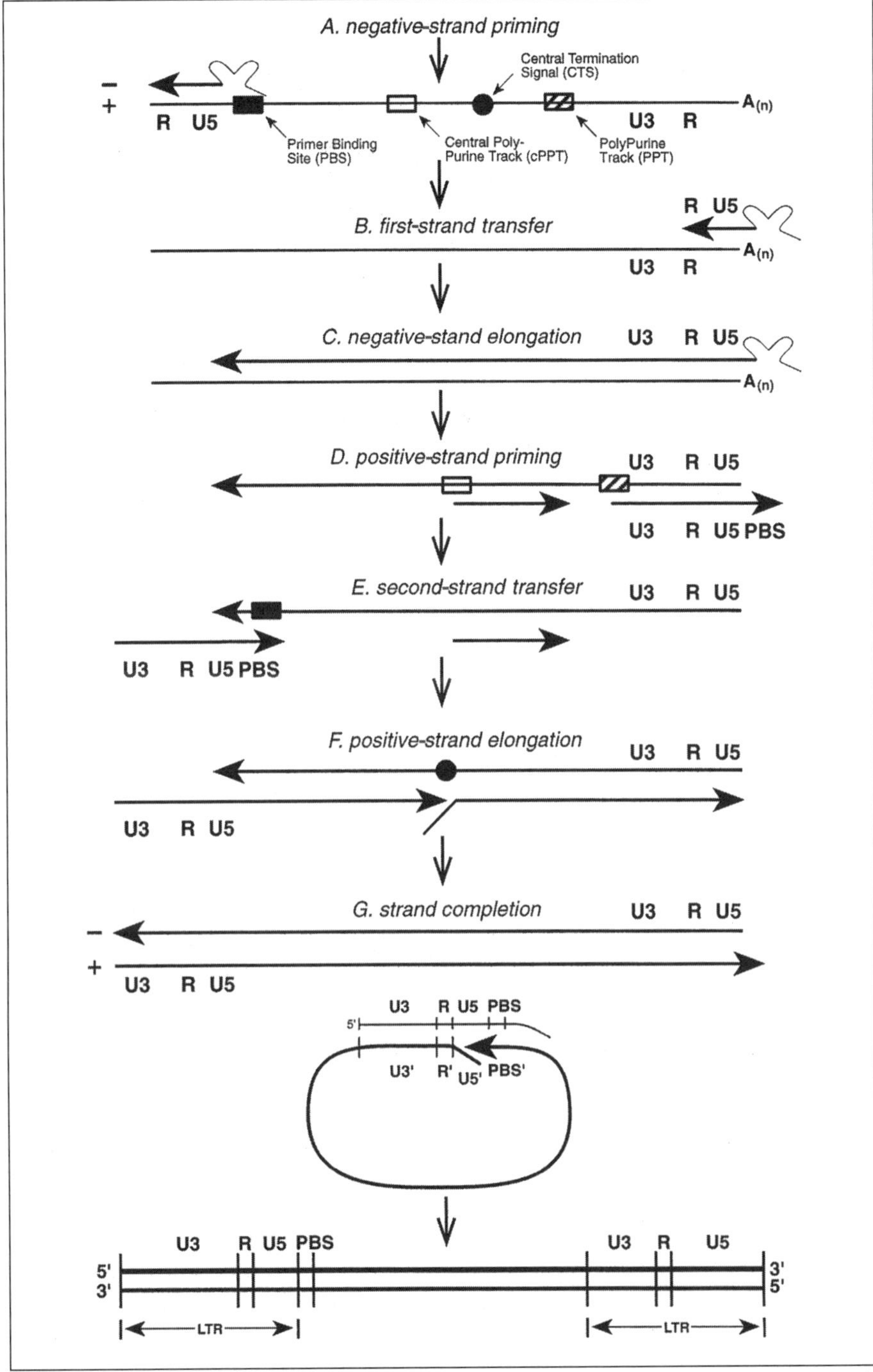

Figure 9. HIV-1 replication: molecular sequence of events leading towards HIV-1 DNA synthesis from HIV-1 RNA (see text for details).

The viral enzymes protease, reverse transcriptase, and integrase are produced by cleavage of the Gag-Pol polyprotein during virion morphogenesis (5). The mature protease is 99 amino acids long, and it cleaves itself out of the Gag-Pol polyprotein. Protease is required for viral replication, and uncleaved noninfectious particles result if this enzyme is inactivated (5). HIV translation products are long polyprotein precursors, which are specifically cleaved to release mature proteins by protease (5). This feature of HIV is economical because several viral proteins may be expressed from the same mRNA. One signal on the precursor can direct several proteins to the assembly site.

Reverse Transcription

All the retroviruses, including HIV-1, carry at least 3 complex enzymes as part of their infecting machinery. The first of these enzymes is called reverse transcriptase. Both reverse transcriptase and related enzymes are encoded by the *pol* gene found in all retroviruses (Figures 8 and 9). All reverse transcriptase enzymes, isolated from various retroviruses, exhibit at least 3 specific enzymatic activities, namely RT, a specific DNA polymerase action, and ribonuclease H activity. The RT activity of the retroviruses allows them to convert themselves into a DNA copy, as the enzyme reverse transcriptase uses viral RNA (or any RNA) as a template to be copied, provided that the action is initiated by a primer at the primer binding site (PBS; see Figure 9). The copy being made is always DNA. The ribonuclease H activity serves to peel away the RNA template from the newly created RNA–DNA hybrid; then the enzyme chews up the original RNA molecule into tiny bits, and only a complementary copy of the viral cDNA stands alone. The single-stranded cDNA molecule (called minus or negative strand) that remains is manipulated by the enzyme once again; this time reverse transcriptase acts like DNA polymerase and weaves a positive or plus complementary strand along the cDNA in order to make a double-stranded cDNA molecule (463–466).

Once HIV-1 has entered the cell (binding/entry described later), the viral particles are partially uncoated to produce a large nucleoprotein complex that resembles the virion capsid. It is believed that the viral coat actually holds or stabilizes the viral relaxed RNA so reverse transcriptase can perform its work more efficiently. A host tRNA primer binds to the RNA template primer binding site near the 5′ end. Synthesis utilizing reverse transcriptase proceeds to the 5′-end R region, which is terminally redundant, forming the minus-strand strong stop DNA. The RNA portion of the RNA–DNA hybrid is digested by RNase H. Hybridization with the R region at the 3′ end of the same, or the second, RNA genome is referred to as the first jump. Elongation continues to a polypurine tract (PPT) at the 3′ end of the RNA. A primer is formed by reverse transcriptase RNase H (PPT primer), and plus-strand elongation continues back to the 5′ end using the minus-strand DNA as template. Meanwhile, minus-strand synthesis continues through the genome using the plus-strand RNA as template. Additionally, plus-strand synthesis continues using RNase H digestion products as additional primers at a number of internal locations along the minus-strand DNA. PPT-initiated plus-strand DNA synthesis stops after copying the annealed portion of the tRNA to generate the plus-strand strong stop product. The tRNA is then removed by RNase H. Annealing then occurs to the PBS on the minus-strand DNA, providing the complementarity for the second jump, and the synthesis continues to completion. The newly formed double-stranded linear DNA is now ready to be integrated into the host genome.

Reverse transcriptase does not have a proofreading function, and therefore it plays a major role in the generation of diverse HIV-1 types. There are several types of errors that can occur during RT: direct misincorporation of a noncomplementary nucleotide can produce a single base substitution; slippage of the 2 DNA strands can lead to repetitive sequences generating a deletion or an addition; or frame shifts can be caused by misincorporation followed by misalignment of the template primer. All of these errors can lead to either a single nucleotide mutation or a mutation incorporating large distances. The mutation rate for HIV-1 reverse transcriptase ranges between 1 per 1700 to 4000 nucleotides, which is quite high compared to other retroviruses. These error mechanisms, combined with antiviral immune responses, provide selective pressure for accumulation of viral variants. Viral variants lead to selection for drug resistance or development of more substrains.

Different types of reverse transcriptase enzymes are found in various types of retroviruses, each having slightly different characteristics because of their different origins. Each was derived from a specific retrovirus that has evolved a particular capsid protein in order to provide a structural milieu within which the enzyme can do its work. Therefore, plus-strand synthesis is profoundly discontinuous in the avian sarcoma virus system with multiple initiation sites, and minus-strand synthesis, although not discontinuous with multiple subgenomic fragments, may not be fully complete until quite late in the RT process (463–469). The synthesis of second-strand (plus-strand) lentiviruses (including HIV-1,) uses 2 primers: a PPT that borders the U3 domain in the 3′ LTR and a central PPT located at the end of the *pol* gene. Most other retroviruses initiate plus-strand DNA synthesis only at the PPT near the 3′ LTR (illustrated in Figure 9). Is this the result of some recombinant event? We do not know yet.

Since HIV-1 and other retroviral virions contain 2 copies of PLUS-RNAs in their core (Figure 8), the possibility that a portion of both of these RNAs is used as template during DNA synthesis by RT is very high. In many conditions, 2 genetically different RNAs from 2 entirely different lentiviruses are co-packaged in a single virion. During RT, portions of each of the RNAs could be utilized—resulting in a new recombinant lentivirus. Recombination can also occur in a single cell infected with more than one type of lentivirus.

There are 2 possible mechanisms of these recombination events. The first is the copy choice mechanism, in which recombination occurs during the first-strand or minus-strand cDNA synthesis. The second mechanism is called the strand displacement-assimilation, where recombination occurs during the plus-strand DNA synthesis. Both of these mechanisms have been shown to take place in nature, but the first one appears to be more prominent (5).

The last major enzyme that is coded by the Gag-Pol polyprotein is the dimer 32-kDa integrase that mediates integration, which is the covalent linkage of linear double-stranded viral DNA created by reverse transcriptase into the host cell genome. The substrate for HIV-1 DNA integration is a linear, mostly double-stranded viral cDNA molecule with terminal direct repeats and blunt ends. To carry out integration, the virus-encoded integrase protein first cleaves 2 nucleotides from each 3′ viral DNA end in a step called terminal cleavage and then joins the newly exposed 3′ hydroxyl groups to phosphodiester bonds in the host DNA. The cDNA is inserted by joining both viral cDNA ends to nearby phosphodiesters on opposite strands of the target DNA. The resulting breaks in the DNA are then repaired by the host DNA repair system. This paired integration of viral DNA is essential; without it, single cDNA integration would result in a branched DNA structure and would be destroyed by the host repair enzymes. Viral integration ensures a stable association between viral DNA and the host-cell chromosome. Integrated viral DNA is then transcribed by host RNA polymerase II to produce the viral RNA genome and mRNAs required for replication. The substrate DNA contains 5′ACTG...CAGT3′ terminal sequences. During the first step of integration, substrate DNA is nicked by integrase on the 3′ side of CA to produce hydroxyl ends that are recessed by 2 nucleotides. Then, translocation of the PIC into the nucleus occurs, mediated by nuclear localization signals in the matrix protein. Once inside the nucleus, the viral DNA is joined to host target DNA after a 4–6-bp staggered cleavage of the target host DNA. The ligation occurs between the hydroxyl ends of the viral DNA and the phosphate ends of the host. The gaps between the hydroxyl and phosphate ends are repaired by either integrase, reverse transcriptase, or host enzymes. The proviral DNA is ready to synthesize viral RNA.

Entry of HIV-1 into cells does not guarantee the integration of HIV-1 into the target cell's genome. A series of studies have demonstrated altered viral replication kinetics in certain nonreplicating cells (455–461). Quiescent T lymphocytes, in cell culture, demonstrate both decreased integration of proviral genomes and partial reverse transcripts after infection with HIV-1, as compared to stimulated and proliferating T lymphocytes (451,455–462,470–474).

The Env glycoprotein 120 molecules on the surface of HIV-1 particles bind to CD4 receptors, located on the plasma membrane of CD4 T cells, monocytes, macrophages, and dendritic cells, and thereby attach virions to cells (5). Upon attachment, Env glycoprotein mediates uptake of virions into cells by fusion of viral and cellular membranes. The CD4 receptor, upon condensing and bringing the virion and cell membranes into close proximity, not only binds the virus but also causes a conformational change in Env glycoprotein that allows for fusion of viral and cellular membranes, a process believed to be independent of pH (5). Certain chemokine coreceptors are also necessary to facilitate the uptake of HIV-1 into the cell (87,126–131,361–364,415,451).

The viral transcript that encodes Env glycoprotein also transcribes the accessory protein Vpu (5). During the late stage of viral replication, the bicistronic mRNA transcribes the Env glycoprotein, which is approximately 850 to 880 amino acids long. The major product of the *env* gene is the heterodimer gp160, which is cleaved to form gp120 (550 amino acids long) and gp41 (about 350 amino acids long). The interaction of CD4 with the Env glycoprotein oligomer promotes dissociation of the gp120 subunit from the gp41 subunit in virion membranes.

Synthesis and processing of the Env glycoprotein occurs in the secretory pathway of the host cell. Cleavage takes place in the Golgi apparatus via a host cell protease. After cleavage, the Env glycoprotein oligomers are directed towards the plasma membrane, utilizing a cellular transport system, where they assemble into virions. The gp120 subunit has a binding domain for the CD4 receptor. The gp41 is required for fusion of the virion membrane with the cell plasma membrane during the entrance of HIV-1 and is also required to serve as an anchor for the Env glycoprotein heterodimer (Figure 10).

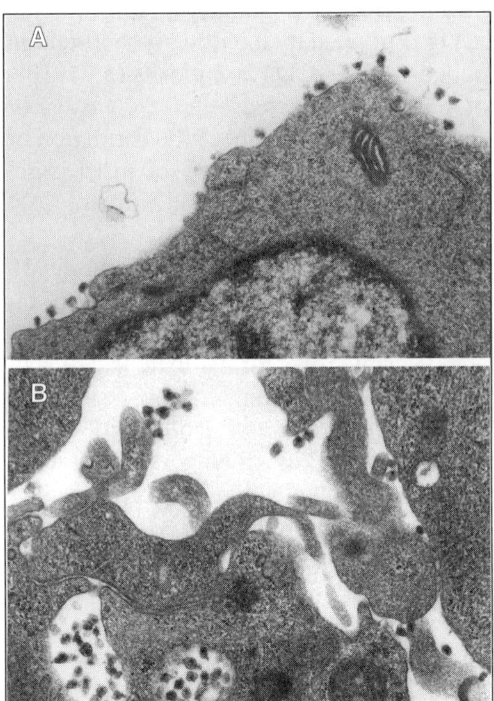

Figure 10. HIV-1 entry and exit from an HIV-1-infected lymphocyte. (A) The attachment process of HIV-1 virion on the cell surface. HIV-1 requires CD4 molecules as well as chemokine receptors for attachment and entry. (B) HIV-1 budding takes places from multiplex membranes of the cell.

Isolates of HIV-1 *env* have the characteristic of extreme heterogeneity. The sequence variation among isolates has shown 5 variable domains interspersed with conserved regions (5,7). The V3 sequence, a variable domain in the gp120 subunit, appears to play an important role in cell tropism, cytopathicity, fusogenicity, and viral infectivity. Up to 25% of the amino acids encoded by *env* may vary in HIV-1 strains. Sequence heterogeneity may be under selective pressure to escape neutralizing antibodies and adaptation to infection of different cell types. In contrast to gp120, gp41 is relatively conserved. However, what role antibodies to HIV-1 play, if any, in protection is doubtful and a matter of controversy (9–14,54–60).

The accessory genes of HIV-1 (*vif*, *vpr*, *vpu*, and *nef*) are exclusive of the *gag*, *pol*, and *env* genes as well as the viral transactivators *tat* and *rev*. Many studies have been performed regarding the phenotypes of all of these accessory proteins and their functions with varying results. HIV-1 Vif is synthesized from an open reading frame encoding 193 amino acid, and accumulates in the cytosol and cytoplasmic membrane of infected cells. While it remains unclear, it appears that Vif could play a role in the infectivity of HIV-1, RT of viral RNA, uncoating and/or internalization of virus, or maturation of the virion. Vpr is a 15-kDa virion-associated protein translated from an open reading frame associated with the nucleocapsid in mature virions. In infected cells it is located in the cytoplasmic membranes and nucleus. Vpr may be involved in viral replication, nuclear localization of the PIC, and/or regulation of viral and cellular gene expression (5).

The open reading frame for *vpu* encodes a protein 81 amino acids in length. The mRNA transcript is bicistronic for both Vpu and the precursor for the Env glycoprotein. Vpu is found in the perinuclear region. Possible roles for Vpu include its involvement in virion release and cytopathicity. Additionally, Vpu is believed to cause a rapid and selective degradation of CD4 in the endoplasmic reticulum. Normally, CD4 is trapped by the Env glycoprotein in the endoplasmic reticulum and produces gp160–CD4 complexes (5,7). This trapping causes down-regulation of CD4, and a decrease in the cleavage of gp160 to gp120 and gp41. By degrading CD4, Vpu reduces the formation of gp160–CD4 complexes and therefore increases the rate of gp160 processing. The 2 phenotypes, enhancement of virion release, and destabilization of CD4 are thought to occur by independent mechanisms (5).

Nef is translated from 2 multiply spliced transcripts of HIV-1 into a 210 amino acid protein. One transcript is monocistronic while the other is bicistronic encoding both the regulatory gene *rev* and *nef*. Nef is localized to the cytoplasm and cell plasma membrane. Possible roles for *nef* include cell activation, which could cause dysfunction of the cell or immunosuppression; acting as a primer in RT, transcription by enhancement of virion infectivity; down-regulating CD4; associating, with a cellular serine kinase, which could signal a transduction cascade; and/or maintaining viral latency by acting as a negative regulator in infected individuals. Of particular importance is the down-regulation of CD4 that causes a cell to be less permissive for reinfection, thereby preventing multiple rounds of superinfection and cytopathology. Recently, the importance of *nef* in the development of attenuated live-viral vaccine has came into the picture and will be described in detail in a later section (5,25,68).

Control of HIV-1 Replication

Control of RNA synthesis involves a complex mixture of viral elements, viral transactivators, and cellular proteins. Viral RNA synthesis occurs in the cell nucleus utilizing the proviral DNA integrated into the host cell genome as a template. The 3 domains of HIV-1's LTRs, U3, R, and U5, all take part in transcription. The 5′ LTR is used for initiation and the 3′ LTR is used for addition of poly (A) tails. Additionally, the regulatory genes *tat* and *rev* control the entire replicative process (see below).

The U3 region of HIV-1's LTR contains the transcriptional promoter consisting of the core that contains the TATAA box, the enhancer that binds $NF_{\kappa}B$, which enhances inducible activation of HIV-1 transcription, and the modulatory domain important for binding cellular factors that governs the structure of the promoter. Viral transcripts are initiated 22 bp down from the TATAA box at the U3/R border. The transactivation response element (TAR), found in the R region, functions in *tat*-mediated transactivation. Downstream from U3 and R is the U5 region, which defines the 3′ end of all viral transcripts (5, 475–485).

Tat augments levels of viral RNA by increasing transcriptional initiation and/or elongation, while Rev regulates splicing and transport of viral RNA from the nucleus to the cytoplasm (5). Tat is a 14- to 15-kDa viral protein translated from a group of multiply spliced transcripts whose role is to increase levels of viral transcripts containing the TAR element (486–513). Tat contains 2 important domains—an activation domain and an RNA binding domain. Tat function is very much dependent on a bell-shaped RNA stem-loop structure, Tat activation domain or TAT, located at the 5′-terminus of all HIV-1 mRNAs. Tat forms a one-to-one complex with TAR, and the mechanism of action is enhanced by interaction of other cellular cofactors. The Tat appears to be required for viral replication, at least in most of the conditions tested in vitro. Any condition that increases the levels of positive regulatory factors will enhance the level of transcription. For example, antigenic, mitogenic, and lymphokine-mediated cell activations are reported to activate dormant HIV-1. Similarly, co-infection with other viruses, many of which can activate HIV-1 LTR, also transactivate HIV-1 (486–496). The Tat protein may be taken up into infected cells in vitro and may enhance transcription of HIV-1 genes, apparently by TAR-mediated activation. There has been a prolonged search for the cellular cofactors to determine the precise elongation mechanism by which Tat performs its function during the enhanced transcription elongation. A cellular protein—a cyclin-dependant kinase called Cdk9—has been identified. A cyclin-related partner, cyclin T, increases the affinity of Tat for TAT (5). The cyclin T gene maps to human chromosome 12 and increases Tat transactivation by 100-fold when expressed (497–513).

The 2 coding exons for the HIV-1 *rev* gene are joined by splicing to produce a 116 amino acid protein localized to the nucleus and nucleolus, which binds to the Rev-response element (RRE) in viral transcripts and shifts the balance from multiply spliced transcripts in earlier stages (i.e., accessory proteins), to both singly and unspliced transcripts in later stages of replication (i.e., structural proteins). Additionally, Rev influences the transport of viral transcripts.

RRE is a 234-bp sequence located within the *env* gene (5,514–516).

There is an expanding body of literature on the various complex and interdependent factors that control HIV-1 replication (516–519). After integration, provirus is transcribed from the single promoter in its 5′ LTR to produce a single primary transcript that spans the complete HIV-1 genome. However, from this single transcript the virus has to express several structural and regulatory proteins (517–529). One of the best characterized and important regulatory and posttranscriptional transactivator proteins is Rev. The product of the *rev* gene appears to regulate expression of the virion, hence the name *rev*. The general agreement among retrovirologists is that one of the functions of *rev* is to allow intron-containing RNAs (unspliced and singly spliced) to be released from the nucleus into the cytoplasm (514–515). Therefore, Rev seems to play a pivotal role in transnuclear transport of unspliced and singly spliced RNAs. In the *rev*-negative or *rev*-defective HIV-1 strains, unspliced and singly spliced RNAs accumulate in the nucleus, whereas multiply spliced RNAs can also be found in the cytoplasm. The mechanism of Rev effects has been explored by a number of investigators (514–515). Their findings indicate that a short segment of the *env* coding region, located within the potential intron that bisects the *tat* and *rev* genes, is a *cis*-acting locus, called RRE. RRE is present in unspliced and singly spliced RNAs and absent in multiply spliced RNAs. RRE is a 240-base region of the HIV-1 transcript that folds into a stable complex RNA secondary structure. The *rev*–RRE complex formation is similar to Tat–TAR interaction and mutations in RRE or *rev* coding segments results in complete elimination of transactivation of HIV-1 in vivo and in vitro (514–515).

The Rev protein consists of an NH_2-terminal domain that mediates RRE-binding, Rev-RRE multimerization, and nuclear localization, and a COOH-terminal leucine-rich domain that contains a nuclear export signal (NES). NES apparently binds a nuclear export receptor, exportin 1, which is related to the inportin-β (karyopherin-β) superfamily of shuttling nuclear transport receptors (5). Mutations in exportin-1 result in inhibition of Rev function. A current model of the Rev mechanism of HIV-1 unspliced RNA transport from nucleus to cytoplasm is depicted in Figure 11. According to this model, the leucine-rich NES of Rev protein interacts with exportin 1 and the Ran guanosine triphosphate (Ran-GTP), an essential nuclear transport factor. This complex is energy-dependent and upon transport of HIV-1 unspliced RNA, the Ran-GTP converts into Ran-GDP. After export of HIV-1 RNA, the complex dissociates and Rev migrates back to cytoplasms. It is hypothesized that cellular cytoplasmic/nuclear GDP/GTP gradient ensures the one-way migration of HIV-1 unspliced RNAs.

Another regulatory gene is *nef; nef,* an acronym for negative factor, was named for its ability to moderately down-regulate transcription from the LTR. Although essential for pathogenesis in vivo, *nef* appears to be nonessential in vitro. The *nef* gene is conserved in all the primate lentiviruses including all SIVs, HIV-1, and HIV-2. Its product modulates the induction $NF_{\kappa}B$

and Spl. *nef* plays a role in facilitating the replication of virus in quiescent cells, which may be accomplished through interaction with cellular kinases. It has been demonstrated that HIV- I *nef* can down-modulate CD4 from the surface of lymphoid cells. Down-regulation of CD4 on the cell surface does not result from a change in CD4 mRNA or protein synthesis, since steady-state levels of the protein and mRNA are maintained. Rather, *nef* induces rapid CD4 endocytosis and lysosomal degradation of the internalized protein (25,68,529). Several live attenuated vaccines that have shown promising results have been produced by *nef*-deleted SIVs (19–20,61–70,333).

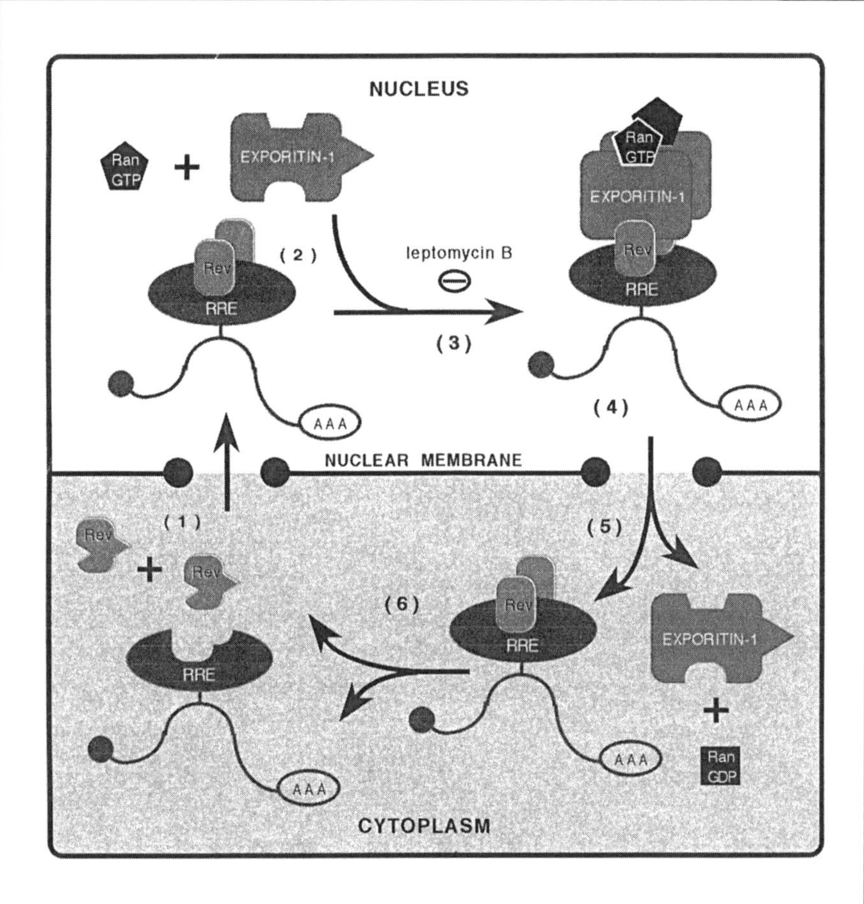

Figure 11. Shuttling function of Rev. Rev nuclear transport function: Rev is synthesized in the cytoplasm and enters into nucleus. Upon entry it binds with RRE, found in the unspliced HIV-1 RNA, in a dimerized form. Exportin-1 and RAN-GTP bind with each other and then cooperatively bind Rev-RRE–HIV-1 RNA complex. This complex is exported to the cytoplasm, where all components dissociate and Rev shuttles back to the nucleus. HIV-1 RNA is packaged or translated into various proteins, which either form the components of HIV-1 virion or perform regulatory functions.

Once the genomic RNA transcripts have been transported to the cytoplasm, the virion is ready to be assembled. The first step in assembly is assumed to be the formation of a complex between Gag-Pol and Gag polyprotein in the cytoplasm and then transport to the site of capsid assembly. Additionally, a packaging element binds to full-length viral transcripts allowing them to enter the virion assembly pathway but excludes the spliced transcripts lacking this element. The polyprotein, RNA, and Vpr all interact to form the nucleocapsid. Finally, an interaction occurs between the matrix protein (MA) of the Gag and the gp41 subunit leading to the extrusion of the nucleoprotein complex through the plasma membrane to produce a virion with a nucleocapsid surrounded by a lipid bilayer membrane that contains oligomers of Env glycoprotein (5, 475–498).

The HIV-1 LTR appears to be an extremely complex control region (490–493). Many of the HIV-1 LTR DNA binding protein motifs appear to interact differently in various cellular milieus. For example, the 3 Sp1 sites appear to be necessary for viral replication only if activated $NF_{\kappa}B$ is not present in a particular intracellular environment (494). The *tat* and *rev* genes are the first genes expressed at the breakdown phase of the latent stage and allow the expression of the structural genes of HIV-1 (495–496).

The Effect of New SIV Strains on Monkeys

SIVs are a family of naturally occurring lentiviruses indigenous in certain wild simian species in Africa. In African monkeys these lentiviruses are completely harmless. Most of these SIVs are more closely related to each other and to HIV-2 than to SIV_{cpz} or HIV-1 (27–49,215,221,223,286,293, 316–334), even though there is one report indicating the discovery of an SIV very closely related genetically to HIV-1 (425). The closest genetic relationship is between HIV-1 and SIV isolated from chimpanzees, which exhibit over 90% homology to each other (33–34). Based on a computer-generated phylogenetic tree, many HIV-1 and HIV-2 viruses may have emerged as recently as 50 years ago (397,425,434–438). It is possible that HIV-1 emerged from recombinant events between various SIVs in the wild or in laboratory culture prepared for an entirely different kind of vaccine, utilizing African green monkey kidney cells infected with various types of SIVs or chimpanzee monkey kidney cells, since both types of animals were readily available to early polio researchers as well as to many other investigators (421,439,518). Endogenous viral sequences with nucleotide homologies to HIV-1 have been identified in the human genome (142–143,154,179–181, 200,202). In addition, the presence of unusually high frequencies of T-cell-mediated response to HIV-1 in HIV-1-seronegative individuals have been reported by various investigators (23–26,182).

As opposed to their nonpathogenic nature within their native hosts, particular strains of SIVs, when inoculated into Asian macaques, result in fatal immunosuppression within 2 months to 3 years (depending on the dose, route of inoculation, and SIV subtype). As mentioned earlier, these AIDS-like symptoms are observed when these monkeys are given relatively high doses of SIV. Also, all strains of SIVs are not pathogenic to Asian macaques, so SIVs from West African sooty mangabeys and many isolates of African green monkeys cause persistent infection but no immunosuppression and no AIDS-like pathology (23–26). Young Asian macaques are more susceptible to SIVs than adults (40,41,72,75,). All species of Asian macaques: rhesus, cynomolgus (longtail), stump-tailed, and pig-tailed, are susceptible to SIVs (40,41,121,186,196–201), to a certain degree.

Interestingly, not all Asian monkeys are equally susceptible to all strains of African SIVs. For example, when SIV from sooty mangabey monkeys (SIV_{sm}), which is nonpathogenic to this species in the wild, is infected into rhesus macaques monkeys, this infection results in a disease very similar to human AIDS. Similarly, when SIV from African green monkeys (SIV_{agm}) is infected into pig-tailed Asian macaques, they also develop a diseases similar in manifestation to human AIDS. However, if rhesus are infected with SIV_{agm} or if pig-tailed macaques are infected with SIV_{sm}, the outcome of these infections is not as severe. These animals do develop immunosuppression but not AIDS per se.

I will discuss in detail the role of initial viral load in predicting the severity of lentiviral infection in various primate species, including humans, in a later section. For now I would like to state that the initial viremia and subsequent course of infection appear to be very important. For example, high primary viremia in experimentally infected Asian monkeys is associated with severity of diseases, whereas low or unmeasurable primary viremia is a good indicator of no or very low grade disease. Therefore, even though pig-tailed and rhesus are phylogenetically closely related, infection with SIV_{agm} causes AIDS-like diseases in pig-tailed macaques and very low grade, if any, diseases in rhesus.

The molecular as well as cellular features of simian AIDS, induced by only limited strains of SIVs, are similar in many respects to HIV-1 infection in humans. For example, SIV infects CD4+ T cells of monkeys (412–422). In both situations, HIV-1 and SIV, infection persists despite a strong humoral and cellular immune response. Several weeks after inoculation the host shows a spike of viremia accompanied by a rash, followed by antibody response. After a few weeks, the animals appear normal and healthy. Then within 6 months to 3 years animals develop CD4+ T-cell depletion and die from complications of immunodeficiency. The most common complications are wasting and diarrhea (517).

The most curious observation in the area of SIV–AIDS is that most of the macaques experimentally infected even with high doses of SIVs isolated with African green monkeys (SIV_{agm}), show no infection or at most very low levels of infection and no disease (29–30,39,43,316,324,–326,329,331, 357,379, 383,390,400,403,517–525). Could it be possible that SIV_{agm} gene sequences are more closely related to New World monkey endogenous retroviruses? Recent data has provided evidence that endogenous type D viral sequences have a high homology to baboon endogenous virus, and related homologous proviral sequences are present in the African green monkeys but not in apes and humans. This may explain why HIV-1 is so pathogenic to humans.

The New World monkeys do not carry SIVs in the wild, but they carry another type of retrovirus, the endogenous type D retroviruses. These are absent in African monkeys (44,30,215–230,335–346). When African monkeys are infected with type D viruses, they also develop AIDS-like illness (335–336).

Humoral Immune Responses

Infected macaques develop strong antibody responses to various SIV proteins (526–543). However, it is important to note that in the SIV model, neutralizing antibodies do not always correlate with immune protection (9–14,41,544,545). It is particularly true in animals infected with SIV by various routes and in animals who were vaccinated with live attenuated vaccines or recombinant vaccines (524,544–547). For example, Joag et al., who infected 8 rhesus macaques with cloned SIV_{mac239}, found that 1 out of 8 animals developed neutralizing antibodies to the virus. However, there was no correlation between the development of antibodies and degree of protection (548). Even in the presence of high titer neutralization antibodies to gp130, which recognized the correct conformational determinants, the monkeys succumbed to SIV infection, while in other cases, even in the absence of neutralization antibodies, animals were protected (544–545). There are too many reports to cite here, but in humans infected with HIV-1, the presence of high titer antibodies to various HIV-1 proteins, including gp120, gp41, gp160, p24, etc., does not correlate with the progression or the outcome of the disease (reviewed elsewhere in this book).

Cell-Mediated Immune Responses

As in humans infected with HIV-1, the majority of SIV-infected macaques mount vigorous CMI responses to SIV antigens (17,18,51,85,414,549–557). More interestingly, a strong SIV *env*-specific T-cell proliferation response was noted in animals exposed to low doses of SIV_{mnd}. These animals did not seroconvert (558–559). Other animals in the same experiment, when infected with a higher dose, seroconverted but showed weak CMI responses (559). CD8+ T cells exhibit a protective role against SIV, as has been shown with HIV-1.

In their natural African primate hosts, all the SIV strains are essentially nonpathogenic. An understanding of the underlying mechanisms that control SIV infection in African green monkeys and in sooty mangabeys may explain why SIVs cause AIDS-like disease when given to evolutionary naive species of Asian macaques. The importance of viral load in the assessment of both the stages and control of HIV infection in humans has become a central theme in recent years (190). However, if one assumes that control of viral load is the measure of success with regard to the "degree of protection" from infection or progression of HIV, this standard cannot be blindly applied to the naturally infected nonhuman primates, who show no sign of disease but in some cases have relatively high viral load. For example, Kaur et al. published their preliminary observations on sooty mangabeys with natural SIV infection, which have high plasma viral loads and yet do not progress to AIDS. In order to understand the immune basis of this protected state, they analyzed SIV-specific cytotoxic T-lymphocyte (CTL) activity in 12 naturally infected sooty mangabeys. They were unable to detect SIV-specific CTLs in fresh PBMCs from 7 of 7 animals, even when tested at high effector-to-target ratios, suggesting the absence of circulating activated SIV-specific CTLs. After ex vivo antigen-specific stimulation they found that the response was heterogeneous. Therefore, they detected vigorous SIV-specific CTL activity in only 4 out of 12 (33%) of the animals. SIV-specific CTL activity remained undetectable or inconsistently present in 5 out of 12 animals and detectable at low levels in 3 out of 12 animals, again confirming that there is no correlation between viral load and SIV-specific CTL activity (559). If one carefully dissects the CMI and HI responses to SIV_{agm} in naturally infected African green monkeys, it fails to reveal any unusually high immune activity in a traditional sense, of either CMI or HI (9–14,331). As a matter of fact, the immune responses of African green monkeys seem to be weaker both qualitatively and quantitatively than immune responses in rhesus macaques and cynomolgus macaques infected with SIV_{sm}, both evoluntionarily naive to SIVs (560). Infected African green monkeys have exhibited almost no neutralizing antibodies against the SIV core protein Gag. Similarly, SIV-specific CMI responses to SIV_{agm} in infected African green monkeys and SIV_{sm}-infected sooty mangabeys have been difficult to demonstrate (125). Despite the absence of any traditionally accepted SIV-specific immune responses (humoral and cell-mediated), and presence of relatively high to moderate plasma viral loads, these animals do not develop AIDS or other AIDS-related illness (561). Even the same experimental manipulations, used to cause rapid disease in rhesus macaques, the African green monkeys, or sooty mangabeys, do not cause immunosuppression or AIDS (562–564).

From the summary of the data digested from hundreds of experimentally and naturally infected monkeys, one can conclude that the level of viral burden in PBMCs or CD4+ T cells in SIV-infected healthy African green monkeys or sooty mangabeys may be comparable to that of a healthy SIV-infected monkey or HIV-1-infected man in some cases (17–26,59–60,63,67, 70–76,102–105,123–125,350–352,358–359). Many virological, immunological, and molecular diagnostic criteria have been used to compare the 3 groups. Not a single obvious difference can be found that can help in deciphering the type of known immune response responsible for the protection.

If neutralizing antibodies as well as SIV-specific T-cell responses do not offer protection—then what does (561–564)?

Surprisingly, after the initial infection, it seems that the viral load is not the determining factor in deciding the fate of the host. The damage caused by the initial viral inoculation dose appears to be the most critical (72–75). The size of this initial exposure determines if the host is able to mount a sufficient defense against a particular retrovirus. In order to do so, this defense must develop before the host suffers irreparable damage to the cells responsible for generating molecular immunity against that retrovirus. Studies comparing SIV_{mac} and SIV_{sm} indicate that Asian macaques were accidentally infected with SIV_{sm} (56,125,196,197,272,297,310,374–383). In the infected animals, SIV was shown to replicate at relatively high rates in both macaques and sooty mangabeys. Macaques developed AIDS in a few months to years after infection (40,41,72,75,131), while the sooty mangabeys remained free from any symptoms. Sooty mangabeys are exposed to very low doses of SIV_{sm} at early stages of their lives. The macaques are not, and are therefore evolutionarily naive to this virus. Exposure to low doses of SIV_{sm} gives these animals the opportunity to prime their cells with specific RNA molecules that protect them against even a high inoculation of SIV_{sm} (58,222,321,335,371,378,384–391). Animals who are naive to the viruses begin producing these RNA molecules when exposed to the virus, but when they are exposed to a high dose, they are unable to prime their cells quickly enough. At this early stage of molecular immunity development, there must be a threshold beyond which this mechanism of protection is no longer effective. Those animals exposed to doses below this threshold can develop protection and be prepared for a subsequent high-dose challenge. I will be exploring these relatively novel intracellular molecular immunity mechanisms in detail and will explain these evolutionary mechanisms which I believe were developed to combat retroviruses.

One may ask how plasma viral load during the course of lentiviral infection correlates with the progression of disease. I believe that measurement of viral load should not be taken as the absolute criteria of disease progression. Since we know that SIVs replicate at a high rate in mangabeys and in macaques, but only one shows signs of disease progression and viral load may vary according to the degree of immune stimulation (455,458–462, 561,562), the evidence is clear that this measurement does not accuately determine disease progression. However, as a general rule, it would be appropriate to state that a low viral load represents a certain degree of "protection" against lentiviruses.

For example, viral load is 1–3 orders of magnitude lower in African green monkeys than in macaques (58,222,321,335,355,378,384–391). This is due to the presence of molecular immunity against a particular substrain(s) of SIV_{agm} in African green monkeys, as compared with macaques. This immunity prevents replication of SIV_{agm} in the majority of the target cells, even though during the normal course of immunostimulation, the activated cells still produce SIV_{agm}. In contrast, in macaques, where the majority of the cells are not primed with the "protective RNAs", a relatively large number of cells are producing SIVs, increasing the viral load, and also more importantly, destroying larger numbers of cells at a given time due to the higher number of cells producing virions (190,559,561).

Chapter 3

Immune Mechanisms Responsible for Inhibiting Retroviral Replication

" ....wild nature and human nature are closely interwoven. I argue that the only way to make complete sense of either is by examining both closely and together as products of evolution."

Edward O. Wilson
In Search of Nature

MOLECULAR IMMUNITY AGAINST RETROVIRUSES

Seroepidemiologic surveys have revealed that wild African primates have high rates of infection with SIVs, whereas Asian primates do not carry these viruses. Up to 25%–50% of captured adult primates of various African species have evidence of SIV infection; these primates are healthy and without evidence of any illness. As with African primates infected with SIVs, chimpanzees naturally infected with SIV_{cpz} or experimentally infected with HIV-1 show no ill effects due to this type of infection. Less complex retroviruses are found in mice, chickens, and cattle without apparently causing any illness to their hosts. I have proposed that this nonpathogenicity is not an intrinsic quality of these viruses but is the result of low-dose exposure to these lentiviruses in the early stage of animals' lives. This acquired resistance, which is limited to a particular strain of SIV indigenous in a specific colony of that species, occurs because a different arm of the immune response is activated after these primates are exposed to a particular strain or subtype of lentivirus. These nonhuman primates get primed with a particular strain(s) of SIV(s) (whatever strain may be prevalent in a particular colony of these primates) as babies, perhaps by breast feeding (392–394). If any member of a particular monkey colony is exposed to other genetically related strains of the lentivirus to which they have been primed previously (nonhuman primates have been known to periodically invade other primate colonies), they will be able to resist this new, but related strain of lentiviral infection. However, if a colony of nonhuman primates is exposed to high doses of a genetically unrelated lentivirus, to which they have no history of previous exposure, then these animals will develop AIDS-like illness or will have some other adverse consequences (depending on the mechanism of pathogenesis of that particular lentivirus). The best example of this would be rhesus macaques being exposed to SIV_{sm} or other related SIVs, or African nonhuman primates getting exposed to type D lentiviruses (44,216–218, 222,322,335,342,565); it is similar to developing a subclinical influenza infection when one has already been exposed to a closely related strain, but, on the other hand, becoming very ill if exposed to a significantly new strain of flu. However, as noted in the preceding chapters, neither HI nor CMI responses appear to play any crucial protective role in the case of retroviral/lentiviral infections (9–14,17–26, 59–60, 63,67,70–76,102–105, 123–125,131,350–352,358–359). An understanding of the underlying immune mechanisms that control SIV infection in African nonhuman primates may explain why SIVs, when given to evolutionarily and immunologically naive species of macaques, cause AIDS-like disease. To explain many of these phenomena I am proposing a new interpretation of previously derived data that I feel is far better at accommodating these observations and provides an explanation as well for the pathogenesis of HIV-1, SIV, and other lentiviral infections.

I postulate that there is a third form of immunity (besides HI and CMI) at work with retroviruses which I call molecular immunity. I hypothesize that this molecular response is akin to both humoral and cell-mediated responses, but it involves a particular virus-specific messenger molecule that delivers to individual cells crucial information about the pathogen in question. This molecule serves both as score and conductor to a whole orchestra of small RNA instruments playing at the molecular level, which must perform in harmony to overpower the discordant genes of the infecting retrovirus (Figure 4). Furthermore, the critical messenger molecule seems to be associated with a specific CD8+ subset of T cells. It is probable that other cofactors and some stimuli (i.e., cytokines/chemokines that regulate the response of these CD8+ cells) may also modulate the course of retroviral infection, particularly during the initial stages of the infection (455,458–462,561,562). Most importantly, the organism can be primed with low doses of genetically related nonpathogenic lentiviral strains, such that the organism can develop a persistent genetic molecular immunity specific to a particular retrovirus. The organism then manifests protective molecular defenses against this retrovirus and genetically closely related pathogenic strains of virus (e.g., HIV-1), with or without the concomitant presence of classical humoral or cell-mediated responses (9–14).

As illustrated in Figure 4, I believe that small endogenous RNAs (i.e., SINES and LINES retroelements) play a pivotal role in blocking the invasion of new retroviruses. Millions of copies of small RNAs of endogenous retroviruses appear to be present in certain subsets of T cells (i.e., CD8+ T cells or NK+ cells) and serve as a repertoire of small RNAs, with all possible sequences found in almost all the retroviruses present in nature (similar to immunoglobulin and T-cell receptor repertoires, which can bind any possible antigen found in nature or designed unnaturally). These RNA repertoires would, upon exposure to a new type of retrovirus, bind the critical portion(s) of the invading retrovirus, inhibiting its entry into the cellular nucleus, stopping it at the PIC (see Figure 12 in Chapter 4 for details). Therefore, these multiple endogenous retroviruses serve as a blocking agent. Evolution has developed the means to amplify the number of copies of the specific RNA which is found to block that particular retrovirus and to distribute it throughout the whole body, hence providing protection to the whole organism. This is in principle similar to other forms of traditional immune responses in which a foreign antigen binds to an immunoglobulin M (IgM) surface immunoglobulin on a B-cell or T-cell surface receptor; that event then initiates a cascade of intracellular events, resulting in the expansion and amplification of that particular cell (now called a clone). Subsequently, the body acquires millions and billions of copies of molecules (immunoglobulins or cytotoxic T cells) that will bind and destroy the agents carrying the particular antigen that initiated the events. Again, this protection is also distributed throughout the body. Therefore, molecular immunity behaves similarly to other arms of the immune system, but the protective agents that defend us against the retroviruses are different from HI or CMI. HI and CMI actually differ radically from each other. For example, with HI, various classes and subclasses of soluble immunoglobulin bind the foreign antigens. They are found in saliva, the GI tract, tears, breast milk, cerebrospinal fluids, blood and other body fluids. CMI is different in that the T cell that originally recognizes the antigen, after expansion, binds the cells or the targets which carry this original antigen, and destroys them. It is possible that a few weeks after exposure to retroviruses, the other types of immune defenses are also activated (i.e., antibodies and cytotoxic T cells; this is a normal physiological response and cannot be stopped), but the real defense exists at the molecular level, and other arms of the immune system play an accessory role, if any (9–14,131). For example, at times when HI does not seem to play any role (as in certain parasitic or viral infections), antibodies to various parasitic or viral antigens are made, but in reality, defense lies in CMI.

The mechanisms that protect the hosts from lentiviral infections have been poorly understood. Even though most AIDS researchers know that neither HI nor CMI mechanisms can protect the host against lentiviral infection, they keep trying to develop new ways to elicit neutralization antibodies or cytotoxic T cells in the experimental nonhuman primates (macaques or chimpanzees; 131). As mentioned earlier, chimpanzees infected with HIV-1 do not develop AIDS, but scientific literature is replete with reports in which these animals are used in AIDS research to develop a vaccine. Absence or presence of anti-SIV or HIV-1 antibodies or cytotoxic T cells does not appear to make any difference in the outcome of the disease (9–14,17–26,59,60,63,67,

70–76,102–105,123–125,131,350–352,358–359). Similar results are obtained with humans infected with HIV-1 (to be discussed below). The problem is that interpreting HIV-1 data through conventional immunologic theory can be compared to sailing a rocky coastline with a map of continental features found on another planet. Meanwhile, the HIV-1 epidemic continues to expand unchecked worldwide, and initially promising intervention protocols result in ultimate failure in nearly every laboratory and every clinical trial (19–23,131). Instead of languishing in this intellectual abyss, we need to explore in earnest new realms in our quest for fundamental understanding of infection by retroviruses. We have established that there may be some other mechanism than the traditionally known HI or CMI, which provides infected individuals protection against the ravages of retroviral infections. Now we will investigate the specific type of cell or cells that may play an important role in protection against HIV-1 or retroviruses.

The Cell Types Responsible for Inhibiting Retroviral Replication

Rapid viral replication during the course of HIV-1 infections is now considered an important factor in the in vivo pathogenesis of this human retroviral disease (190,566). Quantitation of viral burden in plasma, PBMCs, and lymphoid organs have been closely correlated with HIV-1 stage, clinical status, and sometimes with CD4+ T-cell counts (131,567–580). It appears that, from the time of HIV-1 infection until the development of AIDS, the major sites of viral replication are the secondary lymphoid organs (573–575). CD8+ T cells and their anti-retroviral factors from HIV-1-infected individuals, SIV-infected monkeys, feline immunodeficiency virus (FIV)-infected cats, or from uninfected healthy individuals can suppress corresponding retroviral replications (85,126,132–139,575,581–613). This observed suppressive activity is not restricted by the MHC, does not require cell-to-cell contact between effector and target cells, and can be mediated through soluble factors. Therefore, this CD8+ cell-mediated HIV-1 resistance is unique and does not fit into the known concepts of HI or CMI, which require cell-to-cell contact between targets (T) and the effector (E) cells, require a certain E-to-T ratio to be effective, and are MHC-restricted. It appears that CD8+ cell-mediated anti-retroviral immunity belongs to a unique form of natural immunity, distinct from HI and CMI. I wish to present existing data as well as some new data from my laboratory to explore this concept.

During the last 10 years many laboratories have published on the important protective role of CD8+ T cells and associated cytokines/chemokines and their receptors in HIV-1 infection, but I believe that these data are manifestations of only a small part of the picture (85,126,132–139,575,581–613). In the following pages I would like to examine how different methods have been applied to develop a vaccine against HIV-1 and then explore various aspects of the CD8+ T-cell-mediated natural immunity hypothesis, particularly those aspects that are linked to what I have termed molecular immunity and appear to be responsible for controlling HIV-1 replication in humans and other retroviruses in their respective hosts.

First, I would like to discuss in detail why HI and CMI mechanisms are unable to control HIV-1 infection in humans and why all the attempts to boost HIV-1-specific HI or CMI responses have resulted in failure.

Scientific Basis for Current Vaccines

Almost all the current designs for an HIV-1 vaccine are based on one of the following: live attenuated virus, genetically related nonpathogenic viruses, inactivated whole virus; live vector-driven subunit or recombinant subunit virus vaccines; chemically synthesized peptides; viral pseudotypes; or DNA vaccines (12–22,55,94,605–606,614–649). Yet none, except the live attenuated vaccines or in certain cases genetically related nonpathogenic viruses (13,20,67–76,78,79,131), have produced satisfactory results, either in humans or nonhuman primates (reviewed in References 12–14). If partial protection is achieved, it is produced with either low doses of the pathogenic virus itself or with a strain of genetically closely related SIVs with a low pathogenicity (see comments on low-dose infection and activation of natural immunity, in a later section). In addition, inactivated and recombinant approaches to vaccine design leave us with other concerns—can these vaccines prevent the cell-to-cell transmission of HIV-1 or the entry of virions through the mucosal route, since these vaccines do not generally provoke an IgA type response (60,72,385,649–652)?

All of these vaccine designs are directed toward arming the hosts with HIV-1-specific HI or CMI. This focus is due largely to history and momentum. HI and CMI are both well-studied and thoroughly understood immunologic phenomena, and agents stimulating these responses have led to many successful vaccines in the past. However, new data suggest that there are problems in relying upon these approaches for a vaccine against a retrovirus like HIV-1.

The first solution: HI. Most common attempts to develop a vaccine against HIV-1 or SIV (the best existing primate model for AIDS) focus on inactivated virus or various forms of recombinant vaccines (12–22,55,94, 131,605–606,614–649). Despite extensive research, these attempts have yet to yield successful results. If some sort of protection is reported, it is only under very specific conditions (i.e., with small infectious doses or with a secondary challenge with a less pathogenic virus, etc.). With SIV, the numerous attempts to develop protection with viral subunits, whole inactivated SIV, recombinant vectors expressing viral proteins, and various other combinations have met with almost total failure. Even when various vaccines induced high levels of SIV-neutralizing antibodies or CMI, no reliable protection was observed against the pathogenic strain of SIV (SIV_{mac} or SIV_{sm}) (12–22,55, 94,605–606,614–649).

The most recent data in this specific realm have come from a joint effort by a team from Harvard Medical School's New England Primate Research Center and Johns Hopkins', Pittsburgh's and Tulane's primate centers. They evaluated the development of *envelope*-specific antibody responses in macaques experimentally infected with molecular recombinant cloned attenuated SIVs (653). Their conclusion was that HI against SIV-*envelope* matures in about 8 months after infection with the cloned SIV. However, the best known and most investigated concept, the so-called neutralization antibodies, was not a significant component of protection, because, quoting from Cole et al., "a number of the serum samples taken from the unprotected monkeys also contained neutralization levels above 50%" (653). This group also evaluated another component, avidity of anti-SIV antibodies, and found that there was a weak association between the degree of avidity and protection (653).

More recently, Shibata et al. (654) evaluated 3 rhesus macaques who were previously immunized with 2 live attenuated mutant SIV_{mac239} (SIVΔ2 or SIVΔ3) or 2 pristine controls, which were infected with an SIV/HIV-1 chimera virus, SHIV. The previously immunized animals were competely protected from SHIV infection, as measured by the absence of virus by co-culture isolation method and absence of SHIV by RT polymerase chain reaction (RT-PCR) and DNA PCR methods, in the lymph nodes, spleen, lungs, and PBMCs. In these animals no SHIV-specific neutralization antibodies were detected, whereas the control animals mounted SHIV-specific antibody responses and exhibited a very high SHIV viral load in all the areas described above. The previously immunized animals were completely protected as determined by several sophisticated quantitative molecular detection methods, including DNA PCR and RT-PCR. The previously immunized animals showed almost undetectable levels of SHIV, whereas unvaccinated animals exhibited very high viral loads. In these animals the presence of anti-HIV gp120 and gp41 antibodies or anti-SIV antibodies did not provide any protection against SHIV, but absence of these antibodies in the vaccinated animals did not render them more susceptible to SHIV infection either. The key question still remaining to be answered is what happens during the 8 months after the African green monkeys and sooty mangabeys are exposed to SIV in nature? If it takes that long to generate a so-called mature HI to SIV, then why are these animals healthy and not dying from the virus that causes AIDS in experimentally infected but evolutionarily naive animals? What is protecting them during this time period? It takes a few minutes for lentiviruses to enter their target cells, and in a few days they can amplify themselves a billionfold (as all HIV-1 researchers know well, they can grow high titer HIV-1 in human T-cell lines). Obviously, if the host infected with HIV-1 or SIV has to wait 8 months for the correct HI or CMI to come to its rescue, it will not survive. There must be another form of immunity that renders these animals immune to retroviral infection.

More surprisingly, infection of a chimpanzee with HIV-1 results in an initial viremia, but not in the manifestation of any subsequent disease. Somehow this primate possesses a natural ability to prevent replication of HIV-1 and adverse consequences of the infection (17–21,34–37,50–55,73,77,225, 391). However, in various trials, vaccines have failed to prevent this initial viremia in immunized chimpanzees—even in the presence of high HIV-1-specific neutralizing antibodies and CMI responses (17–21,34–37,50–55,73, 77,225,391). Yet other unvaccinated chimpanzees (such as the control animals in the above trials) are able to contain the initial viremia of HIV-1 equally well in the absence of either of these immune responses, and neither the vaccinated nor nonvaccinated animals develop any evidence of the HIV-1 infection (9–14,17–21). The correct interpretation of these observations may hold the key to a successful vaccine against HIV-1.

An even more troublesome problem with the anti-HIV antibodies or soluble CD4+ antibodies is that the development of so-called enhancing antibodies, which actually increase viral replication, has been well documented in both human and animal studies (419,421,540,655–657). Furthermore, in certain animal trials, specific vaccines have resulted in the development of antibodies that markedly enhanced viral replication and disease progression (11,22,421,655–657). Recently, numerous suggestions have been made to target β-chemokines or their receptors (by synthetic or pharmacological agents) to block HIV-1 entry. I believe that such suggestions should be viewed with great caution, since previously soluble CD4+ antibodies have suffered total failure (419,421,655–659). One should also keep in mind that the affinity of gp120 for CD4 receptors in their native form is very strong—the K_a association constant of gp120–CD4 binding is about $2 \times 10^{9-11}$ mol/L. However, the affinity of gp120 to soluble CD4 molecules produced by hybridomas or recombinant antibodies is usually much lower (2–3 log lower; 658). In addition, receptor–ligand interactions are dynamic, and they are always in a state of flux between association and dissociation, allowing the high-affinity HIV-1 to latch onto the target cells and enter the cells if coreceptors are present (87,127–131,361–364,415,423). The magnitude of affinity of HIV-1 gp120 for CD4 molecules is so great that it is difficult to imagine that any monoclonal antibodies against CD4 molecules (or CC5 or CXCR4) would be able to prevent HIV-1 from entering the target cells.

The second solution: CMI. The CMI hypothesis was strongly supported by the late Jonas Salk and his colleagues (226,660) who believed that a protective vaccine against HIV-1 would induce cellular rather than humoral immunity. Salk also hypothesized that HI would not only be unprotective, but that it would actually increase susceptibility to HIV-1 infection (419,421, 540,656–657).

This CMI hypothesis was based on several observations supporting the protective role of CMI. For example, at an earlier stage of the AIDS epidemic, Clerici et al. (23) had shown that a majority of individuals exposed to HIV-1 were still seronegative for HIV-1, and a small percentage of unexposed or low-risk subjects showed evidence of preexisting HIV-1-specific CMI. Lymphocytes (PBMCs) from these individuals released interleukin-2 (IL-2) and exhibited evidence of proliferation when exposed to the gp120 envelope antigen of HIV-1. Furthermore, rhesus macaques (which develop an AIDS-like immunodeficiency upon infection with SIV_{mac}) that are exposed to low doses of live SIV_{mac} usually exhibit CMI responses without producing any antibodies specific to SIV_{mac} or developing any evidence of infection (reviewed in References 17–21,556). On the other hand, all but one of the macaques in this study became infected when injected with high doses of SIV_{mac}, and these animals developed SIV_{mac} antibodies but showed no evidence of CMI. From these observations, Salk et al. deduced that CMI (T_H1) can protect against pathogenic retroviral infections (i.e., HIV-1 and SIV_{mac}) whereas humoral responses (T_H2) make the host susceptible to infection with these types of viruses (660). CMI is divided into 2 types of cellular functions: T_H1 is responsible for the typical cell-mediated events including secretion of IL-2 and IFN-γ, and T_H2 is generally believed to be responsible for helping the humoral arm of the immune system including secretion of IL-4, IL-5, IL-6, IL-10, and IL-13. Tumor necrosis factor alpha (TNF-α), granulocyte-macrophage colony-stimulating factor (GM-CSF), and IL-3 are secreted by both types of cells.

In a nutshell, the CMI hypothesis proposed by Salk et al. (226,660) holds that a patient's fate is determined by which of 2 types of immune effector cells, T_H1 or T_H2, is predominant in responding to HIV-1. According to this hypothesis, HIV-1-infected subjects switch from T_H1 protective to a T_H2 disease enhancing response. Since the above-referenced study was published, Clerici et al. and many others have published several excellent articles in support of this hypothesis (661–668). However, there have also been many studies that do not support the CMI hypothesis. For example, Romagnani et al. (669) tested this hypothesis and failed to confirm the hypothesis of a T_H1 to T_H2 switch during the progression of HIV-1 infection. They did not observe any increase of IL-4, IL-5, or IL-10 production during the progression of disease. Since then it has been documented with HIV-1-infected humans that rapid progressors as well as LTNPs both exhibit good HIV-1-specific HI and CMI, suggesting that neither immunity response provides protection against HIV-1 (669). Furthermore, in chimpanzees and in naturally and experimentally infected macaques, natural protection against HIV-1 can occur in the absence of either HI or CMI responses (17–21,33–37,52–57,72,77,391, 615,670).

More recently, Lemaitre et al. (671) also found no evidence for a shift from a T_H1- to a T_H2-type response in HIV-1 infection. They analyzed IL-2, IL-4, and interferon gamma (IFN-γ) production at the cellular level in PBMCs. To address the question of whether a switch from a T_H1- to a T_H2-type cytokine profile may occur and could be a critical step in the progression of HIV-1 infection, they performed an analysis of cytokine expression at the cellular level after in vitro stimulation with phorbol myristic acetate (PMA) plus ionomycin of PBMCs from HIV-infected individuals at different stages of disease. They utilized immunofluorescence staining by anticytokine antibodies to detect cytoplasmic protein, associated with the identification of cytokine-producing T cells by membrane staining and cytofluorometric analysis, which allowed them to explore the immediate potential of chronically activated memory T cells in 7 LTNP patients, who remained asymptomatic 7–11 years after the diagnosis of infection, and 7 typical progressors. The decreased proportion of IL-2-producing T cells (<15% of PBMCs) paralleled the decline of CD4+ T cells regardless of the stage of disease and was associated with the expansion of in vivo activated CD8+ T cells, which acquired the ability to produce high levels of IFN-γ upon stimulation (>50% of CD8+ T cells). Impaired T_H1-type differentiation was observed at the CD4+ T-cell level in rapid progressors early, during the asymptomatic period of declining CD4+ T-cell numbers, and late in the evolution of the disease in the decline of CD8+ T cells, when T-cell numbers fell below 300 cells/μL, which could be indicative of a defect in the renewal of memory T cells. A shift away from a dominant T_H1 differentiation to a T_H2-type cytokine pattern did not occur in any subject or in any stage of infection, as indicated by the analysis of IL-4-producing T cells, which remained in the range of normal values, <5% of PBMCs (established in seronegative control subjects; 671).

A recent analysis of patterns of progression to AIDS in 2 HIV-1-infected patients who were infected from the same source, has revealed some important information regarding the role of CTLs in these 2 patients (670). One of the patients, a 26-year-old white male, lost 31 CD4+ cells/μL/year during the last 3 years of evaluation but remained essentially asymptomatic. The second patient, a 38-year-old white male, progressed rapidly with a rapid loss of CD4+ cells (175 cells/μL/year) and has had persistent HIV-1 p24 antigenemia and *Pneumocystis carinii* infection within 1.5 years after infection (670). What are the differences between the 2 infections? Briefly, these are the major differences. First, the initial HIV-1 viral loads (both RNA and DNA) in the asymptomatic patient were at least one log lower than in the rapid progressor and remained low throughout the 900 days of the analysis. However, a very interesting observation about this specific report was that the amount of virus produced by both patients was still relatively high. The asymptomatic patient continuously produced virus, ranging from 100 000 to 500 000 viral copies/mL (if one multiplies this with 7–10 liters of body fluid it comes out to be about 1×10^8 copies of virus) and the rapid progressor produced about 10 times that much virus (1×10^9 virus). Second, the HIV-1 quasispecies in the asymptomatic patient developed much more quickly and diversified in a nonlinear manner. At day 887 of the analysis, the *env* fragment populations were over 7% divergent from the quasispecies that had been analyzed on day 735. In contrast, the corresponding variant proviral population in the rapid progressor diverged only about 2% over the same time period (this also casts doubt on the widely held belief among AIDS scientists that a host succumbs because of the rapid development of a variety of quasispecies). Third, the rapid progressor and the slow progressor both exhibited strong HIV-1-specific CTL responses to all 3 groups of HIV-1 antigens, *env*, *gag*, and *pol* at 152 days after the infection. However, at subsequent testing, such responses in the rapid progressor deteriorated, probably secondary to rapid loss of CD4+ T cells, known to be essential for the initiation and maintenance of CTL responses. Thus, it appears that CTLs, even in patients infected from a single source, do not seem to make any difference with regard to protection against HIV-1, at least up to 152 days post-infection (670). Therefore, the only determining factor appears to be the initial viral load, which can potentially tilt the balance either in favor of the host or the pathogenic virus.

Infection of rhesus macaques with SIV_{sm}, which is African in origin, represents one of the best studied animal models of AIDS (653). However, in their natural African primate hosts, none of the strains of SIVs cause AIDS-like disease. In one study, when 12 naturally infected sooty mangabeys, caught in the wild, were evaluated for viral load, it was determined that their blood viral load was not necessarily low, and SIV-specific CTL activity was undetectable, again confirming that there is no correlation between viral load and SIV-specific CTL activity (559). Careful analyses of the SIV-specific antibody and CTL responses to SIVs in naturally infected African monkeys have failed to reveal any unusually high immune activity in a traditional sense (CMI or HI; 331). As a matter of fact, the immune responses of many naturally infected monkeys seem to be weaker, both qualitatively and quantitatively, than the immune responses in experimentally infected Asian rhesus macaques and cynomolgus macaques (560). Naturally infected African green monkeys exhibit essentially no neutralizing antibodies to SIV proteins and no SIV-specific CTLs (125). Despite the absence of any traditionally accepted SIV-specific immune responses (humoral and cell-mediated), and presence of relatively moderate plasma viral loads, these nonhuman primates do not exhibit any AIDS-like illness or immunosuppression (27–49,185–187, 561–564).

From the plethora of published data derived from experimentally and naturally infected nonhuman primates, one can conclude that the plasma viral burden in naturally infected healthy African green monkeys or sooty mangabeys is comparable to that of experimentally SIV-infected Asian macaques or HIV-1-infected humans (17–26,59–60,63,67,70–76,102–105, 123–125,350–352,358–359), and that not a single known traditionally accepted immune response can be shown to be responsible for protection against SIV. If neither neutralizing antibodies nor SIV-specific T-cell responses offer protection, what does (10,561–564)?

In summary, several excellent studies in humans as well as in nonhuman primates have shown that the decline in the initial HIV-1/SIV viremia occurs before either neutralizing antibodies or HIV-1-specific CMI responses appear in the infected individual (672–677).

A THIRD FORM OF IMMUNITY

Viral vaccines work by imitating natural immune responses to pathogens and subsequently clearing the infectious agents from the host's system. However, retroviruses possess a much more complex life cycle than any other infectious agent for which we have previously developed vaccines. We must come to a better understanding of the nature of any unexplored form of immune mechanisms that may exist against retroviruses if we wish to develop an effective vaccine.

First of all, from an evolutionary viewpoint, it is difficult to believe that during the course of evolution, higher organisms did not develop some sort of defense mechanism to protect themselves from the onslaught of retroviral infections. For example, regions between maize plant genes are packed with retroelements that make up more than 50% of the 2 billion base pairs that constitute this plant's nuclear DNA (141). Obviously, if during the course of evolution, higher organisms had not developed some sort of intracellular molecular defenses against retroviruses, they would never have evolved to the mammalian level (this defense mechanism has to be HI- and CMI-independent, since maize plants possess neither of these immune systems). As I mentioned earlier, mammalian cells have accommodated many retroviral genes and even appear to have symbiotic relationships with many retroelements, but they must have developed intracellular defenses to counteract further insertion of such genes. Retroviruses have the ability to acquire and alter the structure of host-gene sequences, leading to altered genes, pseudogenes, and oncogenes in the host species; they have the ability to insert their own genome into the host's germline, potentially making subsequent generations transgenic hosts for this now endogenous virus (179–181,200–202); and finally, the seemingly random insertion of provirus can cause genetic damage to the host, leading to disruptions in the activation or control of specific genes near the site of proviral integration. Therefore, I hypothesize that higher eukaryotes must possess some sort of molecular-based intracellular immunity (which I have named molecular immunity) specifically evolved to combat such clear and present genetic dangers. In fact, there is already a large amount of published data to indicate such immunologic responses exist (19–20,23–26,70,86–87,91–94,97,99–105,10–123,126–139,182,350–353, 545,546,613,672–676). The following is a brief survey of the evidence, selected from current peer-reviewed scientific literature.

Epidemiological Evidence

It is a common belief that the majority of individuals exposed to HIV-1 become infected and develop AIDS. However, there are individuals who remain uninfected with the virus, despite multiple high-risk sexual exposures to HIV-1 (23–26,70,86–87,99–105,350–352). In some cases this may simply be the result of exposure to defective viruses, resulting in abortive or quiescent infection. In other cases, there appears to be clear evidence of resistance to infection. For example, it has been shown that the CD4+ T cells of some individuals resist infection with high doses of virus (about a 1000-fold higher concentration of virus than what is required to establish infection). While in these individuals, a small fraction of cells become infected with such a high viral dose, the viral replication does not take place (23–26,70,86–87, 99–105,350–352). Recently, it has been shown that certain individuals (about 1%) have a homozygous defect in one of the HIV-1 coreceptors, CCR5, which makes them resistant to monocyte-tropic strains of HIV-1 (87,130). However, this observation does not explain why so many of the health care workers who were exposed to low doses of HIV-1 did not become infected with the virus. There are over 2084 health care workers in the US who were accidentally exposed to HIV-1 and were monitored by the CDC (the actual figure may be 10–20 times higher, since most individuals who are accidentally exposed to bodily fluids of HIV-1 seropositive individuals do not inform the CDC). Yet only 4 individuals who had no other source of exposure did become seropositive (99–100), and many of the other exposed individuals had deep percutaneous exposures resulting in visible bleeding from the sites of needle injuries. Recently, more extensive studies indicate that the estimated risk for HIV-1 infection after percutaneous exposure to HIV-1 infected blood is about 0.3% (indicating that 97.7% of these individuals were somehow able to protect themselves against HIV-1). This is a very small percentage considering that this sort of exposure generally involves needle pricks with infected blood. This scenario also does not quite fit into the β-chemokine receptor hypothesis described by Cocchi and others (126–131).

Recently, Cardo et al. from the CDC (672) published a follow-up study on the degree of risk of HIV-1 transmission after percutaneous exposure to HIV-1 infected blood. According to their report, the increased risk of transmission was associated with 3 factors; all were indirectly related to dose of inoculation and included (*i*) deep injury; (*ii*) injury with a device that was visibly contaminated with HIV-1-infected blood; and (*iii*) a procedure that involved a needle placed in the HIV-1-infected patient's vein or artery, indicating that the needle contained undiluted blood. In addition, needle sticks with large hollow bore needles were associated with increased risk, suggesting that a larger dose of blood translated into increased risk. The risk of transmission was higher if the health care worker was exposed to blood from a terminal stage AIDS patient—again higher viral dose increased the risk of HIV-1 transmission. Post-exposure prophylaxis with anti-HIV-1 agents [i.e., zidovudine, or azidothymidine (AZT), appears to be protective in reducing the risk of transmission (by lowering the initial viral load)].

Epidemiological studies indicate that various classifiable subgroups infected with HIV-1 vary considerably in their median incubation period and their susceptibility to HIV-1 infection. For example, the frequency of successful transmission of HIV-1 resulting from a single intercourse with an infected partner is relatively low (0.2%–1%), even though high concentrations of HIV-1 are present in 80%–100% of human semen specimens from HIV-1 infected individuals. Some individuals also lack any evidence for infection with HIV-1 despite multiple sexual contacts with HIV-1 infected partners (350-352,613,672–678). Other epidemiological studies suggest that some individuals are truly resistant to HIV-1 infection (23–26,70,86–87,99–105, 350–352,363,673–676). It has been shown that the rate of infection in individuals exposed to a whole unit of infected blood is about 30% (99–101)—a very high percentage and one that is associated with high-dose exposure.

Furthermore, several investigators have reported isolation of HIV-1 from individuals who remained HIV-1 seronegative and free of disease. Detels et al. (102) have observed that some men with many different partners with whom they practiced receptive anal intercourse have remained seronegative despite repeated exposure. Surprisingly, Bryson et al. (679) documented the clearance of HIV-1 infection in perinatally infected infants, who subsequently remained without a detectable HIV-1 infection for 5 years. More recently, Rouges et al. also documented 12 cases of perinatally infected children who cleared the virus (680). Besides these well-documented cases, several other investigators have also reported evidence of individuals who seroreverted and whose prior infection with HIV-1 was documented by HIV-positive blood cultures, positive serum HIV-1 p24 antigenemia, and in some cases, positive PCR assays (681).

Perhaps most intriguing of all are the reports of the so-called molecular immunity in humans infected with HIV-1 who are LTNPs. The majority of individuals infected with HIV-1 progress to AIDS. The average time from first infection with HIV-1 to death in the progressors is less than 10 years. However, the clinical manifestations of HIV-1-associated illnesses appear much earlier: 4 to 6 years after the infection. In about 5% of individuals infected with HIV-1, the LTNPs, the natural history of HIV-1 infection is altered. These individuals remain healthy, and many of the clinical manifestations of HIV-1 infection are either absent or not as prominent as in the progressors (i.e., low CD4+ cell count, HIV-1 p24 antigenemia, generalized lymphadenopathy, and other AIDS-associated infections, lymphomas, and KS). In recent years, several reports have emerged, some of which indicate that an attenuated *nef*-defective HIV-1 variant may be one of the reasons why these individuals are LTNPs (87; the significance of this is that the infection with a defective HIV-1 strain keeps the initial viral load low). Deacon et al. (123) described a single index case, an HIV-1-infected blood donor, whose blood or blood products were transfused into 6 individuals. All of these recipients have remained free of HIV-1-related diseases after 10–14 years. The analysis of HIV-1 isolates have shown a *nef*-defective gene. In addition, Kestler et al. (682) reported that rhesus monkeys experimentally infected with *nef*-negative SIV_{mac} manifest no signs of immunosuppression. The actual contribution of *nef*-defective HIV-1 in the LTNP of this retroviral infection is still controversial, and several LTNPs do not show evidence of *nef*-defective HIV-1 in their PBMCs (but potential defects at other genetic loci have not been ruled out) (683). In addition, the functional analyses of the *nef*-defective HIV-1 viruses, isolated from 10 LTNPs, have indicated no significant differences in the replication properties of these isolates in vitro (683). Therefore, despite the importance of *nef*-defective SIV strains in vivo, the exact function of *nef* at the cellular and molecular levels still remains to be defined. For example, under standard cell culture conditions, *nef* is dispensable for efficient replication. In contrast, in vivo studies in rhesus macaques have shown that intact *nef* is required for efficient replication and pathogenicity (682). The function of *nef* at the molecular levels has begun to be investigated. For example, it has been hypothesized that *nef* interferes with signal transduction pathways (678). For HIV-1 it has been shown that intact *nef* PxxP motifs bind to the SH3 domains of the tyrosine kinases Hck and Lyn. These motifs are required for the enhanced growth of *nef*-positive HIV-1 but not for the down-regulation of CD4 (678). In the Nef proteins of all known lentiviruses, the amino acid residues that appear to be critically important in the interaction between HIV-1 and the SH3 domain are highly conserved. However, in a recent study, Lang et al. (678) showed that the PxxP motif in SIV_{mac239} *nef* which represents the homolog of the HIV-1 *nef* SH3 binding domain is dispensable for the development of AIDS in rhesus macaques. Therefore, it appears that many factors, including multiple HIV-1 variants with different degrees of virulence and replication capabilities, initial viral inoculation dose, numerous host factors, and environmental influences, can play important roles in the ultimate outcome of infection with HIV-1 (69,224,292,684,685). When analyzing the in vitro data, one also has to keep in mind that most of these data are generated by stimulating the PBMCs with PHA, a lectin that nonspecifically activates T cells in a nonphysiological manner, and such data should be treated with great caution (see Chapter 6).

It appears that there is a race between the rapid replication of the virus and the development of antiretroviral immunity. If an individual is allowed to develop the proper molecular immunity against the virus, the odds may move in favor of the host. I hypothesize that infection with these relatively attenuated viruses or low doses of HIV-1 (as in health care workers), results in the activation of anti-HIV-1 molecular immunity in the infected hosts. A particular point that bolsters this interpretation is that many of the individuals infected with *nef*-defective HIV-1 almost certainly later came in contact with fully pathogenic strains of HIV-1 but remained nonprogressors because of the induction of molecular immunity by the attenuated strains. For example, one of the documented nonprogressors is a hemophiliac and probably has had multiple exposures to virulent strains of HIV-1 (through frequent injection of unscreened Factor VIII in the days before HIV-1 screening was implemented). Similarly, several other nonprogressors are homosexual men and have most likely been exposed to various quasispecies of HIV-1, including the fully virulent strains (69,224,292,682–688). Similarly, experimental infection of monkeys with *nef*-deleted SIV_{mac} has resulted in protection against subsequent infection with the high-dose, full-length, wild-type, virulent strain of the homologous virus (86,96,666).

Other Evidence for Molecular Immunity: No Manifestation of Disease with Other Lentiviral Infections

The various SIVs are the most closely related viruses, and some of these strains cause AIDS-like diseases if they infect evolutionarily naive species of primate. However, there are a number of seemingly anomalous host–virus interactions, and each of these gives clues to how primates deal with lentiviral infection.

As detailed earlier, 36% of African green monkeys, over 70% of talapoins, 34% of sykes monkeys, and 20% of mandrills have been found to contain antibodies to SIVs and it is assumed they have been infected with their respective substrains of SIV in the wild, yet no clinical pathology has been associated to date. (It should be kept in mind that these figures are based on the availability of certain SIV antigens. It is possible that a significantly higher number may be infected in the wild, but we are unable to detect them because of technical limitations.) Similarly, over 50% of sooty mangabeys have been shown, both in the wild and in breeding colonies, to be infected with a substrain of SIV_{sm} (31,41,125,306,381–382,689–692). Like the African green monkey infection, the sooty mangabey infection appears to cause no disease in its native host, even though SIV_{agm} and SIV_{sm} are both known to cause AIDS-like disease in the Asian species of monkey. Somehow, these monkeys have developed a means of controlling these retroviruses. In fact, in the breeding colony of sooty mangabeys where the original SIV_{sm} isolate was discovered, as many as 80% of the animals were infected, some for over a decade, without manifesting any evidence of disease (691). Also, there is a striking homology between SIV_{sm} of sooty mangabeys and HIV-2 (691), and there is correspondingly significant sequence homology between HIV-1 and SIV_{cpz}, which was originally isolated from chimpanzees who were without evidence of disease (33–36,391). Of particular note, chimpanzees experimentally infected with HIV-1 fail to develop overt disease despite establishment of infection as evidenced by transient viremia, development of HIV-1-specific antibodies, and HIV-1-specific cytotoxic T cells (17–21,35,50–55, 77,225,615,670). In many cases, chimpanzees experimentally infected with very high doses of HIV-1, develop neutralizing antibodies to HIV-1 in a year, after viremia has already disappeared, in the absence of HIV-1-specific CTLs (73). Similarly, humans infected with HIV-1 do not fully develop a mature HI or CMI response until after a year or more (671). During this year-long period when the traditional immune responses are being optimized, what prevents HIV-1 from completely destroying the infected individuals? These observations strongly suggest that these primates already have some other immunological means to counter these lentiviruses (i.e., molecular immunity). Why does exposure to these SIV strains , which are nonpathogenic to one species of primate, become pathogenic when other species of primates are exposed to them?

Currently, most investigators still believe that humoral and CTL-mediated immune responses to HIV-1 are responsible for the reduction in the viral load seen after the early rise in acutely infected individuals. Until a few years ago most researchers believed (and many still believe) that the HI responses to HIV-1 were the major anti-HIV-1 protective arm of the immune system (17–21,35,50–55,77,225,615,670). However, after total failure in developing any convincing protection in vaccinated animals possessing strong anti-HIV-1 neutralizing antibodies, the focus has shifted towards development of anti-HIV-1 CTLs, and so far the results are discouraging (reviewed in the earlier section). However, many of these investigators who still believe in humoral or CTL-mediated protection against HIV-1 are keen observers and have reported some unusual observations that cannot be readily explained on the basis of HI or CMI. For example, Koup et al. reported that 1 out of 5 patients they studied exhibited a 100-fold decline in the plasma viral load during acute HIV-1 infection without the presence of anti-HIV-1 antibodies and CTLs (673). Borrow et al. (599) also reported a patient who controlled his viremia in the absence of anti-HIV-1 CTL response. Luzuriaga et al. (673) demonstrated that the 3 children they studied exhibited no HIV-1-specific CTL or humoral responses, but their viral load declined after an initial rise in the plasma viral load. As described earlier, there are numerous reports that demonstrated natural resistance against HIV-1 (19–20,23–26,70,86–87, 91–94,97,99–105,120–123,126,139,182,350–352,363,545–546,613,72– 676). CD8+ T cells have been shown to inhibit HIV-1 replication in vitro. However, more recently, Zhang et al. (613) utilized unique SCID-hu mice to explore anti-HIV-1 protective mechanisms. They utilized SCID/beige mice that were reconstituted with human PBMCs from 2 different multiply exposed but HIV-1-seronegative individuals. These mice exhibited resistance to HIV-1 infection. This resistance was against both macrophage tropic as well as T-cell tropic strains of HIV-1. Mice reconstituted with PBMCs from non-HIV-1-infected individuals became infected with HIV-1. When mice were reconstituted with HIV-1-exposed, uninfected PBMCs depleted of CD8+ T cells, they also became infected with HIV-1. Of note, Zhang et al. also analyzed the CCR5 gene sequences in 6 HIV-1-exposed mice, including the 2 they used in the studies described above, and only 1 of the 6 was heterozygous for the CCR5Δ^{32} mutation; all others were homozygous for wild-type CCR5 (126–131). The PBMCs they used for the above studies were the wild-type for CCR5, which indicates that the molecular immunity is not necessarily related to any of the chemokine receptors (87,127–131,361–364,415,423). However, CD8+ T cells appear to play an important role in the development of molecular immunity.

Recently, Legrand et al. evaluated a potential relationship between specific anti-HIV-1 CTL responses, against structural and regulatory proteins of the HIV-1 LAI isolate, and plasma and cellular viral loads in 17 recently HIV-1-infected patients including 3 who were asymptomatic after the primary infection, which they followed up on for 12 months. Plasma viral load correlated directly with CD8 counts and inversely with CD4 counts. Cytotoxic reactions were observed in all patients and were directed mainly against structural proteins (693). The earliest CTL responses were against Gag and Env proteins detected in 87% and 75% of the subjects, respectively, within the first month following initial infection. Anti-Env and anti-Gag cytotoxic responses were inversely correlated with the plasma viral load. Reactions against the *pol* gene products were thought to be either less involved in or less efficient for the initial decrease of viremia. Responses against regulatory gene products were weak and variable, apart from Nef, which was recognized by half of the subjects. Interestingly, neutralizing antibodies were not detected before month 3, and were found only in 6 patients at subsequent times. Two of the three patients with asymptomatic initial infection had a low viral burden and either a delayed response or one limited to a few protein CTL responses, suggesting that the magnitude of the CTL response depends on the initial plasma viral load (and that CTL responses as well as HI are results of normal physiological responses to foreign antigens and they are controlling the viremia). The third patient displayed viral and CTL parameters identical to those of the patients with symptomatic infection. However, 2 subjects with symptomatic initial infection exhibited similarly low plasma viral loads and moderate CTL responses. These investigators concluded that the CTL responses may not be the sole factor controlling viremia (693).

In humans, this complex pattern of molecular immunity against lentiviruses is also manifested in the clinical expression of other retroviruses, for example, the HFVs (or SVs) that infect humans but that has not been associated with any known disease. This lack of clinical expression persists despite a high prevalence of infection among certain human populations, and infectious virus can be readily cultured from the infected tissue specimens from these individuals (82–83) even though no antibodies to SVs could be detected in these individuals (689). HTLV-II has been shown to be endemic in some native American populations without manifestation of clinical disease (84). In contrast, infection with the similar HTLV-I, in a minority of individuals (<4%), leads to either ATL if acquired in infancy, or a chronic neuropathic disease if acquired late in life (84,85,223,603,694). This virus is spread from mother to child perinatally or by breast milk. In adults, sexual transmission and transmission from infected blood also takes place. This retrovirus also infects CD4+ T cells and cells of the central nervous system. However, this virus does not cause AIDS and, most interestingly, causes disease only in a small percentage of infected individuals. Why? The virus itself is not non-pathogenic, and if some of its genes are introduced into a naive host, they can cause very severe illness. For example, it has a regulatory gene called *tax* (like HIV-1 *tat* gene). This gene is a viral oncoprotein and can immortalize and transform several mammalian cell lines (i.e., NIH-3T3, Rat-1, and human CD4+ T cells). *tax* can induce tumors in transgenic mice and regulates transcription of many cellular and viral proteins, apparently by interacting with p100 and p105 precursors of the p50 subunits of $NF_{\kappa}B$ factors. The point of this discussion is that many individual genes of the retroviruses possess severe pathogenic properties, but in the wild when the evolutionarily familiar hosts are infected with these viruses, they cause no illness (these include human hosts infected with HTLV-I and HTLV-II and foamy viruses).

However, despite many similarities among these retroviruses, there are marked differences in the level of clinical expression. Yet it is apparent by the maintenance of infectious disease processes within these populations that low levels of virions are being produced from the integrated proviral sequences. Interestingly, an apparent exposure to HTLV-I in a naive baboon colony in the Sukhumi Primate Center has resulted in >300 cases of malignant lymphoma. In addition, interspecies transmission of rhesus macaque simian T-cell leukemia/lymphoma virus type I (STLV-I) to baboons has been reported (327,360,377,565,694).

Previously, I gave examples of individuals who were able to clear HIV-1 from their system (678–682): more than 2000 health care workers who were infected with HIV-1-infected material but only 4 have seroconverted (99–100), and numerous individuals who remained seronegative despite their high-risk sexual behaviors (106–108).

It is becoming increasingly apparent that there must be more than HI and CMI protecting more highly evolved animals from the genetic parasites like retroviruses (131). Currently, a great research effort is being directed towards the development of chemokine receptor blockers. I believe that these efforts will prove nothing more than mere distractions and will mirror our failed efforts designed to develop anti-HIV-1 neutralization antibodies and CTL-mediated vaccines (131,695–709). In the next chapter I will define the nature of my proposed natural immunity and then examine what methodologies might be used to enhance this elusive molecular protective immunity.

Chapter 4

The Nature of Molecular Immunity

"When you look back at them, many of the fundamental discoveries of science seem so simple, too absurdly simple. How was it men groped and fumbled for so many thousands of years without seeing things that lay right under their noses?"

Paul de Kruif
Microbe Hunters

MOLECULAR IMMUNITY: A DIFFERENT PROTECTIVE MECHANISM

Most of the research efforts on retroviruses over the past 10–15 years have focused on the mechanisms of disease production by these pathogens. Now it is time to explore the mechanisms by which infected hosts protect themselves, and the potential factors that adversely affect the anti-retroviral molecular immunity. As discussed in the preceding chapters, there is enough evidence that evolution has created a different type of intracellular protective mechanism to specifically battle retroviruses—different from HI or CMI—and that many of the previously anomalous phenomena reported by various investigators can be explained on the basis of this alternative hypothesis. The obvious reason for the evolution of a different protective mechanism is that retroviruses are genetic parasites that penetrate into the host genome much faster than HI or CMI can develop protective barriers. In addition, they appear to be immune to these traditional immune mechanisms. They invade the core of the organism's genes. They integrate into the host genomes and have the potential to significantly damage or change the genotype as well as the phenotype of the host species (3,6,8), but most significantly, retroviruses are very quick invaders. It takes only a few minutes for retroviruses to enter the targeted host cells, reverse transcribe their RNA into DNA, and then integrate into the host's genome. Before even early humoral or cell-mediated responses can be initiated, the retrovirus has already gotten to the host DNA. A few hours after invasion, thousands of copies of the retroviruses can be replicated from a single invaded cell. As we know, it takes 2–3 weeks before the traditional immune systems can respond to viral or bacterial invaders (and takes several months to years to mature; 671,689). If an organism has to wait that long to respond to a retroviral invasion, it will be too late! In this period, the retrovirus can make billions of copies of itself, if it remains unchecked. As a matter of fact, one can see that kind of process going on in a cell culture flask, in which blood cells have been infected with HIV-1 virus, and their molecular immunity has been partially inactivated by stimulating these cells with PHA lectin (455,458). In this case, the blood cells produce billions of copies of HIV-1 virus in few days. Therefore, it is logical for the organisms to develop a more rapid, effective, and efficient protective mechanism against this sort of genetic parasite. Again, nature always has better solutions to problems than those we can muster. It has billions of years of evolutionary experience. Therefore, I believe that the host counters the retroviral infection with a genetic defense of its own. It sends out millions of RNA repertoires to search for the right form of complementary RNA, which forms a triple helix with the crucial gene(s) of the invading retroviruses, blocking its integration into the host and stopping it before it can migrate into the host's nucleus (see Figure 4). This concept may explain many unknown mysteries of our defense capabilities against retroviruses in general and against HIV-1 in particular. For example, it can explain why certain substrains of SIV, which have the same overall genomic organization as the other lentiviruses, cause no known disease in its native host, the African monkeys, but does cause AIDS-like disease in Asian species that are evolutionarily naive to SIVs (as humans are naive to HIV-1). Similarly, it can explain why SIV_{sm} causes no disease in its natural host and yet causes an AIDS-like illness in experimentally infected, naive, rhesus macaques and cynomolgus monkeys. While there are genomic differences between the rapidly fatal variant of SIV_{sm} and other SIV_{sm} subtypes, the differences fail to clearly define the pathogenic moiety of this virus (309–311,324–336). Similarly, neither HI nor CMI responses, alone or together, have been found to be clearly responsible for protection against SIV infection (10–14,45,49,57–59,67–69,78–79, 223,270–271,276–277,281,314– 320,379,382,387–388,525,561,696–709). It is quite clear that an adaptation has taken place between the lentiviruses and the African primates and, despite the high seroprevalence of SIVs among the African primates, there is no evidence that SIV infections are associated with immunodeficiency. Therefore, sooty mangabeys naturally infected with SIV_{sm} show no sign of illness due to this virus; if the same virus is inoculated with evolutionarily naive Asian rhesus macaques, they develop an AIDS very similar to humans. By the same token, endogenous type D lentiviruses common in Asian monkeys and African primates are evolutionarily naive to this lentivirus (44,30,215-230,335-346). When African primates are inoculated with type D lentiviruses, they also develop immunosuppression (335-336). This coevolution of various species of endogenous or exogenous lentiviruses with their respective naturally infected host species is not limited to nonhuman primates. Humans have developed an evolutionary coexistence with certain lentiviruses. For example, HTLV-I, which if acquired in infancy leads to ATL in a very small percentage of infected subgroups (i.e., in less than 4% of the population several years after infection), while in the much larger majority (>96%), the virus remains clinically latent throughout life (84–85,223,603, 693). In certain Caribbean populations, however, infection with this retrovirus tends to occur later in life, and among this population, HTLV-I leads primarily to a neuropathic disease (84,161,694). HTLV-II, in contrast, which is endemic in certain isolated populations throughout the world, causes no known disease (84,161,694). HIV-1, which has devastated certain human populations, is most closely related to SIV_{cpz}, which appears to cause no disease in either naturally infected or experimentally infected chimpanzees (33–36,341). It appears that the final disease potential of retroviruses lies in the complex interaction of the retrovirus with the infected host. I have hypothesized that the survival of the host depends on the rapid development of intracellular defenses that can prime the majority of target cells with the appropriate defenses, outracing the pathogenic effects of the retroviruses. If an immunologically competent host is exposed to very low doses of a pathogenic strain of HIV-1 or exposed to less pathogenic strains of HIV-1 (i.e., *nef*-defective HIV-1) and allowed enough time to develop intracellular molecular immunity, then I believe they can resist subsequent exposure to high doses of pathogenic strains of HIV-1. Therefore, in both the primates and humans, I hypothesize that the defenses are already in place against retroviruses, and it may be that initial dose of infection, replication capacity of the pathogen, coevolutionary history of the infectious agent with host, and environmental factors (which can tilt the balance in favor of the pathogens) play a determining role.

We should learn a lesson from the experiences of nature. As stated above, HTLV-I causes disease in a small minority of patients, leading to either ATL if acquired in *infancy* or to a chronic neuropathic disease if acquired *later in life* (84). From these observations, one can conclude that HTLV-I is not pathogenic in immunocompetent humans, but only causes disease in humans during times when their immune systems are relatively weak or compromised. For example, if adult rhesus macaques are infected with live attenuated SIV_{mac}, it causes no disease, and they are completely immune to very high doses of subsequent infection with the pathogenic strains of SIV (72–75,291,694). However, if neonatal macaques are infected by the same route and same doses as an adult, they get sick and develop immunosuppression (72,291). This problem can be circumvented if neonatal monkeys are infected with very low doses of the live attenuated SIV_{mac} (75). Dose response effect of SIV has been explored by others and shows a clear pattern of protection in vivo if low-dose priming (vaccination) of the animals is performed first. If afterwards these same animals are exposed to high doses of SIV, they are completely protected, which shows the protective role of low doses of pathogenic strains of SIV (121, 291,395–396). Very young and older HIV-1-infected patients have been reported to progress to AIDS much more rapidly than other adults. For example, Veugelers et al. (710) recently characterized the associations of age and progression rates to AIDS-defining neoplasms and opportunistic infections in HIV-1-infected homosexual men. For this purpose, they collected data from 407 homosexual men with documented dates of HIV-1 seroconversion. They analyzed data from 4 participating geographic locations by the Kaplan-Meier and Cox methods. They found that among the 407 participants, 139 (34%) were diagnosed with AIDS, 45 (11%) with neoplasms, and 90 (22%) with opportunistic infections. Older age at seroconversion was significantly associated with faster progression to neoplasms, but not to opportunistic infections. For each 10-year increase in age, the risk for AIDS-associated neoplasms increased 1.65-fold (95% confidence interval). They concluded that increasing age is associated with faster progression to AIDS-defining neoplasms, but not with progression to opportunistic infections. This has not been previously reported and may explain conflicting results in other studies among homosexual men that did not consider the age factor. Such age-related outcome has also been reported in the SIV–AIDS model (72,711).

HIV-1 infection of neonates is typified by a bimodal pattern of disease progression (91–96). Therefore about 20% of perinatally infected infants exhibit a rapid course towards AIDS (91–96), whereas about 80% of children with perinatal HIV-1 infection exhibit a relatively slower development of disease, long-term survival, low viral burden, and limited morbidity with HIV-1 infection (91–98). Many of the perinatally infected children completely eliminate HIV-1 from their system. I believe that such infants were initially infected with very low doses of HIV-1 and developed molecular immunity against HIV-1, thus eliminating the virus or becoming LTNPs (679–681). This point is very clearly demonstrated in the experiment provided by nature with monozygotic twins. Some identical, monochorionic, monozygotic twins, born to HIV-1 infected mothers, show discordant results. This means that one is infected with HIV-1, and the other one is uninfected. In monozygotic, monochorionic fetuses, the blood circulation is unequal, and newly oxygenated blood enriched with nutrients, coming from maternal blood, preferentially supplies more blood to one twin than the other. As a result, the well-nourished baby is red and thin at the time of birth and the malnourished one looks healthy (and fat, due to edema) to an untrained eye. In this situation, the first twin gets exposed to high doses of HIV-1 (if maternal blood contains HIV-1), and the second one gets lower doses of HIV-1. In this case, the first one gets infected while the second one may be vaccinated against HIV-1 (118–120). However, if such twins get infected postnatally, for example by blood transfusion, then the outcome of HIV-1 infection remains the same. For example, recently, Saulsbury et al. (712) reported the course of HIV-1 infection in identical triplets who were infected with HIV-1 at 1 day postpartum via a blood transfusion from a common unit of contaminated blood. The subsequent clinical manifestations of HIV-1 infection in the triplets were remarkably uniform. Also, the CD4+ cell counts declined in a very similar manner. Again, these observations drive home the point that it is the initial viral dose which may be the determining factor. In a recent comprehensive study (712), evaluation of consecutive samples from 324 HIV-1-positive women suggests that the highest risk for infant infection is associated with maternal p24 antigenemia (71% rate of transmission), suggesting that transplacental transmission of HIV-1 is taking place (even though there may be other routes of transmission of HIV-1 from mother to child).

Role of CD8+ T Cells in the Development of Anti-Retroviral Immunity

The pivotal role of CD8+ T cells in the development of the anti-retroviral specific natural defenses has been well documented (85,126,132–139, 575,581–613). Briefly, CD8+ T cells or factors from CD8+ T cells from healthy HIV-1-infected or HIV-1-uninfected individuals can suppress HIV-1 replication without killing the infected cells. These are non-CTL, noncytolytic CD8+ T cells, characterized by their ability to reduce HIV-1 p24 antigen levels and reverse transcriptase levels in the culture fluids of PBMCs infected with all strains of HIV-1 and 2, SIVs, and FIV (85,126,132–139, 575,581–613, 712–717). This anti-retroviral activity does not appear to be restricted by the MHC or require contact between target and effector cells; it occurs at low CD8+/CD4+ ratios; and it is oligoclonal in nature (603). The nature of its anti-retroviral activity is via soluble messenger agents, which are unrelated to any known cytokines or chemokines, though currently this conclusion is controversial. The exact mechanisms of these antiviral effects are still unclear. However, several recent experiments show that CD8+ T cells and their anti-retroviral factors exert their anti-HIV-1 effects by specifically interrupting HIV-1 transcription (137–138,589–590).

Are β-Chemokines the Answer for CD8+ T-Cell Factors?

Recently, there has been a remarkable series of articles demonstrating the coreceptors for HIV-1 in various cell lines (87,127–131,361–364,415,423). It has long been thought that HIV-1 might bind to its primary CD4 receptors but that coreceptors were certainly necessary for the viral entry (127–131). This was determined from data in murine and other animal cell types in which CD4 expression would not permit productive infection. Feng et al. (363) demonstrated that a transmembrane chemokine receptor, Fusin (CXCR4), serves as a cofactor for T-cell tropic, but not monocyte tropic, strains of HIV-1 (now called X4 viruses). Another coreceptor, CCR5, appears to be a major coreceptor for macrophage/monocyte tropic strains of HIV-1 (now called R5 viruses) (362). These coreceptors bind a variety of β-chemokines, i.e., RANTES, MIP-1α, and MIP-1β, and are secreted by variety of cell types. What do these β-chemokines do? Are they the suppressive factors scientists are looking for? It appears that they may not be since their effect is on pre-entry level (127–131,361–364), whereas CD8+ T cells and their anti-retroviral factors appear to work on pre-reverse transcriptase, reverse transcriptase, and/or transcription levels (134,137–138, 589–590,610,717). It has been hypothesized that β-chemokines may serve as blocking agents for their respective receptors and hence as anti-HIV-1 suppressive factors. Recently, it has been reported that analysis of 2 exposed but uninfected people (who have exhibited a significant degree of resistance to high doses of macrophage tropic strains of HIV-1 infection in vitro) has shown that such a resistance is due to the presence of a homozygous genetic defect in the CCR5 receptor (87,130). I believe that CD8+ T-cell factors are different from the β-chemokines described by Cocchi et al. (126) because it has been noted *(i)* that the concentrations of CD8+ T-cell factors and chemokines are independent variables in HIV-1-suppressing culture media; *(ii)* that chemokine-specific neutralizing antibodies do not block the CD8+ T-cell factor activities; *(iii)* that CD8+ T cell factor-susceptible HIV-1 strains are variably sensitive to chemokines; *(iv)* that both T-cell tropic and monocyte/macrophage-tropic strains are sensitive to CD8+ T-cell factors; *(v)* that the levels of chemokines and CD8+ T-cell factors peak at different times, in vitro; and *(vi)* that cell factors have very broad range against several lentiviruses (516,586,609–610, 718–720, and unpublished data). The homozygous defect of CCR5 receptors reported to be present in about 1% of the US population does not explain why the vast majority of health care workers (>97.7%) who got exposed to low doses of HIV-1 did not become infected with the virus (99–101,672). In addition, there are several case reports where individuals with the homozygous genetic defect for CCR5 have developed AIDS, which casts serious doubt on this chemokine theory (721–725). More recent reviews, where antibodies to chemokines have been used in vitro, have shown disappointing results (reviewed in Reference 131).

The Discovery of β-Chemokines and Their Applicability to Vaccine Research

It is very important to explain how the crucial role of β-chemokines as coreceptors for HIV-1 was discovered. An envelope-complementation assay was used to determine the efficiency with which HIV-1 containing various types of envelopes mediates early events in cell entry in different cell types (87,127–131,361–364,415,423). Recombinant HIV-1 was produced by cotransfection of HeLa cells with 2 plasmids, pHXB10Δenv-CAT (which contains an HIV-1 provirus with a deletion in the envelope and a replacement of the *nef* gene with a gene encoding the *cat* reporter gene or other reporter genes like *luciferase* or *lacZ*, etc.) and pSVIIIenv (using different plasmids encoding the envelope glycoproteins derived from a laboratory-adapted HIV-1 isolate, HXBc2, and from macrophage-tropic primary HIV-1 isolates, Br20-4, ADA, and YU2. The recombinant viruses produced in the HeLa supernatants thus contained different envelope glycoproteins, which allowed an assessment of the ability of these glycoproteins to mediate a single round of infection. Transfection with the envelope-defective plasmid, pHXB10Δenv-CAT, served as a control (127–131). HeLa cells transfected with plasmids expressing human CD4 and various 7-transmembrane-segment chemokine receptors were used as target cells. The efficiency of the early phase of virus infection was assessed by measuring CAT activity in the HeLa target cells 60 h following infection. The major problem with such an envelope-complementation assay is that, because the plasmids expressing the cDNAs of a number of chemokine receptors and related molecules were cotransfected with CD4-expressing plasmids into the HeLa cells, the levels of CD4 and other chemokine molecules expressed on the surface of the HeLa cells may not represent the level of expression of these molecules on the cell surface of human PBMCs in their natural environment (i.e., the surface density of these receptors would be artificial). In a natural situation, more than one chemokine receptor may be expressed simultaneously on a single cell type, further confounding the problem. Also, the pseudotypes produced do not represent the naturally occurring viruses, and they may not even express the same conformation of envelope glycoproteins. Similarly, in a modification of this assay, a fusion assay was used. Here, T7 RNA polymerase and envelope glycoprotein were introduced into effector HeLa cells by infection with recombinant vaccinia viruses. Target QT6 cells were transfected with CD4, Fusin (CXCR4: T-cell tropic), or CCR5 (macrophage tropic strain). Both cells were allowed to fuse together and were observed (361–364). Again, these are not viruses fusing with target cells but cells fusing with cells and each cell type, target and effector, is expressing unnatural forms of glycoproteins, in unnatural densities, and unnatural combinations (87,127–131,361–364,415,423).

CD8+ T-Cell Factors are Unique and Different from β-Chemokines

Three years ago, Cocchi et al. (126) published a paper showing that the elusive CD8+ T-cell factors are β-chemokines, RANTES, MIP-1α, and MIP-1β. Since this report, several investigators have shown that chemokines serve as coreceptors for HIV-1 entry into the CD4+ T cells (127–131). At this time, a majority of investigators believe that chemokine receptors could be used to block HIV-1 entry inside the cells, and that the elusive CD8+ T-cell factors are chemokines. I believe that such an assumption is premature and based on laboratory data not representing the natural conditions of host–virus interactions (127–131,361–364). In order to investigate whether anti-HIV-1 factors secreted by CD8+ T cells are β-chemokines, my laboratory, like many others around the globe, has been working on this particular issue. For example, we generated anti-HIV-1 factors from a well-characterized LTNP. The anti-HIV-1 effects of the supernatants from the unfractionated PBMCs, CD8+ T cells, and CD4+ T-cell enriched subsets from this individual were tested on several primary HIV-1 isolates (subtypes B, C, and E, prevalent in various parts of the globe where HIV-1 is prevalent) and various laboratory strains (HIV-1, NL4-3, and 89.6). Ten percent of the final concentration of the suppressive factors showed inhibition of HIV-1 replication up to 76% as determined by reverse transcriptase assay over the period of 12 days (516).

A cocktail of β-chemokines (at 100 ng/mL) was utilized to determine the degree of HIV-1 inhibition of the above HIV-1 primary isolates and laboratory strains. The degree of inhibition of HIV-1 was significantly less (< 40%) than reported previously by Cocchi et al. (126).

We further evaluated the role of β-chemokines in the supernatants we collected from the PBMCs and their subsets ($CD4^+$, $CD8^+$ enriched T cells) from the LTNPs we studied. For this purpose, we utilized specific polyclonal goat IgG neutralizing antibodies against RANTES, MIP-1α, and MIP-β at the final concentration of 150, 50, and 100 μg/mL, respectively. For all the primary HIV-1 isolates, neutralization of the suppressive factor from the unfractionated PBMC ranged from 32%–56% on any given day over the time period of 10 days. No neutralization of CD8+ T-cell factors and CD4+ suppressive factor was observed for the primary HIV-1 subtypes B and C (516).

Our results suggest that the anti-HIV-1 effects exerted by CD8+ T cells and associated cytokines/chemokines are different from the chemokine/chemokine receptor mediated HIV-1 inhibition reported in several recent articles (127–131,361–364).

In addition, Dr. Fauci's group (722) has also demonstrated that only CD8+ T-cell derived factors, but not the β-chemokines, RANTES, MIP-1α, and MIP-1β, suppress HIV-1 replication in monocytes/macrophages. In order to investigate whether a CD8+ T-cell derived soluble factor(s) can suppress HIV-1 infection in a monocyte/macrophage, they infected primary macrophages with the macrophage-tropic HIV-1 strain Ba-L. They also infected CD8+ T-cell depleted PBMCs with HIV-1 IIIB or Ba-L. In addition, they determined HIV-1 expression from the chronically infected macrophage cell line U1 in the presence of CD8+ T-cell supernatants or β-chemokines. They showed that CD8+T-cell factor(s) did suppress HIV-1 replication in the monocytes/macrophages, but β-chemokines failed to do so, and that antibodies to β-chemokines did not neutralize the anti-HIV-1 activities of CD8+T-cell factors. Their findings, like our own, suggest that HIV-1 suppressive activities from the factor(s) released by CD8+T cells may be different from the proposed anti-HIV-1 activities of β-chemokines proposed by Cocchi et al. (126).

Several other investigators, including Dr. Levy's group (who were the first to publish the anti-retroviral effects of CD8+T cells; 132–133) have evaluated the anti-HIV-1 effects of β-chemokines and CD8+ T-cell supernatants, and most of these data suggest that some β-chemokines exhibit anti-HIV-1 activity against certain primary isolates. However, as observed with interferons, IL-8, TGF-β, and TNF-α, these cytokines are not primarily responsible for the non-cytotoxic anti-HIV-1 activity observed with CD8+T-cell-derived factor(s). It has been shown that the level of CD8+T-cell-derived factor(s) is highest in LTNPs and asymptomatic individuals and decreases with progression towards AIDS. RANTES, MIP-1α, and MIP-β are not present in any appreciable amount in CD8+T-cell-derived supernatants from HIV-1-infected LTNPs compared with HIV-1-infected typical progressors (718–724). Also, the anti-

HIV-1 activity of RANTES, MIP-1α, and MIP-β is not as broad as the anti-HIV-1 (and anti-lentiviral) activities of CD8+T-cell-derived factor(s) (718–724). In addition, the targets of the anti-HIV-1 activity of RANTES, MIP-1α, and MIP-1β and CD8+T-cell-derived factor(s) appear to be at different stages of the retroviral life cycle, the former inhibiting entry while the latter block reverse transcriptase as well as integration of the PIC (724). In evolutionary terms, receptor-mediated inhibition (as proposed for HIV-1 via β-chemokines) does not make sense; target cells would express chemokine receptors to different degrees at various stages of the cell cycle, which provides the opportunity for HIV-1 to enter the target cells and defeat the host (131).

Mosoian et al. (725) used herpesvirus Saimiri strain C-488-immortalized CD8+ T cells for screening of HIV-1 inhibitory activity in CD4+ cells utilizing both primary and laboratory-adapted strains of HIV-1. Supernatants with strong activity were tested against the macrophage-tropic strain Ab-I in primary macrophages. They measured β-chemokine levels in these supernatants by ELISA, and they compared the inhibitory activity to that of a mixture of RANTES, MIP-1α, and MIP-1β, each at a concentration of 200 ng/mL, and analyzed the culture supernatants for HIV-1 p24 antigen. Supernatants from CD8+ T cells from infected as well as from a normal donor showed potent inhibitory activity against HIV-1 Ab-I in primary macrophages. The level of RANTES in the supernatants was 5.2–5.6 ng/mL. In contrast, the chemokine cocktail at 200 ng/mL each had little or no activity in the majority of primary macrophage cultures. Increasing the dose to 400 ng/mL had modest inhibitory effects. Their results suggest that the inhibitory activity of the CD8+ supernatants against HIV-1 Ab-I in macrophage was not due solely to a mixture of these chemokines and furthermore that HIV-1 Ab-I interaction with the CCR5 receptor may differ in macrophages compared to lymphocytes.

From some of the statements regarding the nature of CD8+ T cells and their anti-retroviral factors, it might seem that molecular immunity could be similar to the so-called transfer factor (TF), described in the old immunology literature. TF has been described as a less than 10-kDa, dialyzable, cell-free extract of lymphocytes that is able to transfer CMI from antigen-responsive to antigen-nonresponsive hosts. The activity of TF is antigen-specific but generalized immunopotentiation is also achieved. The TF has been reported to be DNase-resistant and heat-sensitive. Many clinical studies to date have employed TF in the therapy of neoplasms, immunodeficiency states, and infectious diseases. It is obvious from the data that CD8+ T cells and their anti-retroviral factor effects described by many investigators (126,132–135,581–613) do not fit into the described effects shown by TF.

Some Cofactors Can Compromise Immunity

I hypothesize that the protective natural defenses against a specific group of retroviruses and genetically closely related viruses can be induced by low-dose inoculation of live attenuated viruses and that such an immunity would be life-long unless untoward events or cofactors adversely affected the anti-retroviral molecular immunity by inducing alterations in the subsets of cells that are involved in molecular immunity (i.e., CD8+ cells, NK+ cells). These cofactors are especially important during the initial stages of infection, at which time they can determine the future course of infection. "Untoward events or cofactors" are of several types, including exposure to low-dose radiation (726), UV light (727), cyclophosphamide (728), steroids (729,730), and protein-synthesis inhibitors (731). Both irradiation and cyclophosphamide have been shown to induce CD8+ T-cell dysfunction in experimental animals (732). Another cofactor is co-infection with another pathogenic virus or exposure to specific viral products, and these other viruses need not necessarily be retroviruses (733–740). A third type of cofactor is temporary immunoincompetence due to abuse of certain substances, such as alcohol (741–750), marijuana (751), cocaine (752–757) or even certain anti-HIV-1 drugs (758)—these latter cofactors may be of particular significance during the initial exposure (759). No doubt there are also unknown cofactors that may interfere with or inactivate the molecular immunity pathways and render the host susceptible to acute retroviral infection. All of these cofactors must exert a common malfunction in the subsets of the cells which are the major protectors against retroviruses.

Factors That Interfere in the Anti-Retroviral Molecular Immunity Pathways

If we have natural defenses against HIV-1 infection, why does infection with HIV-1 result in such devastating consequences for humans? There are 2 main possibilities. I believe that infection with HIV-1 in humans (and other lentiviruses in primates) follows 1 of 2 possible courses.

If the initial single exposure is with a very low dose or a defective HIV-1 retrovirus [for example >2000 health care workers who were accidentally inoculated with HIV-1-infected body fluids (99–101,672); some individuals who got transfused with HIV-1-infected blood but the HIV-1 retrovirus was supposedly defective (70); and naive primates infected with a new type of SIV], the exposure results in the priming of the host's molecular immunity, as has been shown by utilizing SIV-*nef* defective or triple deletion mutation viruses (12,19–21,62,68–71,76–78,187,615,617); this priming subsequently arms the hosts' defenses against HIV-1 or a specific type of lentivirus (i.e., SIV). The host will be resistant to the pathogenic consequences of subsequent infection with high doses of HIV-1 or SIV (in the case of naive primates), after a reasonable lag time (i.e., 1–3 weeks) (12,19–21,62,68–71, 76–78, 187,615,617). Recently, Mellors et al. (759) evaluated 209 HIV-1-infected men and collected several possible variable parameters that may predict the prognosis of these individuals. Collectively, their data indicate that baseline HIV-1 RNA levels (indicator of the initial inoculation dose) were highly predictive of prognosis (759).

If the initial exposure occurs as a high dose of HIV-1, as multiple exposures to smaller doses of HIV-1, or a low dose but at a time when the individual's immune system is transiently compromised (before or during the completion of the priming phase), the exposure will result in the overwhelming of the host's molecular immunity mechanisms, resulting in a susceptible host who will develop the disease or diseases as a result of the pathogenic consequences of HIV-1. Examples of multiple exposures are homosexual men who practiced anal sex that exposed them to variable concentrations of HIV-1 many times over in a short period (429,431,710,727–729), or intravenous drug users who injected themselves with HIV-1-infected needles several times in a very short period (430). If the immune system is transiently compromised because of alcohol, cocaine, other substances of abuse, malnutrition, severe stress, or depression, then even a very small dose of virus may act like a high dose, as has been shown by several investigators, including by our own laboratory (727–737).

This 2-outcome scenario provides an answer to the following problems: *(i)* why primates experimentally exposed to low doses of SIV or exposed to genetically related nonpathogenic SIV develop resistance to high doses of the pathogenic SIVs (12,19–21,62,68–71,76–78,187,615,617); *(ii)* why thousands of health care workers exposed to HIV-1-infected body fluids are still seronegative (99–101,672); *(iii)* why there is a clear-cut difference between 2 groups of pediatric patients, 1 group that progresses rapidly to AIDS within a year after birth and the other group that apparently clears HIV-1 from their systems (91–96,679,680); *(iv)* why patients or primates infected with *nef*-negative or defective virus have done well (12,19–21,62,68–71,76–78, 187,615,617); *(v)* why there is so much variability in the susceptibility of PBMCs infected with HIV-1 or SIV, in vitro and in vivo (45,133, 406,579,704); *(vi)* why some men with many different partners with whom they practiced unprotected receptive anal intercourse have remained seronegative, despite repeated exposure (1,2,23–26,80–82,117); *(vii)* why certain identical (monozygotic) twins, born to HIV-1-infected mothers, show discordant results (760–764); *(viii)* why infection with HTLV-1 in the majority of individuals leads to no adverse consequences; and *(ix)* why all the primates infected with a various strains of SIVs in the wild exhibit no clinical signs of AIDS or other related illnesses (84), but if exposed to different strains do get sick (though only if they are exposed to very high doses of SIVs) (84,161). The explanation of this phenomenon, if we accept the hypothesis, is that primates get primed with low doses of SIVs in utero or during an early period of their lives, making them immune to that particular strain or to related strains of SIVs. The reason African nonhuman primates do not develop AIDS or immunosuppression when infected with SIVs is because they carry various strains of SIVs in their systems. A low level of virus is always present in their systems, ensuring the survival of that particular strain or strains, which coexist with a particular primate colony, and it also keeps the molecular immunity activated and alert against certain lentiviruses. This low-grade replication of lentiviruses ensures that the next generation of this monkey colony will also be primed and will survive if exposed to genetically related SIVs, which commonly occurs in the primate life cycle when they are either attacked or attacking other primate colonies.

I would also suggest that any conditions such as an immature immune system, a naturally immunocompromised state like old age (72–75,291), exposure to chemical agent(s) or other biological agents (e.g., radiation), or stress or depression, which induce certain dysfunctions in CD8+ T cells, may lead to inactivation in the arm of the immune system that is responsible for molecular immunity. Stress releases steroid hormones and thus induces dysfunctions in the CD8+ T cells (732), which then activates lentiviral replication. Also, any agent(s) that nonspecifically stimulates T lymphocytes [e.g., T-cell mitogens like PHA, concanavalin A (ConA), PMA, etc.] may induce alterations in the anti-retroviral immune mechanisms (455,471,717).

WHAT FACTORS INACTIVATE MOLECULAR IMMUNITY?

Several experiments by various investigators have provided information regarding these events. Zack et al. (455) evaluated the molecular events after HIV-1 entry into CD4+ cells. After entry into unstimulated human PBMCs, the HIV-1 genome is blocked from completing RT by some unknown host factor(s). Even though viral RNA and incomplete reverse transcripts of proviral DNA may persist for a short period of time, the researchers found that these viruses were labile and were degraded by host factor(s). Stimulation of PBMCs with a T-cell mitogen (PHA) results in the breakdown of this natural defense system against HIV-1.

In a different series of experiments, Bukrinsky et al. (471) examined the PBMCs from HIV-1-seropositive individuals for the presence of HIV-1 provirus. In their studies, they observed that in the resting (quiescent) T cells from asymptomatic individuals, HIV-1 existed as unintegrated full-length HIV-1 but not as an integrated form. This observation suggests that certain naturally occurring host factors may be preventing the integration of HIV-1 provirus. However, when the PBMCs were activated with a mitogen (like PHA) in vitro, HIV-1 provirus integrated into the host genome. The same authors further noticed that in AIDS patients, the percentage of integrated HIV-1 was higher and was associated with HLA-DR+ T cells (activated subsets of T cells).

Recently, Sonza et al. (717) showed that in fresh PBMC monocytes, HIV-1 replication is blocked prior to the RT and integration steps. They isolated PBMC monocytes from HIV-1-seronegative individuals' buffy coats and enriched them by the plastic adherence method. These PBMC monocytes were found to be resistant to productive HIV-1 infection after they were infected with monocyte-tropic strains of HIV-1. They were unable to detect any HIV-1 cDNA by the PCR method. However, if the monocytes were activated with PHA, they completed the HIV-1 RT reaction and produced HIV-1 p24. In the quiescent cells the HIV-1 existed as extrachromosomal virus.

Early Viral Load in Primates

As we discussed in detail earlier, infection of African nonhuman primates with SIVs, the most closely HIV-related lentiviruses, causes no harmful effect in their natural hosts. However, if Asian strains of monkeys are infected with SIVs from the other monkey species, in many cases this results in AIDS-like disease (reviewed in References 19–21,56–57). These animal models have played a pivotal role in our understanding of the pathogenesis of HIV-1 in humans. In a recent study, Watson et al. (765) investigated whether early events in macaques infected with a cloned SIV (SIV_{smE660}) could predict the ultimate outcome of the infection. For this purpose, these investigators infected a group of macaques with a cloned SIV and observed them for 2 years. As in numerous prospective studies conducted in humans, when macaques were infected with SIV, the plasma SIV loads at 6 weeks postinfection were predictive of progression to AIDS in the experimentally infected macaques (765).

Early Viral Load in Humans

In humans, the progression to AIDS, rate of progression, and outcome of the illness depend on the early infecting dose. Since this kind of experiment cannot be carried out in humans, the next best thing is to measure the early viral load in individuals when they enter a study and follow them for several years and see what the outcome is. Mellors et al. (759) did exactly that. For 10 years or more, they followed 209 HIV-1-infected gay or bisexual men who entered a major university hospital during 1984–1985. These patients were followed through progression to AIDS and death. None of these individuals had received anti-retroviral drugs by the time of entry, and only 41% received anti-retrovirals at any time during follow-up. The HIV-1 RNA at the time of entry ranged from less than 500 copies/mL to about 3 million copies/mL. They correlated the relationship of HIV-1 RNA viral burden at the time of entry to progression to AIDS by utilizing Kaplan-Meier survival curves. Subjects who had very high viral load at entry progressed to AIDS within 3.5 years, and those with the lowest progressed to AIDS in >10 years (and thus were LTNPs). The median time of death of individuals who had HIV-1 RNA burden >10 000 copies/mL at the time of entry was 6.8 years, whereas the individuals whose viral burden was below 10 000 copies of HIV-1 RNA/mL at the time of entry had survival rates significantly higher. In fact, only 30% of these individuals had died within 10 years (759). In summary, individuals with initially high HIV-1 RNA viral load and individuals with persistently high viremia were at increased risk of developing AIDS within a short period after seroconversion. As I have already mentioned, the initial viral load seems to play an important role in predicting the severity of lentiviral infection in various primate species, including humans. For example, high primary viremia in experimentally infected Asian monkeys is associated with severity of diseases, whereas low primary viremia is a good indicator of no or very low-grade disease. Shibata et al. (654) demonstrated that in macques previously vaccinated with live attenuated mutant SIV_{mac239} and then infected with SHIV, the immunized animals were completely protected from SHIV infection, as measured by the absence of virus by various methods. On the other hand, the control animals (unvaccinated) exhibited a very high SHIV viral load. The previously immunized animals with the mutant virus were completely protected as determined by several sophisticated quantitative molecular detection methods, including DNA PCR and RT-PCR. In humans, the initial inoculation dose of HIV-1 has been shown to play a pivotal role (672). Therefore, the potential transmissibility of HIV-1 was directly associated with the degree of severity of injury and inoculation dose of HIV-1.

Siliciano et al. (766,767) analyzed the total body load of latently infected cells using novel molecular and cellular assays in HIV-1-seropositive individuals. Their results indicated that the fraction of latently infected CD4+ T cells carrying integrated HIV-1 DNA was extremely low (<0.01%), was not different in blood and lymph nodes, and remained at a stable steady state with declining CD4 counts. An average of 25% of the integrated provirus was replication-competent, indicating that even in HIV-1-seropositive individuals and some of the AIDS patients, molecular immunity is still functioning. The dominant form of provirus, present in a 200-fold higher number of copies than integrated HIV-1 DNA, was a full-length, unintegrated species that is not blunt ended, again suggesting that molecular immunity is keeping the HIV-1 virus in unintegrated form in the majority of cases (possibly at the PIC level). They estimated that total body loads of resting and activated CD4+ T cells with integrated provirus were 6.7×10^6 and 1.2×10^7 cells, respectively. Virus load in lymph node and alveolar macrophages was also determined. The frequency of lymph node macrophages with integrated provirus was <0.1% with even lower frequencies in macrophages in the lung. These results indicate that HIV-1 infection persists and progresses even though only minute fractions of the susceptible cell populations are stably infected (<0.01%). The surprisingly small size of the latent reservoir confirms the notion that an extremely small fraction of cells actually gets infected, while the rest of the cells carry the virus as a PIC that only gets integrated (and completes the infection process) when the cells are activated. That brings us to the explanation of why, even in LTNPs, the HIV-1 RNA levels still can be measured (760,761). As described above, Mellors et al. (759) showed that even 3- to 5-fold differences in plasma HIV-1 RNA levels are associated with rapid disease progression. Therefore, protection against HIV-1 does not necessarily mean that viral load is unmeasurable. It only means that the majority of the cells are protected, and only a small fraction of cells, which get activated during the normal physiological course of immune activation, are responsible for the viral load. As a matter of fact, if asymptomatic HIV-1-infected patients are vaccinated against pneumococcus (by pneumococcal vaccine), it leads to a rapid and significant increase in viral burden in the majority of the patients (768), although transiently. The magnitude of these increased viral loads correlates with the extent of the antibody response to the vaccination (768–770). Therefore, antigenic stimulation in vivo as well as mitogenic stimulation (as with PHA lectin) in vitro breaks down the protective molecular immunity in the individual cells. This transient increase in viral burden after exposure to a stimuli, either chemical, physiological, or psychological, is inevitable and may be beneficial, since such an increase would also be forthcoming if the host were exposed to a retrovirus and needed up-regulation of molecular defenses. However, this is part of the evolutionarily designed normal physiological response of molecular immunity. This process guarantees the survival of the host and the invading retroviruses, and explains why in African nonhuman primates infected with SIVs, there is no illness due to these viruses even when they exhibit varying degrees of viral burden. The same scenario holds true for nonhuman primates naturally infected with SIV and for LTNP humans infected with HIV-1.

How Molecular Immunity Relates to Identical Twins

Because twins share an in utero environment and genetic relationships, similarities and differences between them can provide insight into the epidemiology and natural history of infectious agents, especially HIV-1. As described earlier, some identical, monochorionic, monozygotic twins born to HIV-1-infected mothers show discordant results. This means that one is infected with HIV-1 and the other is not, because in these situations, the blood flow is not equal. One actually gets more blood than the other; thus, the first twin gets infected while the second is in effect vaccinated against HIV-1 (118–120). Recently, Goedert (760) summarized 2 cases of discordant HIV-1 transmission and AIDS-free survival in 2 sets of identical twins. His analyses showed that infected identical twins in one set had intermingling of each infant's HIV-1 quasispecies, whereas in the second set, each twin had its own distinct cluster of quasispecies around a maternal sequence. In each set of twins, one child went on to develop AIDS, while the other remained without symptoms. I believe this is a typical example of the dose response effect mentioned above. Duliege et al. (761) assessed concordance, birth order, route of delivery, and other factors for HIV infection in 115 twins born to HIV-infected women. They reported that infection with HIV occurred in 35% of vaginally delivered first-born (A) twins, 16% of cesarean-delivered A twins, 15% of vaginally delivered second-born (B) twins, and 8% of cesarean-delivered B twins. Among A twins, 52% of the transmission risk was related to vaginal delivery (which received the highest dose of HIV-1). Comparing vaginally delivered A twins (infants most exposed to vaginal mucus and blood) to cesarean-delivered B twins (infants least exposed). Infected B twins had reduced risk of HIV-1 infection. HIV-1 replication biological and genetic variability is a prominent feature of HIV strains, especially in tropism, syncytium formation, and replicative capacity. Identical twins are not identical in their susceptibility to HIV-1 because of factors other than initial viral load, hypothesized above.

The next question we should ask is whether the host has some sort of natural resistance against HIV-1. The answer to this question comes from another series of experiments reported by Chang et al. (762). To determine whether there were variable host cell effects on HIV replication in monocytes, these investigators utilized 3 different strains of low-passage-number monocytotropic blood isolates of HIV-1 and 1 laboratory-adapted strain, Ba-L. They inoculated these strains of HIV-1 into panels of adherent monocytes drawn from 44 different donors and compared the peak extracellular HIV p24 antigen titers. The primary clinical HIV-1 strains showed patterns of either moderate or low-level replication in most donor monocytes (20 to 4000 pg/mL). However, within this range there was marked variation in peak titers in most donors. They measured replication of 21 clinical blood-derived strains of HIV in blood monocytes and monocyte-derived macrophages from pairs of identical twins and they compared age-matched unrelated donors of the same sex. In all of the 7 pairs of identical twins, the kinetics of replication (measured by extracellular HIV p24 antigen) of panels of 4 clinical HIV-1 isolates in monocytes were similar within pairs, no consistent genetic linkage of HIV-1 replication pattern with HLA-DR genotype was observed. Hutto et al. (763) reported viral growth pattern differences in a pair of nonidentical twins. Bex et al. (764) evaluated the potential transfer of immunity by adoptive immunity. This immunotherapy by adoptive transfer of lymphocytes was attempted in identical twins, one of whom was virus-free while the other was infected with HIV-1, at the stage of AIDS. The noninfected twin was vaccinated by priming with a recombinant vaccinia virus expressing the envelope glycoprotein of one of his brother's viruses and boosting with the same purified gp160 adsorbed on alum. Vaccination elicited MHC class I-restricted CD8+ cytolytic T cells specific for HIV-1, but no antibody response. The diseased brother, a 38-year-old homosexual who had developed repeated opportunistic infections since 1990 and had a CD4+ T-cell count reduced to practically zero, was treated by infusions of lymphocytes collected from the vaccinated brother by lymphopheresis. After a transfer of the whole lymphocyte population, no changes were observed. As it would be predicted from the hypothesis forwarded here, the transfer of lymphocytes would not make a difference in the outcome of the disease, once the initial damage to the host's immune system had taken place (see Figure 4).

What are the Molecules of Molecular Immunity?

For the last several years, the author's laboratory has analyzed the nature of anti-HIV-1 protective mechanisms in acutely infected PBMCs. As mentioned above, several other laboratories have also been involved in deciphering the mechanisms of protection against murine and avian retroviruses. Best et al. (771) reported a gene, *Fv1*, an endogenous Gag-related gene found in certain strains of mice, which makes the mice resistant to MuLV. The *Fv1* gene is one of a series of mouse genes originally identified by Lilly et al. (772) in 1973. These genes reportedly control the susceptibility of mice to leukemia induced by FLV. The *Fv1* gene was found to be cell-autonomous, and cell lines derived from *Fv1*-resistant animals were resistant to viral infection; in vitro, however, the mode of action of this gene had remained unclear until recently (771). The *Fv1* gene product, identified by Best et al. as a Gag-related protein of an endogenous retrovirus-like element (771), is able to block virus in the early phase of the viral life cycle. The course of infection is blocked after reverse transcriptase but before the establishment of the integration of provirus in the host genome. The location of the anti-retroviral action of *Fv1* (cytoplasm or nucleus) is still undetermined. There are 2 major naturally occurring *Fv1* alleles among inbred strains: the $Fv1^{n}$ allele, found in NIH Swiss mice, which allows replication of small plaque-forming N-tropic strains of retrovirus and blocks large plaque-forming B-tropic strains of retrovirus; and the $Fv1^{b}$ allele in Balb/c mice, which allows replication of B-tropics and inhibits replication of N-tropics. A null allele (termed $Fv1^{0}$) is present in wild mice that are completely susceptible to both N- and B-tropic retroviruses (773,774). Interestingly, retroviral resistance is present in genetic crosses, and therefore the heterozygous animals are resistant to both B- and N-tropic retroviruses. The inhibition to viral replication in either of these tropic viruses is not absolute, but nevertheless very effective, resulting in low viral burden. From these data one can infer that mice immune to N- and B-tropic strains are pre-exposed to the reciprocal viruses in utero, allowing them to develop resistance to these viruses, and this is probably why the heterozygous strain $Fv1^{n/b}$ is resistant to both types of retroviruses. More curiously, as would be predicted from the hypotheses outlined above, the inhibition of replication of these retroviruses is not absolute but relative, meaning a moderate viral load is present for a short time during the primary phase of infection (allowing a short period for the RNA molecules of molecular immunity to reach the majority of the target cells); after this initial phase, a low viral load is present for a long period of time. Live attenuated viral vaccines that inhibit development of AIDS-like symptoms in macaques do not inhibit infection (775). Most interestingly, retroviral replication is blocked at a particularly crucial step in the course of infection: after the RT step of the RNA genome but before entry into the nucleus or integration into the host DNA (764). It is proposed that a Gag-like protein acts as a dominant negative mutant, binding incoming retroviral Gag and blocking its movement into the cellular nucleus (776). We have experimental evidence from my laboratory which shows that this is one of the major steps at which molecular immunity exerts its anti-viral effect on retroviruses.

The author's laboratory has been examining the fate of HIV-1 and the possible block(s) in the intracellular life cycle of HIV-1 after it enters into CD4+ T cells. In order to test the above-described hypotheses and determine the effect of factors released from the PBMCs exposed to very low doses of HIV-1 or relatively high doses of HIV-1, we took PBMCs from 13 HIV-1-seronegative individuals and infected them with various concentrations of HIV-1, starting from tissue culture infectious dose 50 ($TCID_{50}$) to $TCID_{0.0005}$, and then isolated the supernatants from these cells. The supernatants from each experimental variable were collected and filtered through 0.22-μm syringe filters to remove HIV-1 and any cellular material. Freshly isolated PBMCs were exposed to these supernatants for various time periods (4–10 days to determine the optimal priming time). These so-called primed PBMCs were infected with very high doses of HIV-1 (with $TCID_{50}$ of cell-free HIV-1 virions). Four different types of HIV-1 subtypes were used (301660, 93IN101, CMU10, NL4-3, representing primary HIV-1 subtypes B, C, E, and a common laboratory strain, respectively). After overnight incubation all the PBMCs were washed to remove unbound HIV-1. These PBMCs were cultured for 15–18 days in a complete medium (CM = RPMI-1640 medium containing 10 U/mL of native IL-2). Media were changed every third day and fresh CM was added to each well. These cells were cultured for 15–18 days. The PBMCs from all 3 HIV-1-seronegative individuals pre-exposed to cell factors from low doses of HIV-1 (ranging from $TCID_{0.005}$ to $TCID_{0.0005}$) exhibited significant blockage in replication of HIV-1, as compared to cells that were pre-exposed to cell factors isolated from the PBMCs that were infected with high doses of HIV-1s. These PBMCs were analyzed by DNA in situ PCR (DNA ISPCR) for the subcellular localization of HIV-1 *gag* sequences. The HIV-1 PICs were present in the cytoplasms and were unable to enter the double membranes of the nuclei, as determined by ISPCR. Figure 12A shows the absence of HIV-1 *gag* sequences in the PBMCs from a negative, uninfected specimen (negative control). Figure 12B shows that in PBMCs pre-exposed to factors from $TCID_{0.005}$-infected HIV-1, over 90% of the PBMCs showed HIV-1 PIC signals in the cytoplasm. Figure 12C shows that in PBMCs pre-exposed to factors from $TCID_{0.05}$-infected HIV-1, over 50% of the PBMCs showed HIV-1 signals in the cytoplasm. In Figure 12D of the PBMCs pre-exposed to factors from $TCID_{50}$-infected HIV-1, over 80% of them showed HIV-1 signals in the nucleus. Figure 12E shows that the majority of the PBMCs exposed to medium alone show signals in the nucleus. The supernatants were also collected every third day and were measured for HIV-1 activity by HIV-1 p24 ELISA and reverse transcriptase activity. If the supernatants were pretreated with RNase, the observed "protective" effect was completely abrogated.

The presence of the aborted integration of HIV-1 provirus was detected by the double LTR, as determined by DNA ISPCR. The following pairs of primers were used: sense, 3′-CAGATCCCTCAGACCCTTTTAG; antisense, 3′-CAGGGATCAGATATCCACTGAC. This primer pair results in 170-bp product. A biotinylated or fluorescein-isothiocyanate (FITC)-labeled, 47-bp probe: 3′-CCTTGATCTGTGGATCTACCACAACAAGGCTACTTCCCT-GATTGGC was used for in situ hybridization. Color was detected by 3′ amino 9′ ethyl carbazole (AEC), which gives a reddish-brown color for positive cells. As shown in Figure 12E, HIV-1 integrated when the PBMCs were exposed to only medium instead of supernatants from low-dose primed PBMCs. Figure 12F shows the HIV-1 double LTR in the cytoplasms of cells that were pre-exposed to CD8+ T-cell derived factors (CAF). Figure 12G shows that when we utilized an integrase mutant HIV-1 virus (as control), and PBMCs from an HIV-1-negative volunteer were infected with integrase mutant HIV-1, the HIV-1 double LTR signals were detected in the cytoplasm. Figure 12H shows that when the same cells were exposed to the CAF from a LTNP overnight and infected with wild-type HIV-1, NL-4-3, multiple HIV-1 double LTR signals were detected in various areas of cellular cytoplasmic compartments, indicating that integration was prevented. This provides evidence for an HIV-1 integration block at the molecular level (766,767). Figure 13 shows data from a representative experiment on the optimization of molecular immunity.

What Factors Interrupt Molecular Defenses?

One of the crucial questions that should be asked here is whether any of the antiviral agents currently being used activate the immune system. If they do, they may be helping on the one hand and causing harm on the other (765–767,777). These issues should be considered. Presently, I will discuss various nonspecific T-cell activators, which may be part of our normal social habits and diet, that are known to activate the immune cells and increase the viral load. Several investigators have provided information regarding the potential inhibitions in HIV-1 life cycles after entry of HIV-1 into CD4+ T cells. As mentioned earlier, Zack et al. (455) evaluated the molecular events after HIV-1 entry into CD4+ cells; these events indicated that in unstimulated human PBMCs the HIV-1 genome was blocked from completing RT by some unknown host factor(s). However, activation of PBMCs with a T-cell mitogen (PHA) resulted in the breakdown of the observed block. Similarly, Bukrinsky et al. (471) examined the PBMCs from HIV-1-seropositive individuals for the presence of HIV-1 provirus. In their studies, they observed that in the quiescent T cells from asymptomatic individuals, HIV-1 existed as unintegrated full-length HIV-1 but not as an integrated form. Again, if the PBMCs were activated with a mitogen (i.e., PHA) in vitro, HIV-1 provirus integrated into the host genome. Sonza et al. (717) have shown that in fresh PBMC monocytes, HIV-1 replication was blocked prior to the RT and integration steps.

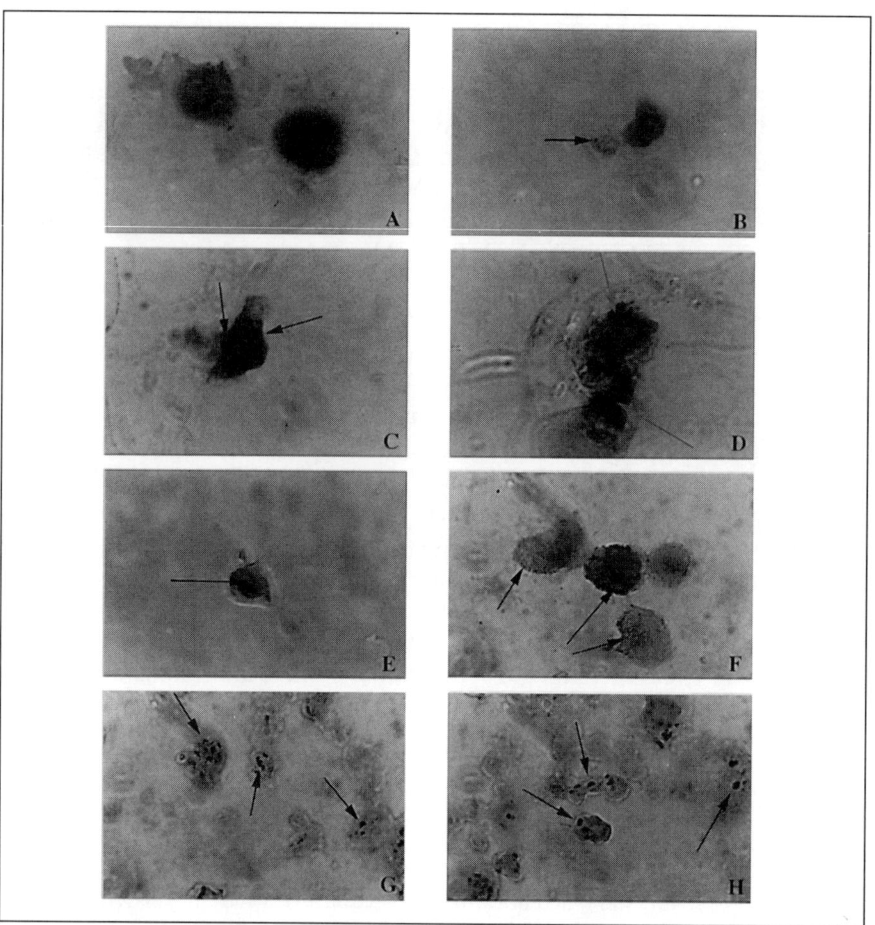

Figure 12. Major effect of molecular immunity. PBMCs were analyzed by ISPCR for the subcellular localization of HIV-1 PICs, which were present in the cytoplasms and were unable to enter the double membranes of the nuclei. (A) Absence of HIV-1*gag* sequences in the PBMCs from a negative, uninfected specimen (negative control). (B) PBMCs pre-exposed to factors from LD 0.005 infected HIV-1; over 90% of the PBMCs showed HIV-1 PIC signals in cytoplasm. (C) PBMCs pre-exposed to factors from LD 0.05 infected HIV-1; over 50% of the PBMCs showed HIV-1 signals in cytoplasm. (D) PBMCs pre-exposed to factors from LD 50 infected HIV-1; over 80% of the PBMCs showed HIV-1 signals in nucleus. (E) The majority of the PBMCs exposed to medium alone (no factor) show signals in the nucleus. Double LTR circle in the aborted integration determined by ISPCR: for the presence of aborted integration of HIV-1 provirus was detected by the double LTR. The following pairs of primers were utilized: sense; 3′-CAGATCC-CTCAGACCCTTTTAG, antisense; 3′-CAGGGATCAGATATCCACTGAC. This primer pair results in a 170-bp product. A biotinylated or FITC-labeled, 47-bp probe (3′-CCTTGATCTGTGGATCTACCACAA-CAAGGCTACTTCCCTGATTGGC) was utilized for in situ hybridization. Color was detected by AEC, which gives a reddish/brown color for positive cells (areas indicated by arrows throughout the figure). (E) HIV-1 integrated when PBMCs were exposed to only medium instead of supernatant from CD8+ T cells exposed to low-dose concentration of HIV-1 (CAF). (F) HIV-1 double LTR in the cytoplasms of cells that were pre-exposed to CAF. (G) When we utilized an integrase mutant HIV-1 virus (as control) and PBMCs from a HIV-1-negative volunteer infected with integrase mutant HIV-1, the HIV-1 double LTR signals were detected in the cytoplasm. (H) When the same cells were exposed to the CAF from LTNP overnight and infected with wild-type HIV-1, NL-4-3, multiple HIV-1 double LTR signals were detected in various areas of cellular cytoplasmic compartments, indicating that integration was blocked at the PIC level.

In summary, there is growing evidence that neither the humoral immune responses nor the traditionally understood virus-specific CTLs play any important role in the inhibition of HIV-1 replication in vivo. The majority of the HIV-1 vaccine strategies that have received the greatest attention to date, including the use of recombinant HIV-1 Env glycoprotein immunogens, live vaccinia virus subunits, and many vaccine approaches attempting to elicit virus-specific CTLs, have given disappointing results. I believe that the real natural defense against HIV-1 lies inside the CD8+ and NK cells. Our preliminary evidence shows that molecular immunity is mediated by RNA repertoires that block the integration of retroviruses into the host genome. Understanding the mechanisms by which this intracellular molecular

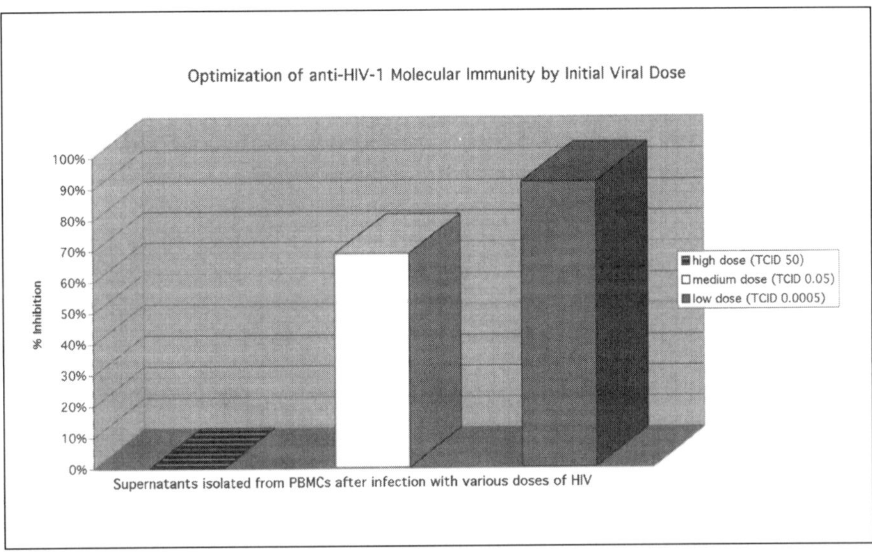

Figure 13. Activation and optimization of anti-HIV-1 molecular immunity. To test the molecular immunity hypothesis, PBMCs were obtained from HIV-1-seronegative individuals. These PBMCs were infected with 10-fold dilution of cell-free HIV-1 virions; ranging from $TCID_{50}$ (tissue culture infection dose 50: 3 ng/mL) to $TCID_{0.0005}$. After overnight incubation, these PBMCs were vigorously washed to remove any unattached virion particles. After another 6-h incubation, the PBMCs were washed again to remove any additional virions that might have been released from the dead cells or by any other mechanism. After multiple washes, the PBMCs were cultured for 4–5 days in RPMI-1640 containing 10 units of IL-2, 10% fetal calf serum, 50 mM L-glutamine and antibiotics. Supernatants from each experimental variable were collected and were filtered through a 0.22-µm syringe filter, to remove any virion particle. The protective role of these supernatants against HIV-1 replication was tested by utilizing 4 different types of HIV-1 isolates, US92301660, 93IN101, CMU10, and NL4.3, representing subtypes B, C, E, and a common laboratory strain, respectively. Briefly, freshly harvested, unstimulated PBMCs from 3 different HIV-1-seronegative individuals were incubated with the supernatants (10% final concentration) from each experimental variable, for 4 days. Following this "priming period", PBMCs were infected with high doses of HIV-1 (3× $TCID_{50}$). After overnight incubation PBMCs were washed vigorously as above to remove unbound virions and maintained in complete medium for 15–18 days. Supernatant from uninfected PBMCs with complete medium served as negative control. Supernatants were collected every third day and replaced with equal volume of fresh complete media. These supernatants were assayed for HIV-1 activity by HIV-1 p24 ELISA and RT activity.

immunity precisely operates would provide us with the tools we need to fight HIV-1. The potential anti-HIV-1 vaccine would be radically different from what has been tried so far. In the next chapter I will describe how we can utilize our knowledge, though limited, to develop a vaccine against HIV-1.

Chapter 5

Hypothesis of Molecular Immunity

"We acquire many notions unconsciously, without abstracting them and reasoning on them."

Charles Darwin
Charles Darwin's Notebook, 1836–1844

THE THIRTEEN POSTULATES OF MOLECULAR IMMUNITY

I would like to present 13 postulates on how I believe molecular immunity against retroviruses actually works, and then I will discuss data that I feel support these postulates.

(*i*) **Initial Exposure:** Upon initial exposure to a retrovirus, the host organism requires a brief lag period to fully activate its molecular responses. This short period is required so that the small RNA or RNAs that serve as blocking agents against the specific invading retrovirus can be amplified in the CD8+/NK+ cells and then reach other target cells so the maximum number of cells can be protected from damage.

(*ii*) **Initial Viral Activity:** During the lag period, the retrovirus may actively replicate in non-CD8+ cells or infect some cells and then become dormant, depending on the nature of the retrovirus (i.e., depending upon the kinds of receptors that particular retrovirus binds to and the sorts of cell types it binds and how avidly). Therefore, the number of cells a retrovirus initially infects is the property of that specific retrovirus. If the replication capacity and the pathogenicity of a particular retrovirus is high, it will infect and damage a large number of cells during the lag period. The number of cells infected initially may ultimately determine the final outcome of the infection. More cells infected at an early stage may translate into a higher viral load, a greater degree of damage, and a worse outcome. If a host is evolutionarily naive to a particular retrovirus, and does not possess an active repertoire of mRNA to block the integration of the invading retrovirus at the PIC level, then many cells and a potentially large variety of cells would be infected before the end of the lag period. This would initiate a vicious cycle, where more cells would be producing virus and more cells would be infected. Subsequently, more cells would be destroyed per day than the body could replace with healthy cells—resulting in immunodeficiency (86,122).

(*iii*) **Lag Period of Host:** During the lag period, myriad intracellular defense mechanisms become activated, and these responses have evolved over time to block the replication of the retrovirus at every important step of its life cycle. These mechanisms do not primarily use cytokine or chemokines as protective mechanisms but use intracellular nucleic acids and certain proteins directed against infecting retroviruses or lentiviruses (134,516,744).

***(iv)* Virus-Specific Messenger Molecule:** Following the lag period, which seems to last 3–5 days in healthy, immunologically competent and mature individuals, retrovirus-specific small RNA messenger molecules are produced by the host's PBMCs (i.e., CD8+/NK+ cells). These molecules relay specific information to uninfected cells, probably forming a triplex with the provirus, stopping its activity at the preintegration level. This molecular immunity against a particular retrovirus seems to be persistent over the long term (similarly to HI and CMI).

***(v)* Cascade of Molecular Responses:** The messenger molecules are highly specific to the particular retrovirus in question, and they activate a cascade of events in the uninfected cells that allows these cells to arm themselves against infection by that particular retrovirus.

***(vi)* Immunity Against Genetically Closely Related Viruses:** Although this immunity is highly specific to the retrovirus that initially infects the host, molecular immunity also inhibits infection by retroviruses that are genetically closely related. Therefore, immunity against one subtype of HIV-1 would be effective against other naturally occurring HIV-1s, but may not be as effective against laboratory created HIV-1 (i.e., HIV-1 IIIB, or NL-4-3, created in the lab) or HIV-1 clades that may be genetically too dissimilar (126–131,361–364).

***(vii)* Late Evolutionary, Ontogenic Development of Molecular Immunity:** The development of molecular immunity seems to have occurred relatively late in evolution, and consequently it matures relatively late in the ontogenic development of the organism. For humans, molecular immunity seems to fully mature between the ages of 0.5 to 1 year of age. Prior to this maturation, infection of a young host with a retrovirus of relatively low pathogenicity or a low-dose infection with a pathogenic retrovirus may prove uncontrollable or fatal [this explains why macaque neonates exposed to adult doses of defective SIV develop infection (72)]. However, lower dose exposure to SIV protects these neonatal macaques the same way it protects the adults (75,333).

***(viii)* CD8+/NK+ Lymphocytes Are the Basis of Response:** A subset of CD8+/NK+ lymphocytes initiate the molecular response to retroviruses, and these cells also dispatch the mRNA molecules to various cells in the organism, including CD4+ cells, monocyte/macrophage cells, and cells of the central nervous system [i.e., neurons, astrocytes, oligodendrocytes (778)]. These small RNAs are designed to inhibit the early steps in the life cycle of retroviruses, such as reverse transcriptase, RNase H, and integrase activities. However, the most efficient of all the inhibitory molecules seems to be the ones that form a triplex with the double-stranded viral DNA, blocking it at the PIC levels (779,780). Upon exposure to the messenger signals, the recipient cells become protected from that particular invading retrovirus or from genetically related retroviruses. Interruption or dysfunction of the primary responder cells—namely, specific CD8+/NK+ lymphocytes—can result in unchecked replication of the retrovirus (455,471,717).

How do we know that the HIV-1 PIC potentially contains the triplex of viral double-stranded DNA and the protective host defense the small RNAs? We do not know the answer to this question yet. Currently, my laboratory is conducting experiments to confirm this mechanism of protection. However, indirect proof has come from a laboratory in the Salk Institute (451). A group of investigators have studied the organization and function of HIV-1 PICs. They showed that when they isolated the HIV-1 PICs from cells and used them in vitro, the PICs were capable of carrying out the integration process (after they were purified and digested). They found that, surprisingly, the ends of the HIV-1 cDNA were not digested by exonucleases (*Exo*III) but were protected. Since *Exo*III required a double-stranded DNA for a substrate, a triple helix at the ends would be protected. One of the possibilities was that the ends of HIV-1 cDNA contained single-stranded DNA, which would be then protected from the digestive effect of *Exo*III. This possibility was ruled out by incubating the HIV-1 cDNA with mung bean endonucleases, which digest single-stranded DNA. Another possibility was that there were proteins present at the cDNA ends, or it could be due to triplex formation, which would also protect the cDNA ends from exonuclease digestion. This concept and the other hypotheses are illustrated in Figure 4.

(ix) **Cofactors Can Compromise Immunity:** Protective molecular immunity against a specific strain of retrovirus and genetically closely related viruses would be life-long unless untoward events or cofactors adversely affect the functions and intracellular mechanisms of protection of the subsets of lymphocytes that are involved in molecular immunity (particularly CD8+/NK+ cells). These cofactors are especially important during the initial exposure and during the lag period, at which time they can determine the future course of infection. Untoward events or cofactors are of several types, including exposure to low-dose radiation (726,732), UV light (727), cyclosporine (728), cyclophosphamide (728,732), steroids (729–730), certain anti-HIV-1 agents (731), protein synthesis inhibitors (731), co-infection with another pathogenic virus or exposure to specific viral products (733–740), or certain substances of abuse (e.g., alcohol, cocaine). These factors appear to directly or indirectly affect the normal functions of molecular immunity by adversely affecting the functions of CD8+ T cells. No doubt there are also unknown cofactors that interfere with or inactivate the molecular immunity pathways and that will render the host susceptible to acute infection by retroviruses (741–757,760–764).

(x) **Low-Dose Inoculation Can Provide Molecular Immunity:** A low-dose inoculation of a pathogenic retrovirus will result in the development of

protective molecular immunity against the specific retrovirus or against genetically closely related retroviruses, provided cofactors do not interfere excessively in the initial immunologic response. This is akin to a subclinical infection in which low-dose exposure to a pathogen results in the development of protective immunity without overt signs or symptoms of the disease.

(xi) **A Genetically Related Nonpathogenic Lentivirus:** Similarly, exposure to an HIV-1 genetically closely related nonpathogenic live lentivirus should provide immunity against HIV-1 (12,19–21,62,68–71,75–78,187, 615,617–618,621–623). The degree of success in developing molecular protection is directly proportional to the degree of genetic relatedness of the challenging retroviruses and inversely proportional to the degree of pathogenicity and replication ability of the inoculating retrovirus.

(xii) **Active Replication Necessary for Effective Vaccine:** The activation of molecular immunity requires exposure of primary target cells to live retrovirus. A heat-inactivated, formalin-fixed whole virus, virion subunits produced by recombinant vectors, peptides and subunits produced by bacterial or baculovirus expression systems, or any other form of a vaccine in which the virus is unable to form a PIC would not be able to bring molecular immunity to its full potential and thus would not protect the host. In other words, the very mechanisms of retroviral infection—not the antigenic nature of the virus itself—elicit the molecular response that leads to protective immunity. This is why the only reliable and consistently successful protection thus far in the nonhuman primate models and in humans has been achieved by utilizing a live attenuated SIV vaccine (12,19–21,23–26,62,68–71,75–78,187, 615,617–618,621–623).

(xiii) **Possible HIV-1 Vaccines:** The hypothetical vaccines that should produce protective immunity against HIV-1 are the following live-virus vaccines (in descending order of desirability): *(i)* an engineered replication-defective HIV-1 virus (i.e., *env, vif, nef*, or multiple accessory gene defective virus); *(ii)* very low doses of a genetically closely related, nonpathogenic lentivirus, such as an attenuated form of SIV_{cpz}; *(iii)* low doses of a nonpathogenic HIV-1 virus, such as a particular *nef*-defective strain or known HIV-1 clades with very low pathogenicity (which can be determined on the basis of epidemiological data, but not on the basis of in vitro data. I believe that the thousands of individuals in sub-Sahara Africa who carry nonpathogenic strains of HIV-1-related viruses—many of whom were originally inoculated with live-experimental polio virus—carry a potential vaccine for AIDS in their blood cells.); or *(iv)* a controlled, extremely low-dose inoculation with fully pathogenic HIV-1 in combination with effective doses of an appropriate anti-HIV chemical agent, preferably an integrase inhibitor, to reduce replication of HIV-1, thus creating very low-dose exposure conditions, similar to those existing in thousands of health care workers accidentally exposed to HIV-1-infected blood (obviously this method would require very stringent conditions).

Role of Triplex Formation in Gene Regulation and Transcription

Regulation of expression of specific genes by antisense RNA is a naturally occurring phenomenon in prokaryotic systems. Antisense RNA has been shown to decrease expression of specific genes when injected into frog oocytes and *Drosophila* embryos. Inhibition of the expression of artificially introduced genes has been demonstrated by transient expression of antisense RNA constructs in mammalian cells and plant protoplasts, and by stable expression of the endogenous, developmentally regulated gene for polygalacturonase in the stably transformed tomato expressing antisense RNA (reviewed in References 359 and 360). In recent years particular attention has been directed towards a unique form of antisense system found in various promoter regions of eukaryotes. Simple repeating d(GA:TC)n sequences are frequently found at eukaryotic promoters, and in some cases they have been shown to be nucleosome-free in vivo, and make up about 0.4%–0.5% of the total mammalian genome (reviewed in References 359,360,779,781). These sequences exhibit a high degree of structural polymorphism and show a fold-back triple-helix structure (359,360). Sequence-specific recognition of the major groove of DNA at homopurine–homopyridine sequences [i.e., d(GA:TC)n] shows a special type of antisense homopyridine oligonucleotide (359,360,779,781). Many areas of HIV-1 and other lentiviruses contain an even more particular type of homopurine nucleotide, including both ends of the LTRs of HIV-1 (unpublished data). Therefore, it is possible that small RNAs form triple helices at different portions of HIV-1 RNA and DNA and especially at the terminal ends of the LTR promoter regions, and block HIV-1 cDNA at the preintegration step (451). There are numerous recent reports that strongly support this notion (779–781). This potential mechanism is currently being evaluated in the author's laboratory (Figure 14).

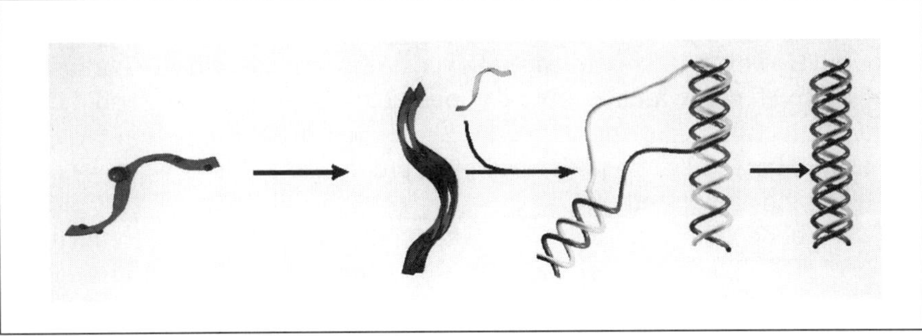

Figure 14. A proposed model of triplex formation between HIV-1 provirus (or any retroviral provirus) and the protective RNA. Left to right: HIV-1 RNA enters the cellular milieu of the host which had already received the protective RNAs from the "primed" CD8+/NK+ cells. Upon RT, HIV-1 cDNA is formed. The complex reactions of PIC formation are interrupted by the protective RNAs, which form triple helices with the HIV-1 cDNA. Hence, blocking the integration of HIV-1 and intercepting it before it gets into the nucleus. Also see Figure 4.

Chapter 5

EVIDENCE FOR THE EXISTENCE OF MOLECULAR IMMUNITY

Studies have already been conducted with humans, primates, and other experimental animal models that provide convincing evidence for the existence of anti-retroviral molecular immunity. I have already described much of this evidence in detail but would like to briefly reiterate and put the evidence into proper perspective. For the sake of clarity, I have divided various aspects of the evidence into separate sections.

Cross-Protection

As I stated previously, exposure to a nonpathogenic live retrovirus provides an immunity against genetically closely related pathogenic retrovirus. The degree of molecular protection is directly proportional to the degree of genetic relatedness and inversely proportional to the degree of pathogenicity of the retrovirus in question.

Travers et al. (68) reported on the existence of significant protection against HIV-1 in individuals who were pre-exposed to HIV-2. A team of investigators went to West Africa where HIV-2 is endemic and followed HIV-2-infected, high-risk women for several years. The individuals infected with HIV-2 had a significantly lower incidence of HIV-1 than did women who were seronegative for HIV-2, with a relative risk of 0.32 ($P = 0.008$), and this protection was independent of CD4+ cell count. These investigators concluded that this type of HIV-2-mediated protection provided about 70% protection from subsequent HIV-1 infection (see below).

Analysis and comments. HIV-2 and HIV-1 appear to have some common ancestry, according to several reports (38,48,123,197–199,201,270,324,398, 425,437,624). They have a 40%–70% genetic homology [depending on which genes are being compared and by what methods (see Figure 2)]. Therefore, it is not surprising to see some degree of protection when the molecular immunity system is primed with this other retrovirus of lower pathogenicity. However, if the sequence of exposure is reversed (the individual first exposed to HIV-1, which is more pathogenic to its human hosts, and the secondary infection occurring with HIV-2), no significant protection would be seen. This is what the hypothesis would predict, and this is what was concluded in the above study (68).

One other conclusion can be drawn about the difference between the initial doses of HIV-1 and HIV-2 viruses. The initial inoculation dose for priming the cells for protection from HIV-2 was most probably very low (due to the relatively low pathogenicity of HIV-2 and low viral loads in the blood and other body fluids), and hence served as vaccine. On the other hand, the initial inoculation dose of HIV-1 was high (since the level of HIV-1 viremia is much larger than HIV-2, in relative amount of antigen), and did not serve as vaccine.

As shown in Figure 2, the most genetically closely related lentivirus to HIV-

1 is SIV_{cpz} (33–36). Since it may not be appropriate to immunize humans with SIV_{cpz} at this time because of our lack of knowledge about this lentivirus (however, development of a defective SIV_{cpz} is not out of question; see below for alternatives), another logical step would be to examine a homologous cross-protection in a simian model (e.g., between HIV-2 and SIV_{mac} or SIV_{sm}). One could infect cynomolgus macaques with HIV-2, which is not pathogenic in this species, and then subsequently challenge them with SIV_{mac} or SIV_{sm}, both of which cause an AIDS-like pathology in this species of monkey.

Fortunately, this experiment has already been done. Recently, Putkonen et al. (74,624) reported protection of cynomolgus macaques against high doses of SIV_{sm} (10–100 monkey-infectious doses of pathogenic SIV_{sm}) after they were infected with genetically closely related HIV-2 (which has a genetic homology of about 90% to SIV_{sm}). The vaccinated group of cynomolgus macaques were protected against very high doses of pathogenic SIV_{sm}, and they did not develop SIV-induced immunosuppression or AIDS-like pathology during more than 5 years of follow-up. However, all the unvaccinated control animals died within 2–26 months after the infection from AIDS-like disease. I believe this report is one of the landmark works supporting the existence of molecular immunity, even though it appears that these investigators did not think in these terms (21,74,624,782,783).

It should be noted that if one immunizes the animals with recombinant vaccine and then infects them with a live heterologous but closely related virus, no protection is achieved. For example, Girard et al. (21) wanted to determine if the HIV-1-specific HI elicited against one type of HIV-1 might prevent infection by a strain of HIV-1 from a different part of the globe. For this purpose, they immunized 2 chimpanzees with a recombinant vaccine rgp 160-MN/LAI (prepared from subtype B) and then challenged them by an intravenous inoculation of a comparable dose of a subtype E HIV-1 from Central Africa. Both animals became infected with the subtype E virus, indicating that intraclade antibody mediated protection does not protect against different variants of HIV-1. These results also weigh against a protective role for neutralizing antibodies, as described in the previous chapters.

Naturally Occurring Protection Against Lentiviruses in Primates

African green monkeys are classified into 4 distinct species (commonly termed vervet, grivet, sabaeus, and tantalus monkeys), all of which are known to be infected with SIV_{agm} in the wild. Sequence analysis of partial *gag* and *env* regions recently indicated that geographically diverse SIV_{agm} isolates cluster according to their species of origin. Each of the 4 African green monkey species thus harbors a phylogenetically distinct SIV_{agm} subtype, indicating that African green monkeys have been infected with SIV_{agm} for an extended period of time. A significant percentage (up to 70%) of African monkey species held in captivity in various zoos and 19 primate centers in the

United States have been demonstrated to have antibodies to SIVs (23,30,37,43–45). In addition, a large percentage (>40%) of animals caught in the wild also have antibodies to SIVs (27–49). In all cases, various strains of SIVs are carried by their natural host as a harmless infection in their natural conditions (27–47). The species specificity of SIV for each of their respective monkey species strongly suggests these primates have had an opportunity to fully activate their molecular immunity against their respective strains of SIVs. This is, as I suggested earlier, due to their coevolution with these viruses and due to low-dose exposure with these viruses during childhood (e.g., in utero exposure, breast feeding, kissing, bites during playing, etc.). This does not mean that these lentiviruses are dormant in their bodies; some of these primates may carry measurable viral loads during certain periods of their lives, but because of the activation of molecular immunity, these viruses do not integrate into the majority of their lymphocytes (559,717, 784–789). The studies of Kaur et al. (559) showed that sooty mangabeys newly caught in the wild with natural SIV infection exhibited measurable plasma viral loads and yet did not progress to AIDS. To understand the immune basis of this protected state, they analyzed SIV-specific CTL activity in 12 naturally infected sooty mangabeys. They found that SIV-specific CTLs were not detectable in fresh PBMCs from 7 of 7 animals, even when tested at high effector-to-target ratios. Therefore, like the African green monkey infection, the sooty mangabey infection causes no disease in its native host. In a particular breeding colony of sooty mangabeys where the original SIV_{sm} isolate was discovered, as much as 80% of the colony was infected (some for over a decade) without any evidence of disease (31,124,276,381–382, 560,691). As shown in Figure 2, there is a striking homology between this SIV of sooty mangabeys and HIV-2. As mentioned earlier, there is a significant sequence homology between HIV-1 and a simian immunodeficiency virus, SIV_{cpz}, which was originally isolated from chimpanzees who were without evidence of disease (17–21). Of particular note, chimpanzees experimentally infected with HIV-1 fail to develop overt disease despite establishment of infection as evidenced by transient viremia, development of HIV-1-specific antibodies, and HIV-1-specific cytotoxic T cells (17–21, 34–37, 50–55,73–77,225,391). These observations strongly suggest that these primates already had a natural molecular immunity to these lentiviruses, similar to the other African nonhuman primates infected with various SIVs.

Since 1991, there have been 388 vaccine development trials utilizing various nonhuman primate models of AIDS. Of these, 49 have used chimpanzees and 339 have used macaques (19–21,56,75–78). Eighteen different kinds of vaccine strategies were utilized including killed/inactivated, infected or transfected cells, attenuated live virus, whole inactivated virus, recombinant vector, recombinant products, subunits, synthetic peptides, genetic immunization, plasmid DNA, enriched or concentrated viral products, passive antibody, virus-like particles, toxoid preparation, and cell-derived factors, among many others. In addition, several gene therapy clinical trials have been approved by the FDA for near future experimentation. None of the vaccine strategies except live attenuated virus have resulted in consistently high levels of protection following challenge with pathogenic or nonpathogenic genetically related virus, and this protection was not provided by HI or CMI.

The vaccine efforts using nonhuman primates have shown quite clearly that if the monkeys are first infected with a nonpathogenic lentivirus, then challenged with a genetically closely related pathogenic variety, they do not develop disease (12,19–21,62–71,75–78,187,615,617–618,621–623). However, if they are first infected with a pathogenic variety that is genetically unrelated to any prior lentivirus infection, then the monkeys do develop AIDS-like disease. For example, rhesus macaques raised in the wild have no previous SIV infection. If they are inoculated with the SIV_{sm} strain of SIV, which is pathogenic in this species, they developed an immunodeficiency syndrome which closely mimics the clinical features of HIV-1 infection (125,185,371,384,385, 555,558,562). Similarly, cynomolgus monkeys that appear not to have been previously infected with SIV are quite susceptible to experimental infection with SIV_{sm}, and they rapidly develop an immunodeficiency syndrome with an AIDS-like disease (14,74,521,542–543,557,768–769,790–795).

At this point, I would also like to mention that some recombinant vaccine trials in primates have shown partial success with animals exposed to their brand of vaccines. Some of these studies should be viewed with reservation because experimental animals kept in captivity do get exposed to low doses of SIVs (from animal bites and accidental inoculations or exposure; 314). Therefore, if these animals are exposed to live, high doses of homologous SIVs, they may show protection. There are numerous studies claiming success, but this outcome could not be confirmed in other laboratories. I believe that at least in some cases these animals were exposed to low doses of genetically related lentiviruses, and in some other cases they were actually infected with a very low dose of virus, since viral infectivity is not a precise science and inoculation doses used to infect animals are usually derived from tissue culture infections ($TCID_{50}$) or are prepared as stock, frozen at -70°C, and then used later. In the freezing conditions, viral particles may become less infectious after a period of time. Also, the freezing process can inactivate viral infectivity if not properly handled. Finally, some Asian macaques are infected with endogenous type D viruses that are known to share sequence homologies to various infectious SIV substrains (221,223,227,322,342–343). All of these factors confound the vaccine trials in the nonhuman primates and explain why diametrically opposed claims of success have been made in the past regarding vaccines against SIVs. I believe low-dose exposure may provide the explanation for these discrepancies (121,291,395–396).

Evidence of Molecular Immunity in Humans

HFV (or SV), a retrovirus originally isolated from patients with various neoplastic and degenerative diseases, has yet to be clearly associated with any disease in humans, despite the fact that it is prevalent in certain geographical areas and can be readily cultured in explanted tissues from these individuals (78,79). Like other retroviruses, this virus also encodes 3 structural genes, *gag*, *pol*, and *env*, and an additional region containing 3 open reading frames, *bel-1*, *bel-2* and *bel-3*. Bel-1 activates transcription of its LTR as well as the LTR of HIV-1. Recent genetic analyses of the HFV genes (i.e., *bel-1*), by inserting parts of HFV into mouse embryos and developing transgenic mice, show that it causes progressive degenerative diseases of the central nervous system. Obviously, this virus causes no known illness in humans, but even a small portion of HFV genes expressed in evolutionarily naive species (i.e., mice) causes severe pathology (78,79,80). The expression of HIV-1 genes in various transgenic rodents has produced variable results. We do not know what kind of evolutionary relationship exists between certain rodent species and a particular HIV-1 gene. For example, utilization of SCID-hu mice provides a window from which we can observe various evolutionary mechanisms. The SCID-hu mice are prepared by implanting human fetal tissues (i.e., bone marrow stem cells, liver, thymus, or lymph nodes) into the immunodeficient C.B.-17 SCID mice. It was assumed that human implants would proliferate in the immune-deficient environment of SCID mice and, by the same token, that the SCID mouse and the human cells would become tolerant of each others' incompatible genes. Therefore, multilineage human stem cells derived from the fetal liver would differentiate, and a mature, single, positive T-cell progeny might then migrate into implants of human lymphoid tissue, creating a chimeric mouse with a human immune system. Amazingly, this model has worked very well. SCID-hu (referred to as Thy/Liv) mice transplanted with human fetal liver and thymus demonstrated long-term multilineage human hematopoiesis, and SCID-hu mice appeared to be less immunodeficient. This model has been successfully used to analyze the effects of exogenous species-specific cytokines and various other cofactors. However, as would be suspected from the molecular immunity hypotheses, infectious HIV-1 isolates from tissue cultures were noninfectious to human cells in the SCID-hu mice (due to the priming of human cells to murine retroviruses, many of which may share homologous sequences with HIV-1). Certain primary human HIV-1 isolates were infectious but completely nonpathogenic in the SCID-hu animal models. Transgenic mice stocks prepared for the analyses of whole HIV or a specific HIV-1 gene function, have proved completely unreliable (reviewed in References 81 and 82). For example, a transgenic mouse containing an HIV-1 provirus without all 3 structural genes developed extensive lymphoid depletion in the thymus, spleen, and lymph nodes. However, in this animal model, despite high expression of viral genes early in life, cell death did not become evident until about the time of full lymphoid maturation (83). In another transgenic mouse, a KS-like disease appeared in the animals. We know now that KS and HHV-8 have a close association (83). Therefore, I believe that because of so many dissimilarities between the human and mouse immune systems and our different evolutionary histories with regards to retroviral exposure and coexistence, the transgenic mouse models would not be appropriate for use in HIV-1 research; they will give results that cannot be applied in preparing a vaccine against HIV-1.

HTLV-II is endemic in certain American Indian tribes without causing clinical disease (84,161,782). As with HFV, when the *tax* gene (equivalent of HIV-1 *tat* gene) is introduced into mouse embryos, the transgenic mice exhibit various forms of tumors. Obviously, a pre-exposure in evolutionary terms appears to play an important role in the development of resistance to disease. Interestingly, a species of monkey has been known to be infected with a similar virus in South America, without any apparent illness (796–798).

HTLV-I appears to be a relatively new introduction, in evolutionary terms, and humans have learned to accommodate this retrovirus. However, it can still cause illness in the very young and very old (72–75,291).

Despite many similarities among HTLV-I, HTLV-II, and HFV, there are marked differences in the level of clinical expression, and it is apparent by the maintenance of infection within these populations that some level of infectious progeny virus is generated from the integrated proviral sequences [similar to what was mentioned earlier regarding the viral load in the sooty mangabeys caught in the wild or in humans infected with HIV-1 (559)].

Even within human populations infected with HIV-1, there is substantial disease variability (21,87,96,682,685,679–681), from LTNPs (who remain asymptomatic for >10 years after HIV-1 infection) to patients who rapidly progress to immunodeficiency in a matter of a few years (95,418,445–446, 566). Some pediatric patients clear HIV-1 infection (679–681). Many other so-called anomalous observations are the reported isolation of HIV-1 from individuals who remained HIV-1 seronegative; the observation that some men with many different partners with whom they practiced receptive anal sex still remain seronegative; rapid decline of HIV-1 viremia after the primary exposure without HI and CMI; and that CD8+ T cells seem to be the major factor in this apparent molecular immunity (23–26,70–71,86–87, 91–97,99–105,120–123,126–139,182,350–352,545–546,613,672–676).

Analysis and comments. If one accepts the hypothesis that evolution has created molecularly based intracellular protective mechanisms to specifically battle retroviruses, then many of the previously anomalous phenomena reported by various investigators can be explained on the basis of the hypothesis presented in this book. For example, it can explain why so many lentiviruses prevalent in myriad species of African nonhuman primates cause no known illness in their native hosts, whereas the same lentiviruses cause AIDS in Asian nonhuman primates. While there are no clear genomic differences between the rapidly fatal variant of SIV_{sm} and other SIV_{sm} subtypes, the differences fail to clearly define the pathogenic moiety of this virus (10–16,27–49,51–60). However, if one species of monkey gets infected with

SIV from the other monkey species, variable outcomes can occur, depending on the degree of genetic relatedness of the infecting SIV to the SIV prevalent in their own colony and their evolutionary history with the new SIV type and the initial inoculating dose. Cross-species transmission of primate lentiviruses has caused several outbreaks in the captive primates (reviewed in Reference 270). For example, accidental introduction of SIV_{mac} and SIV_{stm} have caused immunodeficiency indistinguishable from human AIDS in the Asian rhesus and stump-tailed macaques (215–230,270). Similar results were obtained when these Asian macaques were experimentally infected with high doses of SIV_{mac} and SIV_{stm} (215–230,270). One may raise the question that perhaps African nonhuman primates are genetically immune to retroviruses. However, if African nonhuman primates are exposed to type D retrovirus (SRV-1), for which they are evolutionarily naive, they develop AIDS-like diseases (215–230,270,335). Accidental infection with this virus is responsible for 99% of spontaneous AIDS-like disease in captive primates in the US (270,370–371). Therefore, naturally occurring primate lentiviruses are not naturally nonpathogenic, but they are nonpathogenic only because of their coevolution with their respective hosts. Similarly, the host species are not intrinsically immune to SIV-induced disease—only if they have coevolved with that particular strain of lentiviruses and have been exposed to small doses of that particular lentivirus early in life. Nonhuman primates get their initial exposure to very low doses of the SIVs predominant in their particular colony during early neonatal life, through breast feeding, childhood playing, and biting during fighting. Breast milk has been reported to contain retroviruses (392–394), and horizontal transmission of such viruses is well documented (58,355). This initial exposure to low doses of SIVs vaccinates the newborns with specific molecular immunity against that particular type of SIV.

When Molecular Immunity Does Not Work

If a host is infected with a harmless lentivirus (with which it has coevolved) and then comes in contact with a genetically unrelated type of lentivirus, the host can be infected with this entirely different lentivirus, and molecular immunity does not provide protection against this different type of virus. There is experimental evidence that such an exposure with a relatively high dose of virus (at least in experimental conditions) can break down the natural defenses altogether, at least transiently. An example of this is that HIV-1 and HTLV-I/II dual infections occur in at least 5% of HIV-1-infected patients in many urban areas (84,161,796–800). There is evidence that dual infection may be associated with unique immune phenotypes and altered progression to AIDS. Also, HTLV-I-associated neurological diseases are becoming recognized in dually infected patients. It is possible that some of these features may be explained by enhanced HTLV-I/II gene expression. To test this hypothesis Beilke et al. (799) isolated PBMCs obtained from 24 co-infected patients and 13 patients with HTLV-I/II infection alone and cultured them to detect HTLV-I/II viral antigens, by RT-PCR, in order to test for the presence of HTLV-I/II Tax/Rex mRNA in uncultured PBMCs. Tax/Rex mRNA was detectable in at least 16 of 24 (67%) patient samples with dual infections, compared with only 2 of 13 (15%) PBMC samples from those singly infected with HTLV-I/II alone (67% vs. 15%; $P < 0.01$). Viral antigen detection was more frequent in samples obtained from dually infected individuals (42% vs. 23%; $P > 0.30$). The agreement between the PCR assay and culture result was 70% (Kappa score = 0.40). These data suggest that in the case of dual infection with a genetically unrelated virus, molecular immunity may be even further weakened, since up-regulated HTLV-I/II virus expression occurs in many dually infected patients. The molecular mechanisms that explain this phenomenon may be that the RNA molecules responsible for protection against one type of virus (say HIV-1) may be getting nonspecifically quenched by HTLV-I/II or vice versa, causing up-regulation of one or both types of viruses.

In another series of experiments, investigators inoculated 7 juvenile rhesus macaques with cultured HTLV-I-infected cells obtained from a patient with tropical spastic paraparesis and polymyositis, which led to seroconvertion and viremia (as detected by viral antigen detection in PBMC cultures) in 7 of 7 and 6 of 7 animals, respectively. The first animal developed a steroid responsive myopathy and arthritis at the peak level of antibody production and virus antigen expression, after which viral antigen detection became negative. Subsequent co-infection with SIV-ΔB670 was associated with a decline in HTLV-I antibodies and the reappearance of HTLV-I antigens. A second HTLV-SIV co-infected animal sustained HTLV-I antigen expression in the face of weak antibody response (800). Dual infection with various unrelated lentiviruses in primates and in humans have been reported (216,801–803). These observations suggest that SIV co-infection may blunt anti-HTLV-I protective immunity, thus raising levels of HTLV-I virus expression.

Maturity of the Molecular Immunity

Intracellular molecular immunity is not optimal during early infancy or in old age. It is similar to HI and CMI, which peak after 6 months of age. Therefore, if humans are exposed to certain lentiviruses during these vulnerable phases, even a relatively less pathogenic virus could cause disease. For example, HTLV-I infection, if acquired in infancy, leads to leukemia (ATL) in a small minority of the population (84). HTLV-I leads to a neuropathic disease if acquired in old age (84–85,223,603,693,782). (This is very similar to susceptibility of young and old individuals to *Mycobacterium tuberculosis*.)

Analyses and comments. It appears that the final disease potential of retroviruses lies in the complex interaction between the virus and the immune status of the host. Therefore, the survival of the host depends on the rapid development of an intracellular molecular immunity that can prime the majority of target cells with the appropriate defenses, outracing the pathogenic effects of the retroviruses. However, if the host's immunity is weak, as in the neonatal period or old age, a less pathogenic virus or a lower dose of pathogenic retrovirus would be able to induce disease. In both human and nonhuman primates I hypothesize that the defenses could be raised by exposing the host to very low doses of the pathogenic virus. The potential low dose of virus would come from LTNPs with the *nef*-defective HIV-1 strains mentioned earlier. The replication capacities of *nef*-deleted strains isolated from many of the LTNPs are 100 times poorer in PBMC cultures than are *nef*+ HIV-1 strains (21,87,96,682–685,679–681,804). This suggests that the viral load produced by these strains would be lower upon initial infection and would allow molecular immunity to develop before the virulence of the virus can destroy the natural defenses.

Defenses could also be raised by exposing the host to a closely genetically related nonpathogenic strain of the retrovirus first before any exposure to a genetically related pathogenic strain of the virus. This concept is similar to the low-dose theory, because a less pathogenic virus will replicate poorly and cause a relatively low initial viral load. Reports of molecular immunity in various African monkey species against relatively pathogenic SIVs can be explained on the basis of this hypothesis. Since primates are exposed to various types of lentiviruses in the wild, they may be protected against a wide range of lentiviruses. On the other hand, Asian primates who are evolutionarily naive to SIVs (or various primates raised in captivity or naive for certain lentivirus strains) would be susceptible to even relatively mild types of lentiviral infection. Similarly, neonates and young humans or primates exposed to even relatively mild pathogenic strains of lentiviruses or small doses of pathogenic SIVs/HIV-1, would develop immunodeficiency, due to late maturation of this molecular immunity system (72,75,121,291,396). As mentioned above, Baba et al. (72) reported that an attenuated SIVΔ3 induced a lethal AIDS-like disease in 2 of the 4 macaque neonates infected orally, but the infection remained attenuated in the adult after intravenous infection. The question remained whether the neonate would tolerate a low dose of SIVΔ3. If so, then the low dose/high dose hypothesis regarding the pathogenesis of HIV-1 would be verifiable (805).

Wyand et al. (75) addressed this issue. These investigators exposed newborn rhesus monkeys to 3 different dilutions of SIVΔ3 by placing droplets containing various concentration of SIVΔ3 in such a way that it would mimic the natural exposure of human infants during vaginal delivery. They also exposed 18 neonatal monkeys with the SIVΔ3, 2 of which had high levels of viral load and developed AIDS-like diseases. Both of these infants had received the highest dose of virus; infants who were exposed to less concentrated SIVΔ3 remained disease-free. In addition, 4 female rhesus monkeys were exposed to high doses of SIVΔ3 during the second trimester of pregnancy to determine whether this mutant strain of SIV could be transmitted transplacentally or cause fetal damage, or could protect the fetus from SIVΔ3. None of the infants born to pregnant mothers who received SIVΔ3 during the second trimester were infected at birth, nor did they develop disease after birth. From these observations, one can conclude that mutant/defective SIV (SIVΔ3 in this case) will induce molecular immunity against full-length SIV and will require a complete cycle of replication. Molecular immunity develops later during ontogeny, and therefore neonates are relatively susceptible to even lower concentrations of low-virulence retroviruses; molecular immunity can be potentially initiated during the fetal lifetime (if the dose is small enough or if the virus is a less pathogenic mutant). In the case report by Ho and Cao (791) mentioned earlier, a baby born to an HIV-infected mother died although the mother was still symptom-free 12 years later (122). The analysis of her HIV-1 virus showed that it was attenuated, which explains why she had remained symptom free, but exposure to even attenuated virus caused disease in the infant, which confirms the hypothesis that much smaller doses of attenuated virus(s) would be needed when we subsequently decide to use live attenuated vaccine in humans to protect them from the ravages of HIV-1 infection (72,75).

If someone is exposed to a live but replication-defective (or some other gene-defective) virus (e.g., *nef*-deleted virus), would that live virus become more virulent after the immune stimulation of a host, as has been suggested previously (451,791,795)? Recently, Dittmer et al. attempted to answer this question. They vaccinated juvenile macaques with an attenuated SIVΔ*nef*, which conveyed protection against pathogenic SIV. Then they infected these macaques with vaccinia virus, which broadly stimulated their immune system, as was evident by expression of CD25/CD69 in 80% of their lymphocytes. This super-stimulation did not result in the increased activation of SIV (795). This question should remain open though, because we still do not know at what stage immune stimulation may become harmful and what types of stimulation may be harmful and why (767–770).

How *nef*-Deleted SIV (or HIV-1) Works

A natural experiment has been described by Deacon et al. (123) who reported on the transfusion from a single blood donor infected with HIV-1 to a cohort of 6 recipients of blood or blood products and have reported that all the recipients have remained free of HIV-1-related disease after 10–14 years. This HIV-1 isolate was defective at the *nef* gene, very similar to SIVΔ3 described above. Another such experiment has been described by Travers et al. (68) who followed the HIV status and health of 756 "commercial sex workers" for 9 years in Dakar, Senegal. They tracked the spread of HIV-1, as well as the spread of HIV-2, in this cohort of prostitutes. They found that of 187 women who were pre-exposed to the less pathogenic strain of HIV (HIV-2), only 7 became infected with HIV-1. However out of 618 uninfected with either type of HIV, 61 became infected. This reported existence of significant protection against HIV-1 in individuals who were pre-exposed to HIV-2 again points towards activation of molecular immunity.

The absence of cross-protection between HIVs and the HTLVs also exhibits a certain pattern (84,161,796–800). These 2 classes of retroviruses are genetically unrelated (as a matter of fact, they are entirely different forms of lentiviruses: endogenous vs. exogenous), and humans infected with one type of virus could be infected with other type (84,161,796–800).

I hypothesize that molecular immunity could be raised in immunocompetent hosts against a pathogenic strain of lentivirus, such as HIV-1 in humans under the following circumstances.

(*i*) If the host is vaccinated with a genetically closely related virus that is nonpathogenic to the host; for example, if a human is infected with live but defective SIV_{cpz} (similar to SIVΔ3 attenuated vaccine in macaques), it should provide very good protection to the vaccinated host.

A study by Travers et al. (68) was described above where a significant protection against HIV-1 in individuals who were pre-exposed to HIV-2 was observed. We also know that, compared to HIV-1 infection in Senegal, incidence of which has increased 26-fold over an 8-year period, the incidence of HIV-2 in the same cohort over the same period had remained the same (806). Maternal or neonatal transmission of HIV-2 also appears to be less efficient than that of HIV-1 (807). HIV-2-infected individuals suffer a very low rate of clinical symptoms, and most importantly, the HIV-2 viral load is very low, as compared to HIV-1. I believe that a very low virulence strain of HIV-2 could be made and should be tried as vaccine initially in an appropriate primate model and then in human volunteers.

(*ii*) Molecular immunity could be raised by exposing the host to attenuated pathogenic lentivirus (e.g., SIVΔ3). However, the attenuated virions must be able to complete RT for the molecular immunity to be completely activated.

(*iii*) The host could be immunized by exposure to a very low dose of the pathogenic lentiviruses in conjugation with anti-HIV-1 pharmacological agents. Examples of the development of such lentivirus-specific protection comes from various sources. Baba et al. reported a summary of their experiments with pathogenic Rauscher murine leukemia virus (RLV). In the first series of experiments, they pretreated the mice with antiviral therapy, which essentially keeps the viral load to a minimum, and then they inoculated the mice with a high dose of RLV. Subsequently, most of the animals resisted rechallenge with the same high dose of RLV, this time without any antiviral therapy. It is my hypothesis that a low dose of retrovirus induced molecular immunity because antiviral agents kept the early viral load to a minimum. In a second series of experiments, Baba's group inoculated naive mice with low doses of RLV. These mice were not given any antiviral therapy whatsoever. The mice without viremia from this low dose were rechallenged with high doses of RLV, and 21% of these mice were found to be immune, suggesting that during low-dose exposure there seems to have been a race between the development of molecular immunity and the spread of infection by the pathogenic virus to a larger percentage of cells, reaching a threshold resulting in damage to the host. If the host is allowed to develop molecular immunity, the defenses will be up and the infected host will be safe.

In addition, the example of attenuated SIVΔ3, which in high doses is pathogenic to some of the neonate rhesus monkeys but offers protection for these neonates in lower doses, further strengthens the validity of the hypothesis.

(*iv*) Vaccination may also take place by exposure to a genetically engineered HIV-1 strain that only goes though one cycle of replication. If HIV-1 strains are developed that only go through one cycle of replication, I hypothesize that that will be sufficient to activate HIV-1-specific molecular immunity. This type of virion has to be engineered in such a way that it does not destroy the cells it infects, and its replication is limited to only one growth cycle. Such experiments have been started in my laboratory and the preliminary results are very encouraging.

Role of the CD8+ T Cell in the Development of Anti-Retroviral Molecular Immunity

As opposed to nonhuman primates naturally infected with SIVs, humans infected with HIV-1 show a gradual decline in the number of CD4+ T cells or possibly a dysfunction of this cell type. However, it has yet to be clearly determined how HIV-1 causes the gradual depletion of CD4+ T cells. In 1992, my laboratory, utilizing an ultrasensitive method—ISPCR—was the first to show that in HIV-1-infected individuals the number of PBMCs infected was much higher than previously believed, and the number of CD4+ T cells infected with HIV-1 in AIDS patients could be as high as 69% (457,808). In 1995, David Ho and George Shaw used mathematical models to show that about 100 billion new HIV-1 virions (viral particles) are produced daily and 1–2 billion CD4+ T cells are destroyed each day, in an HIV-1-infected individual, regardless of his or her HIV-1 status. These data proposed that CD4+ T-cell turnover was extremely high in HIV-1-infected individuals. In both of these studies, the investigators used the data from a very small number of AIDS patients and all the measurements were by indirect mathematical calculations (462,809,810). In our studies, we analyzed the PBMCs from 56 individuals, and there was a clear difference in the percentage of PBMCs infected in the AIDS patients versus the asymptomatic individuals (189,457,566). Frank Miedema's group challenged Ho's and Shaw's data a year later (811). They also estimated CD4+ T-cell turnover by measuring changes in the length of the T cells' telomerase. They found no significant difference in the telomeric length from HIV-1-infected versus uninfected individuals. In the academic realm, this CD4+ T-cell turnover rate has sparked a new series of discussions. However, the question remains—what keeps HIV-1-infected individuals alive for so many years (up to 18 years in some cases)? What are the mechanisms, at both the cellular and molecular levels, that can keep an infected person symptom-free for several years? In recent years, CD8+ T cells have gained a special attention; some of this information has been discussed in preceding chapters. Now I would like to present most of the relevant information in capsular form.

The pivotal role of CD8+ cells in the development of the anti-lentiviral-specific molecular immunity has been mentioned earlier. Briefly, CD8+ cells from healthy HIV-1-infected individuals can suppress HIV-1 replication without killing the infected cells. These are non-CTL, noncytolytic CD8+ cells, characterized by their ability to reduce HIV-1 p24 antigen levels and reverse transcriptase levels in the culture fluids of PBMCs infected with all strains of HIV-1 and 2, SIV, and FIV. This anti-retroviral activity is not restricted by the MHC, does not require contact between target and effector cells, occurs at low CD8+/CD4+ ratios, and is oligoclonal in nature (85,126, 132–139,575,581–613,641,685,713–725). The nature of the anti-retroviral activity of CD8+ cells is via soluble messenger agents that are unrelated to any known cytokines or chemokines, though currently this conclusion is controversial (718–724). The exact mechanisms of these antiviral effects are unclear. However, recently, experimental evidence has been reported that shows CD8+ cells exert their anti-HIV-1 effects by specifically interrupting HIV-1 transcription. Using in situ hybridization, our laboratory was the first to demonstrate that anti-HIV-1 activity of CD8+ cells can modulate the expression of HIV-1 RNA (134). In order to evaluate the status of HIV-1 replication at a molecular level, we performed in situ hybridization of cultured cells with an HIV-1 *gag* probe. The unfractionated PBMCs infected with $TCID_{50}$ of HIV-1 exhibited the presence of HIV-1-specific RNA only in 1:1000–1:3000 cells. When CD8+ T cells were removed from the PBMCs and infected with HIV-1, a significantly larger percentage of cells, up to 52%, were actively transcribing HIV-1-specific RNA. A significant number of cells were also being destroyed by HIV-1 infection. Reconstitution of syngeneic CD8+ T-cell-depleted PBMCs inhibited the HIV-1-specific RNA production. In these wells, the fraction of cells exhibiting HIV-1-specific RNA varied from 1 in 600 to 1 in 850 (134). Recently, several investigators, using different approaches, illustrated the anti-retroviral activities of an unknown substance(s) secreted by the primed CD8+ T cells that arrest the viral replication at the level of transcription (581–583,794–796).

Recently, Kootstra et al. (812), a research group from the Netherlands, further analyzed the CD8+ T-cell-mediated noncytolytic suppression of autologous and heterologous primary HIV-1 isolates. They reported that the CD8+ T-cell factors harvested from LTNPs and progressors showed that the former possessed much higher levels of the protective factors as compared to the latter. However, 4 out of 6 progressors to AIDS also possessed the same amount of the CD8+ T-cell factors, even in the face of increasing viral load. Surprisingly, CD8+ T cells from uninfected PBMCs and even from cord blood from uninfected fetuses exhibited the CD8+ T-cell factors that protected the PBMCs from HIV-1 infection, which supports the conclusion that the CD8+ T-cell factors are already present as a protective repertoire in our systems and get amplified when exposed to a certain specific retrovirus. Therefore, when these investigators examined the anti-HIV-1 activities of the CD8+ T-cell factors isolated from the PBMCs from individuals at 2 months before seroconversion and at 3 and 14 months after, they found that the CD8+ T-cell factors were able to completely suppress the HIV-1 replication, irrespective of the time at which they were isolated. In addition, they found relatively high levels of the anti-HIV-1 factors from 2 out of 3 LTNPs they tested. My laboratory showed several years ago that the anti-HIV-1 CD8+ T-cell factors can be harvested and amplified from HIV-1-seronegative healthy PBMCs (134).

The anti-HIV-1 activity of CD8+ T cells is mediated by soluble factors (137–138). CD8+ T cells from HIV-1 seronegative as well as from HIV-1-infected individuals can significantly suppress viral replication in vitro (134,137–138). This antiviral activity is not restricted to HIV-1. The CD8+ T-cell-mediated inhibitory effects have been reported in SIV-infected sooty mangabeys, in HIV-2-infected primates, in SIV_{agm}-infected primates, in FIV-infected cats, in retrovirus-infected mice, and in HIV-1-infected chimpanzees (575,582). However, these CD8+ T-cell factors are virus-specific and do not cross species in a significant way (which is predicted in the hypotheses described above; unpublished data).

The Role of CD8+ T Cells in the First Year of Life in Perinatally Infected Babies

Recently, Pollack et al. (813) explored the role of CD8+ T cells in suppression of HIV-1 in perinatally infected infants. For this purpose, they evaluated the anti-HIV-1 CD8+ T-cell-mediated HIV-1 in vertically infected infants by analyzing such activity 45 times during the first year of life, correlated with viral load (HIV-1 p24), CTLs, production of antibody in vitro, and clinical outcome. They demonstrated the CD8+ T-cell-mediated anti-HIV-1 activities in 11 out of 16 infants in the first year of life and in some as early as 3 weeks after birth. Infants who exhibited CD8+ T-cell-mediated anti-HIV-1 activities had a significantly lower viral load and survived longer ($P = 0.003$). However, the infants who lacked CD8+ T-cell-mediated anti-HIV-1 activities were rapid progressors, and they had higher viral loads (0.094 vs. 0.639×10^6 copies/mL) and shorter survival times (4 out of 5 died before 2.5 years of age). The CD8+ T-cell-mediated anti-HIV-1 activities appeared before or at the same time as anti-HIV-1 antibody production. No CTL activity was detected in any of several hundred T-cell clones generated on 6 different occasions from 2 infants with strong CD8+ T-cell-mediated anti-HIV-1 activities. These data are in agreement with the previous studies of Mackewicz et al. (581) in which they found a correlation between detection of CD8+ T-cell-mediated anti-HIV-1 activities at the time of seroconversion in adults and a decline in viral load. Why did some infants develop anti-HIV-1 CD8+ T-cell-mediated immunity (molecular immunity) and others did not? The answer to this question, I believe, lies in the initial dose of viral infection. The most consistent correlation with vertical transmission is increased HIV-1 p24 antigenemia. Even asymptomatic HIV-1-seropositive women with a CD4 count below $500/cm^3$ and p24 antigenemia are 10-fold more likely to transmit HIV-1 to their children than women without p24 antigenemia (814). In this study, the viral load of mothers during gestation correlated with the survival of the babies would have been very informative. Currently, my laboratory is carrying out this analysis.

Can the Use of Protease Inhibitors Vaccinate HIV-1-Infected Individuals?

At the time of this writing, there is a good deal of excitement, both in HIV-1-infected individuals and in the mass media, over the possibility that newly FDA-approved anti-HIV-1 agents called protease inhibitors can turn the tide against the scourge of AIDS. It is hoped that use of protease inhibitors in combination with other anti-HIV-1 agents (i.e., AZT and 3TC, reverse transcriptase inhibitors), called triple therapy, can cure or at least turn infection with HIV-1 into a chronic illness. Numerous studies have shown that this triple therapy cocktail can reduce the blood viral load to very low levels (815,816). As proposed in this hypothesis, a low viral load can potentially vaccinate the infected individuals by priming the target cells with the protective RNAs, but only if viral load is low at the initial stage of HIV-1 infection (759). In this case, treating HIV-1-infected individuals at a very early stage after exposure to the virus should induce the appropriate anti-HIV-1 immunity. However, the answer to this question is not available yet and may not be so simple. We do not know if treating HIV-1-infected individuals who already have reached a threshold number of productively infected cells, can turn the tide, but it is unlikely (767,817,818). At present we do not know if these protease inhibitors interfere in the development of molecular immunity pathways. Since these agents interfere with numerous molecular events inside the cells and affect RNA and protein synthesis, it is possible that these very actions also cripple the development of intracellular antiviral events leading to the development of molecular immunity. We know that AZT exerts numerous toxic effects on the cells, and its actions are limited to its inhibitory effects on the reverse transcriptase enzyme. Therefore, it might interfere with the molecular vaccination steps. In my opinion, combination therapy in which AZT and 3TC are combined with protease inhibitor(s) may be helpful if given at a very early stage of HIV-1 infection, before the virus infects a threshold number of PBMCs and establishes itself in the host system (before HIV-1 has entered a certain number of target cells—high enough to maintain a relatively modest viral load). The toxic effects of AZT and 3TC are well documented (758). Recently, reports have emerged that certain protease inhibitors induce sudden hyperglycemia, which could potentially result in death if it occurs during sleep or goes unnoticed. In addition, a number of reports have emerged that indicate resistance of HIV-1 to triple therapy (817–820).

Can Retroviral-Based Gene Therapy Create a New Kind of AIDS Epidemic?

Retrovirus-mediated gene delivery has become one of the most widely applied methods for the introduction of genes into primary cells. This method has already been used in several clinical trials (reviewed in References 111,112). Attractive features of retroviral vectors include the ease with which the variety of coding sequences can be transferred, the relatively high transduction efficiency, and the stability of the proviral genome once integrated into a host cell chromosome. The greatest concern about the use of retroviral vectors for clinical applications has been their potential to induce or contribute to neoplastic transformation. This concern was enhanced by the development of rapidly progressive, fatal lymphomas in 3 nonhuman primates subjected to autologous transplantation with retrovirus-transduced bone marrow cells. The disease pattern, latency period, and high titer of replication-competent retroviruses in the sera of these animals are highly reminiscent of the features of retrovirus-induced lymphomas in rodent species (791).

However, the much greater concern is that exposure of humans to new types of retroviruses, to which we are evolutionarily naive, may start a dangerous new epidemic. We have to realize that although many of the new, genetically engineered retroviral vectors have been used in primates or rodents and found safe in these animals, we should not necessarily interpret them as safe for human clinical trials. Evolutionarily speaking, the exposure history of either of these types of animals to certain retroviruses may not coincide with the exposure history of humans (616,797). Great care must be taken in approving any retroviral vector for human use, and all humans already exposed to any type of retroviral vector in the past should be monitored for the potential development of some new pathogenic form of recombinant retrovirus.

Currently, the packaging cell lines that constitutively synthesize retroviral vectors have been derived from components of various proviral genomes. Packaging lines that yield viruses with ecotropic specificity are based on components of the Moloney MuLV, whereas amphotropic packaging lines are engineered with the *env* gene from the 4070A virus, a naturally occurring murine retrovirus with amphotropic host range. The retroviral vectors and packaging components used to develop producer clones for clinical applications have been designed to minimize the potential for mutational events that could give rise to a replication-competent retrovirus. However, emergence of replication-competent viruses has been common with packaging cell lines. For example, Donahue et al. (787) reported that rapidly progressive T-cell lymphomas were observed in 3 of 10 rhesus monkeys several months after autologous transplantation of enriched CD34+ bone marrow stem cells that had been transduced with a retroviral vector preparation containing replication-competent virus. The animals with lymphoma appeared to be tolerant of retroviral antigens because their sera lacked antibodies reactive with viral proteins and contained 10^4–10^5 infectious virus particles/mL (791). By molecular cloning and DNA sequencing, the investigators demonstrated that the serum from 1 of the monkeys contained a replication-competent retrovirus that arose by recombination between vector and packaging encoding sequences (vector/helper recombinant) in the producer clone used for transduction of bone marrow stem cells. Southern blot analysis demonstrated that 14 or 25 copies of this genome per cell were present in 2 animals. The genome of a second replication-competent virus was also recovered by molecular cloning; it arose by recombination involving the genome of the vector/helper recombinant and endogenous murine retroviral genomes in the producer clone. Twelve copies of this amphotropic virus/mink cell focus-forming virus genome were present in tumor DNA of 1 animal, but it was not found in tumor DNA of the other 2 animals with lymphoma. Southern blot analysis of DNA from various tissues demonstrated common insertion site bands in several samples of tumor DNA from 1 animal, suggesting clonal origin of the lymphoma. These data were consistent with a pathogenic mechanism in which chronic productive retroviral infection allowed insertional mutagenesis of critical growth control genes, leading to cell transformation and clonal tumor evolution. Some of the most disturbing data has recently come from a report by Purcell et al. (790). These investigators analyzed, by direct RNA-PCR, the T-cell lymphomas that developed in rhesus macaques during a gene therapy experiment. Their analyses revealed the presence of multiple recombinant MuLVs in the lymphoid tissues. The most common recombinant virus was designated $Mo_{LTR}Ampho_{env}$, in which the amphotropic envelope of the helper packaging virus has recombined with the LTR of the vector derived from the MMuLV. An additional copy of an enhancer acquired from the vector LTR is thought to have increased the replicative capacity of the $Mo_{LTR}Ampho_{env}$. Also, 2 different types of mink cell focus-forming MuLVs that arose from endogenous retroviral sequences of the packaging cell line were also found in the macaques and were very highly expressed. In addition, murine virus-like VL30 sequences were also present in the monkeys' lymphomas. The presence and expression of these new viruses are matters of great concern. The emergence of new viruses, which do not exist in nature, from exposure to retroviral vectors could wreak havoc in human communities.

A similar serious concern is related to our inadvertent exposure to other retroviruses. Currently, the number of individuals suffering from heart, kidney, or lung failure is in the millions. The demand for suitable donor organs to fill the urgent medical need is impossible to meet; therefore, xenotransplants from transgenic nonhuman primates and pigs are being evaluated. The recently publicized cloning technology, where a lamb was cloned from a single cell of an adult sheep, demonstrated the power of cloning. There is no doubt that cloning is of practical importance; it can be used to produce a large number of identical animals that can provide clinically useful proteins (e.g., factor IX for hemophilia patients). The utility of cloning technology in organ transplantation is enormous (821). However, as with any new technology, one should also be cautious. It is likely that transgenic pigs would be better candidates than lambs for organ transplantation since they are more suitable donors of cells, tissues, and vascularized organs (due to a variety of practical reasons). Recently, Patience et al. (791) examined whether pig endogenous retroviruses could be infectious to human cells in culture. They co-cultured 2 pig kidney cells, which spontaneously produced type C retroviruses, with human 293 cell line. These pig endogenous retroviruses infected human cell lines and resulted in a broad range of human cell infection. Upon passage into human cells, pig endogenous retroviruses could rescue a Maloney retroviral vector and acquired resistance to lysis by human complement (791).

As mentioned earlier, inoculation of attenuated HIV-1 into already infected individuals may not bring any benefit to them; we already know that such attenuated viruses will recombine with preexisting full-length HIVs (214). It is important that we carefully evaluate the possible side effects of transgenic animals' retroviruses and their potential long-term harmful effects, before we make an error that could result in an another AIDS-like global pandemic.

Chapter 6

Factors That Break Down Molecular Immunity Pathways

"It is quite likely that no single factor explains the control of infection in all long-term nonprogressors. Indeed, some of these individuals may have been infected with a virus of limited replication competence, pathogenicity, or both. However, many long-term nonprogressors appear to have been infected with pathogenic viruses that they have controlled. Indeed, in many of these individuals, viral burden is very low."

William E. Paul
Cell 82:177, 1995

SUBSTANCES OF ABUSE AND IMMUNITY

If molecular immunity is so effective and has been able to keep many lentiviruses at bay for thousands of years, even though these lentiviruses have the potential to cause severe disease in humans (e.g., HTLV-I), why has HIV-1 had such a serious impact on our society? If we have molecular immunity against HIV-1 infection, why does infection with HIV-1 result in such devastating consequences for humans when several primates, including our closest evolutionary relative, the chimpanzee, is able to resist clinically significant infection with HIV-1 and its related viruses (i.e., SIV_{cpz})? There are 2 possible answers. First, HIV-1, as opposed to other lentiviruses, is naturally more pathogenic for humans than for primates. Second, humans have factors in their diet and social habits that adversely affect that arm of the immune system specifically responsible for defense against retroviruses, i.e., molecular immunity. The answer could also be some combination of these possibilities.

We know that HIV-1 possesses several genes that have a scenario of pathogenic consequences. We also know that our history of exposure to HIV-1 appears to be very short—only about 50 years (19,32,47–49,354,356,434–439). We have come to understand that evolutionarily we are a naive host for this virus. The main reservoir for this class of virus is African nonhuman primates; therefore, it would not be surprising that once we are exposed to relatively high doses of this virus, we can suffer fatal consequences (as do Asian macaques). However, I believe there is another factor (or to be precise, there are other factors) that adversely affect the arm of the immune system that is responsible for activating molecular immunity, namely, the CD8+/NK+ cells. These factors are substances that most of us use as a normal part of our daily lives without paying any special attention to their adverse effects on our body. Importantly, nonhuman primates do not consume alcohol, cocaine, or prescription drugs.

In this section, I would like to provide some information regarding the immunomodulatory effects of substances of abuse as well as other prescription drugs. This is important because if any chemical agent(s) exerts an adverse effect on the CD8+/NK+ cell functions, which appear to have the most pivotal role in controlling retroviral infection, the balance between host and HIV-1 may tilt in favor of the invading retrovirus (90,609).

Both epidemiological and biological data support the idea that certain chemical agents may adversely affect the functions of CD8+ T cells. For example, an increased incidence of AIDS has been associated with increased use of substances of abuse (429–431). Alcohol ingestion has been associated with significant depletion of CD8+ equivalent subsets in animal models and in humans (744–746,748–750,752–754). Consumption of alcohol has also been reported to significantly decrease resistance to HIV-1 in vitro (748–750,752–754). Several in vitro studies and in vivo studies in experimental animals exhibit clear similarities between immune dysfunctions caused by excessive alcohol and cocaine consumption and those observed after HIV-1 infection (745–747,822–825). A transient immunosuppressive-like environment caused by alcohol consumption in which CD8+ T-cell functions are impaired might provide an environment in which HIV-1 could replicate faster than in an intact immune system (744,746,748–750,752–754, 822–825), increasing the initial viral load over a certain minimum threshold, resulting in the development of AIDS. Epidemiologic studies have also suggested an association between alcohol and cocaine abuse during sexual activity and an increased incidence of AIDS (744-750).

Molecular Mechanisms of CD8+ T-Cell Functions and Certain Drugs

In a rodent model of chronic cocaine abuse, my laboratory has shown that cocaine consumption induces profound modulations in immune systems. The most significant effect of cocaine in vivo, in the animal model of chronic cocaine abuse, has been observed on CD8+ cells (822,826). Chaisson et al. (430) reported that intravenous cocaine use significantly increases the risk of HIV-1 infection with a seroprevalence of 35% in daily cocaine users (as compared to non-cocaine users, among the high-risk populations). Sterk has also published a slightly higher prevalence in a study with a smaller group of cocaine abusers (756). Immunomodulations caused by exposure to cocaine might render the immune system more susceptible to HIV-1 infection and provide a favorable environment for HIV-1 dissemination.

However, I would also suggest that any agent(s) that decreases certain functions in CD8+/NK+ cells may lead to nonspecific activation of the immune system (827,828). This results in the release of control by T-suppressor cells over B and T lymphocytes, which results in polyclonal activation of T and B cells (reviewed in Reference 44). Both alcohol and cocaine have been shown to induce CD8+ T cell-mediated nonspecific activation of the immune system, resulting in polyclonal activation of T and B cells (752,822). As described earlier, I have hypothesized that such activation results in the weakening of molecular immunity against HIV-1, as suggested by the data of Zack et al. (455), Bukinrinsky et al. (458), and Sonza et al. (717), all of whom showed that in normal conditions, human PBMCs are able to keep the HIV-1 replication at minimum levels and that some unknown intracellular factors interrupt the viral replication pathways. However, if these cells are exposed to a lectin called PHA, a nonspecific stimulator of T cells, the intracellular defenses are broken down and are no longer able to protect the cells from productive infection. Therefore, CD8+ T-cell dysfunction alters some of the anti-retroviral immunity pathways (752,822). It is interesting to note the similarity between AIDS patients and individuals who abuse alcohol and cocaine, with both groups demonstrating hyperimmunoglobulemia, resulting from alterations in CD8+ T-cell functions (741–743,745–746, 822–825).

Our observations in experimental models of alcoholism and cocaine abuse, as well as other indirect evidence, suggest that the CD8+ cell is the most sensitive subset of lymphocytes to alcohol and cocaine abuse (752,822). These observations become more interesting in light of recent evidence in a large body of literature that CD8+ T cells play a pivotal role in the inhibition of HIV-1 in vitro and in vivo (described in detail in an earlier section; 132–139,581–613). Even more striking is the fact that one can isolate HIV-1 or other lentiviruses from the PBMCs or other tissues by using various agents that affect CD8+ T cell function, the most common being PHA lectin, which nonspecifically stimulates the T cells and breaks down the normal functions of the CD8+ T cells. Other agents that are known to break down the CD8+ T-cell functions include exposure to low-dose radiation (726), UV light (727), cyclosporines, cyclophosphamide (728), steroids (729–730), co-infection with some other pathogenic viruses (733–740), products of certain viruses including pathogenic lentiviruses, and temporary immunoincompetence due to certain substances of abuse, e.g., alcohol, cocaine, or even certain antiviral drugs (741–757).

Therefore, I have suggested that cocaine and alcohol abuse, and possibly the consumption of other immunomodulatory drugs, may play an important role in the development and expression of AIDS (827). For example, T lymphocytes seem to be extensively altered by ethanol. A transient immunosuppressive state induced by moderate alcohol consumption might support an environment in which HIV-1 could replicate faster than in an intact immune system. It is possible that transient CD8+ T-cell dysfunction may indirectly release the regulatory controls over the immune system and act as a stimulant for CD4+ lymphocytes (reviewed in Reference 826). This has been demonstrated to occur in vivo after chronic ethanol abuse in experimental models of alcoholism (829). Both alcoholics and patients with AIDS also exhibit increased levels of serum immunoglobulins, presumably caused by CD8+ T-suppressor lymphocyte dysfunction, resulting in a lessening of control over B lymphocytes (826).

Various groups have evaluated the anti-retroviral effects of CD8+ T cells (described earlier). Several investigators have demonstrated that progression to AIDS from the asymptomatic stage in HIV-1-infected individuals is associated with the loss of CD8+ cell function. Margolick et al. (830) analyzed CD8+ subsets and reported that increases in the CD38+ CD8+ subset was associated with rapid progression to AIDS, whereas the CD38- HLA-DR+ CD8+ subset was associated with asymptomatic disease. Fong et al. reported a case study in which an alcoholic patient rapidly progressed to AIDS only 3 months after seroconversion (746). PBMCs from this patient exhibited no CTL activity against HIV-1 antigens. These authors suggested that the rapid course of this patient was the result of ethanol abuse, which suppressed his T-cell functions and stimulated HIV-1 replication.

A failure in the HIV-1-specific T-cell responses and the amplification of CD8+ T cells due to defects in cytokine production, especially IL-2, may result in increased risk for HIV-1 infection after exposure to alcohol. Several studies suggest the existence of such adverse outcomes. For example, Avins et al. (745) observed a substantial prevalence of HIV-1 infection among heterosexual individuals in San Francisco's alcohol treatment programs. They reported that the overall prevalence of HIV-1 infection was 5%, most of which was not associated with intravenous drug use. These authors also suggested the role of alcohol in suppressing the T-cell functions, which subsequently results in increased prevalence of HIV-1 infection. Several epidemiological studies have suggested an association between alcohol abuse during sexual activity and an increased incidence of AIDS (reviewed in Reference 753), although this was not universal (831). Of note, in one study, approximately 33% of HIV-1-seropositive adult hemophiliacs (22 years or older) developed AIDS within 6 years after HIV-1 seroconversion, whereas only about 5% of HIV-1-infected younger hemophiliacs developed AIDS within the same period (832). There are various explanations for such differences in the incidence of progression to AIDS between the 2 age groups. However, it is conceivable that the lower incidence of alcohol consumption in the younger group might play a role. Watson et al. (829) have reported that mice infected with murine AIDS (MAIDS; a retrovirus which causes an AIDS-like immunosuppression in mice) and given 36% of their calories from an ethanol-containing diet, exhibited a significantly lower survival rate (8.6% after 25 weeks) compared to controls who were given no ethanol (45.0%).

It is still unclear whether normally functioning CD8+ T cells or an intact immune system are important in resisting an initial HIV-1 infection or in the maintenance of asymptomatic states in individuals already exposed to HIV-1. In recent years, information has accumulated that suggests an increased viral load in adult HIV-1-seropositive patients correlates with CD8+ T-cell dysfunction and disease progression (132–139,581–613). Also, HIV-1 grows well in a CD4+ cell line free from CD8+ cell effects. As a matter of fact, these are the conditions in which the first large-scale HIV-1 was grown to prepare HIV-1 antigens for the development of ELISA tests. In addition, it is almost standard practice today to isolate HIV-1 from patients or from SIV-infected primates by depleting CD8+ T cells from the PBMCs (132–139,581–613).

My laboratory was the first to consider the possibility that alcohol consumption might affect the outcome of HIV-1 infection. In several reports, we demonstrated that the susceptibility of PBMCs to infection with HIV-1 was significantly increased in patients who consumed alcohol or who were given intravenous infusion of ethanol. This increased HIV-1 viral replication was also associated with concomitant deficiencies in CD8+ T-cell function, as well as in T helper and monocyte/macrophage functions. In one of our previous studies in which 60 volunteers were asked to consume various amounts of alcoholic beverages, we analyzed the percentage of PBMC subpopulations, including CD4+, CD8+, and B lymphocytes plus monocytes, which demonstrated significant alterations in the functions of these cells after ethanol exposure versus before ethanol exposure (833). Although this is not proven, the data from these studies and from many other investigations (see below) suggest that these associations may be causally related. Together, these observations suggest that CD8+ T cells in the HIV-1-infected but otherwise healthy individual may provide protection against the further spread of HIV-1 to CD4+ T cells and/or monocytes, and ethanol potentially interferes with one or more of the CD8+ T-cell-mediated protective mechanisms. This might adversely alter the natural protective balance between the host's antiretroviral capabilities and the virus' degree of virulence. These data suggest that exogenous agents may alter HIV-1 replication in vivo. As such, various environmental stimuli may affect the natural history of HIV-1 infections (reviewed in Reference 833). In addition, the recent study in which we infused volunteers with ethanol intravenously is unique because it eliminates the role of condiments and nonalcoholic components of alcoholic beverages in inducing adverse effects on the immune system. These studies may provide an explanation for the reported high incidence of HIV-1-seropositive individuals in various alcohol treatment programs and the rapid progression to AIDS after HIV-1 seroconversion in alcoholics. These experiments extend our previous findings that exposure to ethanol may influence the initial stages of HIV-1 infection and possibly alter the delicate balance between host and virus in asymptomatic individuals. Ethanol may, as well, increase the likelihood of HIV-1 infection in an individual who has consumed a moderate amount of alcohol, if it occurs prior to or during exposure to HIV-1, for example, at times of high-risk sexual activity or intravenous drug use. Recently, Barker et al. (685) showed that CD8+ cells isolated from the long-term survivors infected with HIV-1 for 10 years or more have a threefold greater ability to suppress HIV-1 replication than the CD8+ cells from rapid progressors. They also demonstrated that exposure of CD8+ cells to IL-2 potentiated the anti-HIV-1 activities of these cells, whereas exposure to IL-4 or IL-10 reduced such activity. We have demonstrated that individuals who consumed a moderate amount of alcohol or were exposed to low levels of ethanol demonstrated a significant reduction in their ability to secrete IL-2 (833).

In the following sections I would like to review in detail some of the published aspects of various substances of abuse.

LINK BETWEEN ALCOHOL INGESTION AND HIV-1 INFECTION

The immunosuppressive effects of alcohol, the most common substance of abuse, have been documented since the time of Robert Koch who, in 1884, reported that alcoholics were the most common victims of cholera. Since then hundreds of carefully conducted studies in humans and in animals have documented various adverse effects of alcohol abuse. One earlier, well-documented study by Tennenbaum et al. (reviewed in Reference 834) reported that chronic administration of alcohol led to significant impairment of the immune response in the rat. Since then, alcohol has been shown to induce alterations in immune responsiveness in the host, including a functional impairment of granulocytes, macrophages, and lymphocytes. Human alcoholics have an increased risk of developing serious infections, including pneumonia and tuberculosis and neoplasms of the head and neck—a phenomenon that could be, at least in part, related to alcohol's effect on the immune system (834).

The medical community has recognized the association between alcohol abuse and increased episodes of infection, but the cellular and molecular mechanisms underlying these observations have remained elusive.

Alcohol, CD8+ T-Cell Dysfunction, and HIV-1: An Historic Perspective

Since the beginning of the HIV-1 epidemic, my laboratory noted the moderate HIV-1 inhibitory effect of CD8+ T cells. Fortunately, at this time, my laboratory, while working on an animal model of chronic alcoholism, discovered that alcohol exerts an adverse effect on the CD8+ T-cell function. In our initial studies (834), we showed alcohol-induced immunomodulations on various subpopulations of T cells, B cells, and macrophages, and we have assessed primary B-cell response to helper T-cell-independent and T-cell-dependent antigens in a chronic alcohol animal model (Sprague-Dawley male rats) originally described by DeCarli and Leiber. This research design allowed us to assess CD4+, CD8+, and B-cell responses in animals before they were given ethanol and during the course of their chronic alcoholism. Briefly, functional and numerical analysis of T-cell subsets and B-cell and macrophage populations during the course of chronic alcoholism strongly suggested that the T-suppressor cell subset (CD8+ equivalent in rats) function was most sensitive to the effect of chronic alcoholism, while T-helper cells (CD4+ equivalent in rodents) and finally B-cell function subsequently become influenced by the adverse effect of chronic alcohol consumption. T-cell subset enumeration, using FITC-labeled monoclonal antibodies revealed that a sequential T-suppressor, T-helper cell loss occurred several days following dysfunction of these T-cell subsets. There have been numerous observations in patients and in experimental studies that support our observations. Conversely, our data provided further explanation of otherwise unexplained information from other investigators. For example, Smith et al. (741) reported decreased total PBMCs and T cells in patients with histological evidence of liver damage. These patients also exhibited increased levels of serum IgG, IgA, and IgE, and enhanced antibody response to pneumococcal polysaccharide antigens (similar to SIII, used in our studies). Theoretically, the weakening of suppressor T-cell control over the immunoregulatory T-cell network could produce such a result. Drew et al. (823) reported polyclonal B-cell activation in alcoholic patients with no evidence of liver dysfunction. Such alterations in the concentration of serum immunoglobulins are well-recognized features of alcoholism (as well as AIDS). Autoantibodies are also detected more frequently in patients with alcoholic liver disease than with other forms of chronic liver disease (825). Antibody responses to immunization with various vaccines are increased in these patients. Titres of serum antibody to measles and rubella viruses are significantly increased in chronic alcoholics, presumably due to the release of T-suppressor cell control over B cells (reviewed in Reference 834).

Our observations in experimental models of alcoholism and much other indirect evidence (834) indicate that the T-suppressor cell is the most alcohol-sensitive subset. This notion becomes more intriguing in light of the overwhelming evidence that CD8+ T cells play a pivotal role in protection against HIV-1 and other retroviral infections in vitro and in vivo (132–139,581–613).

At the time of the research discussed above, I began to develop the idea of molecular immunity and started to consider whether primates and humans might have developed an immune system directed against retroviruses and whether this system might be regulated by a certain subset of CD8+/NK+ cells.

Molecular mechanism(s) by which CD8+ cells can potentially inactivate retroviruses became the focus of our work. The mechanism by which CD8+ cells destroy their target was limited; however, I observed that CD8+ cells can inhibit the expression of HIV-1 in acutely infected PBMCs in vitro. For this purpose, we utilized an in situ hybridization technique (134). I hypothesized that higher organisms, i.e., eukaryotes, may have developed an immune defense mechanism(s) that either digests retroviral nucleic acid upon its introduction to the host system or blocks HIV-1 RT or integration by some intracellular mechanism(s). I was surprised to learn that there were some hints in the previously published literature that provided clues into such mechanisms. For example, in 1983 DesGroseillers and Jolicoeur (115) published an article that described the differences in the host range of MuLVs. These host ranges were originally designated N-tropic and B-tropic because they replicated preferentially in vitro on NIH and BALB/c fibroblasts, respectively. It was later found that N-tropic MuLVs were in fact restricted in BALB/c cells, that B-tropic MuLVs were restricted in NIH cells, and that both viruses were restricted in (BALB X NIH) F1 cells. A single gene, *Fv1*, with 2 alleles, $Fv1^b$ and $Fv1^n$, determines this dominant restriction. They also reported that a virus-encoded protein seemed to carry the viral host range determinant that was recognized by the *Fv1* gene product. In order to map the viral DNA sequences encoding this determinant, they constructed viral DNA recombinants in vitro between the cloned infectious viral DNA genomes from BALB/c N-tropic and B-tropic MuLVs. Infectious recombinant MuLVs were recovered by microinjecting these recombinant DNAs into murine Fv1-SC-1 cells and were subsequently tested in vitro for their host ranges (N- or B-tropic). They found that a short 302-bp 5′-end fragment was necessary and sufficient to confer a specific host range to a recombinant. Furthermore, their sequencing data revealed that this fragment coded for amino acid sequences in *gag* p30. They also showed that only 2 consecutive amino acid differences, glutamine–arginine and threonine–glutamine, in p30 were responsible for the N- and B-tropic host ranges of the BALB/c MuLVs, respectively. Therefore, it appears that the $Fv1^b$ and $Fv1^n$ gene products can discriminate between these p30 amino acid sequences. The series of experiments described in an earlier section led to further elucidation of the molecular immunity and its role in the anti-retroviral immunity.

Effect of Alcohol on CD8+ T-Cell Function

In a different area of investigation, my laboratory started to explore the potential role of alcohol on the replication capacities of HIV-1, and a combination of in vivo and in vitro experiments were designed. In the preliminary experiments, 2 blood samples were taken from 6 volunteers, the first following at least 1 week of abstinence from alcohol, the second on the morning after drinking an average of 4 beers. The PBMCs were isolated from the whole blood and were infected with HIV-1 in vitro. In my mind there was already a suspicion that T-cell mitogens (i.e., ConA and PHA) might be toxic to PBMC cultures in vitro (since they have been known to be extremely toxic to animals in vivo and to induce granulomas the size of golf balls if injected into the peritoneum cavities of the experimental animals). I had to devise a new method to keep the PBMCs alive without adversely affecting the natural immune responses. A new method was envisioned that mimicked the natural conditions of PBMCs in vivo; PBMCs were incubated in 6–10 units of IL-2 without mitogens (748). This had to be devised and perfected months before the experiments regarding the effect of alcohol on the HIV-1 replication could be carried out. The problem with PHA stimulation of PBMCs has been that they nonspecifically stimulate various T lymphocytes in a nonimmunological manner and can destroy the natural immune pathways (at that time I had speculated on this fact but had yet to prove it). The in vitro replication of HIV-1 was found to be markedly increased (P>0.001) in the PBMCs from the volunteers following alcohol consumption, as compared with the parallel controls (each person served as his or her own control), and the susceptibility appeared to persist for 24 to 36 h. The results of the initial pilot experiments involving 6 normal adults were published before repetition because of their potential importance. They revealed depression of the ability of PBMCs to produce IL-2 and soluble immune response suppressor (SIRS), 12 to 15 h after a single ingestion of moderate amounts of an alcoholic beverage by nonalcoholic healthy adults. This depression is predominantly of CD4+ and CD8+ T-cell functions, which lasted for 1.5 to 4.5 days. It was associated with the development of susceptibility of their PBMCs to infection with HIV-1 (748).

Susceptibility to infection was demonstrated by prolonged incubation of the unstimulated PBMCs with high concentrations of free virus and by assay for productive infection using an indirect syncytia-formation assay and an antigen capture immunoassay (ELISA) of HIV-1 p24 in culture supernates (748).

The results of the pilot study needed to be confirmed and extended with a relatively large number of volunteers. In addition, it was important to know if small amounts of alcohol (e.g., 1–2 beers) would have the same degree of adverse effect as an alcohol binge, so I designed an experiment and recruited 60 volunteers. The pilot experiment was confirmed with this large group of volunteers. Each volunteer was placed into a group based on total 2-day consumption of alcoholic beverages as follows:

Light	1–2 beers or equivalent
Moderate	3–6 beers or equivalent
Heavy	7 or more beers or equivalent

Each volunteer was advised to completely abstain from drinking any form of alcoholic beverage (and each person was tested by a sensitive biological assay to make sure that they complied). PBMCs from each volunteer were isolated before they were allowed to drink alcohol and then 12–15 h after alcohol ingestion. All PBMC specimens were coded, and assays were performed in a double-blinded manner. The specimens were tested for HIV-1 replication after culturing the donor PBMCs with cell-free virus in $TCID_5$ and $TCID_{50}$ doses of HIV-1, and we measured the ability of the cells to induce syncytium formation on overnight incubation with SUP-T_1 cells after 20 days of culture and for the production of HIV-1 p24 in culture supernate, on days 10,15, and 20.

Significant generation of syncytium-forming cells occurred only on incubation with the higher dose of virus ($TCID_{50}$). As shown in Figure 15, syncytia were generated in this system by only 3 of the 60 subjects prior to alcohol ingestion and then only 1–7 syncytia per well. This was consistent with previous assumptions that infection of CD4+ T cells with HIV-1 requires activation by mitogens, antigens, and other agents. On the other hand, syncytia were recorded in the PBMCs of 56 of 60 subjects with ingestion of alcoholic beverages, even those consuming less than 3 beers or the equivalent in 2 evenings. The difference between pre- and post-alcohol specimens was highly significant (P<0.001).

The degree of HIV replication in PBMCs infected with $TCID_{50}$ of HIV-1 was indicated by HIV-1 p24 levels in culture supernates after 10, 13, and 20 days of culture (Figure 15). Even after 10 days of culture, there was significant replication of HIV-1 in the cultures established after ingestion of alcoholic beverages. After 20 days of culture there was also very significant HIV replication in cultures established from PBMCs taken after alcohol ingestion. No syncytia were observed in cultures infected with the $TCID_5$ dose of HIV-1 (low dose), due to the apparent insufficiency of the infective viral dose or

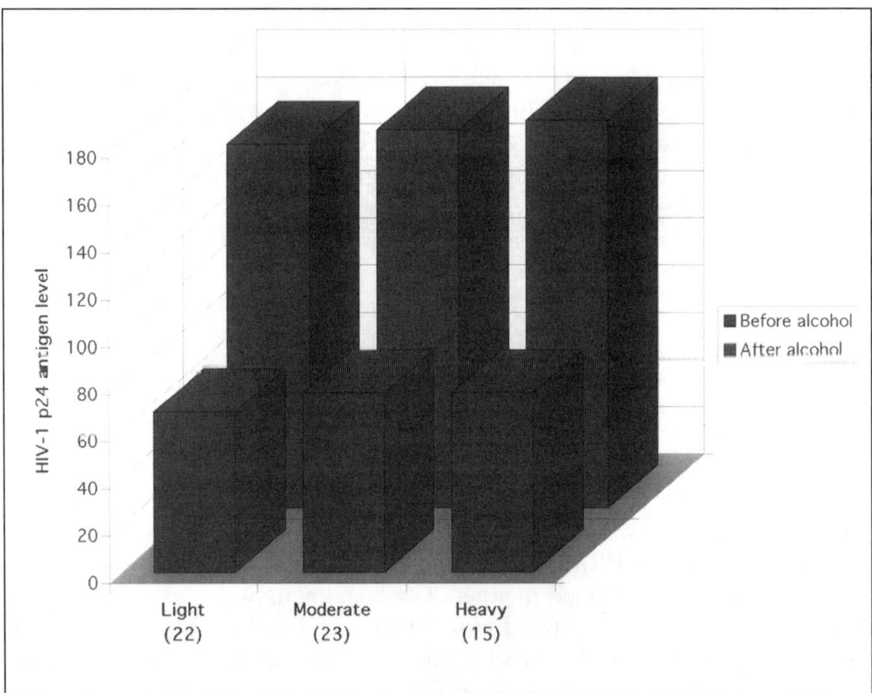

Figure 15. HIV-1 replication in PBMCs isolated from 60 individuals who ingested alcohol, compared to their own PBMCs before they ingested alcohol. PBMCs were cultured for 20 days after HIV-1 infection with tissue culture infectious doses ($TCID_{50}$) of HIV-1.

activation of intracellular molecular immunity. No correlation was evident in the post-alcohol cultures between the amount of p24 produced and the numbers of syncytia generated. A significant increase in HIV-1 p24 antigen levels were observed in PBMCs infected with the $TCID_5$ of HIV-1 dose (Figure 16). Significant reduction in the ability of CD4+ T cells and CD8+ T cells to secrete IL-2 and SIRS, respectively, was also recorded. No significant reduction in the pre- and post-alcohol PBMCs was observed with regard to γ-interferon production (Figure 17).

Our studies showed that alcohol ingestion significantly increases HIV-1 replication in PBMCs isolated from 60 volunteers who drank various amounts of alcohol. Further studies were necessary to determine whether the increased replication of HIV-1 observed after alcohol ingestion was due to unknown factors released from the GI tract during alcohol ingestion or by certain metabolites produced by intestinal flora that degrade alcohol. In addition, cellular mechanisms involved in the increased replication of HIV-1 after alcohol exposure also needed to be evaluated. For this purpose, 12 healthy, HIV-1-seronegative individuals were recruited. All individuals with a history of chronic alcoholism, smoking, substance abuse, any active

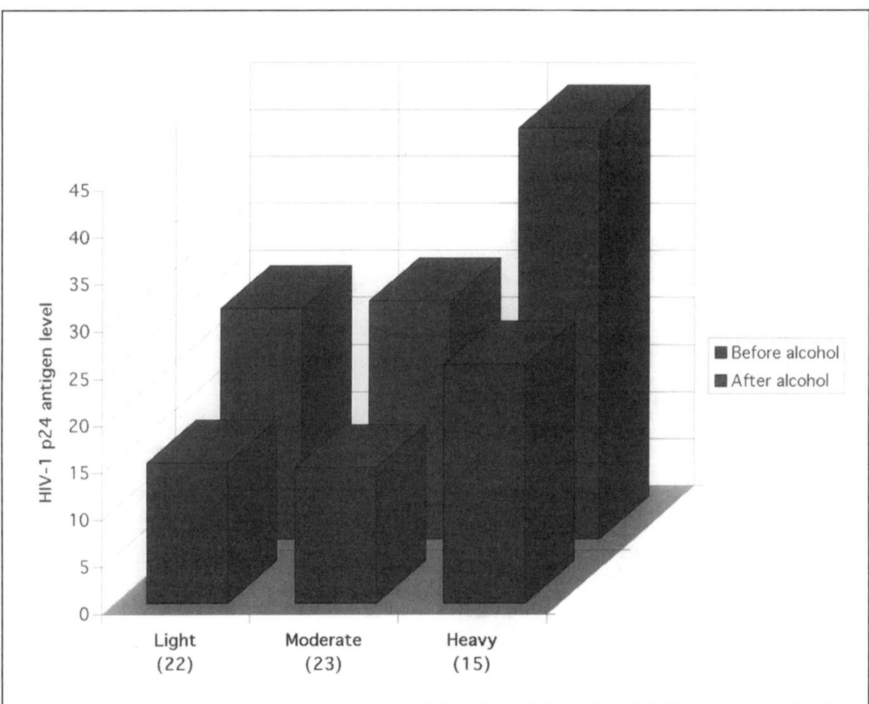

Figure 16. HIV-1 replication in PBMCs isolated from 60 individuals who ingested alcohol, compared to their own PBMCs before they ingested alcohol. PBMCs were cultured for 20 days after HIV-1 infection with $TCID_5$ (LD_5) of HIV-1.

autoimmune disease, diabetes mellitus (both type I and type II), amyl nitrite use, and known recent viral infection were excluded from the studies. Any individuals being treated with anti-inflammatory medications were also excluded from participation in the studies. All volunteers were serologically negative for HIV-1 infection, as evaluated by HIV-1 antibody ELISAs. None were heavy users of alcohol. The subjects were asked to abstain from alcoholic beverages for at least 10 days prior to the study. They were then admitted to the Clinical Research Center overnight. Venous catheters were placed in both arms, one for infusion and one for periodic blood samples. Twenty milliliters of blood were drawn at -30, +30, +60, and +120 min, and 24, 48, 72, and 120 h. After the first day, all the blood samples were drawn between 8:00 and 9:00 AM, so the effects of circadian rhythms, corticosteroids, and other unknown factors on the immune system could be reduced.

Nine individuals were infused with 500 mg/kg ethanol (7.5% at 20 mL/kg/h) in saline for 30 min, and 3 were infused with saline alone. Blood specimens were presented to the Retrovirology Laboratories in a blinded fashion. PBMCs were separated on Ficoll®/metrozoate (Amersham Pharmacia Biotech, Piscataway, NJ, USA). All PBMC specimens were divided into 6 aliquots, coded, and frozen at -70°C (in 50% fetal calf serum, 10% dimethyl sulfoxide). Specimens (both pre-ethanol and post-ethanol) were thawed after

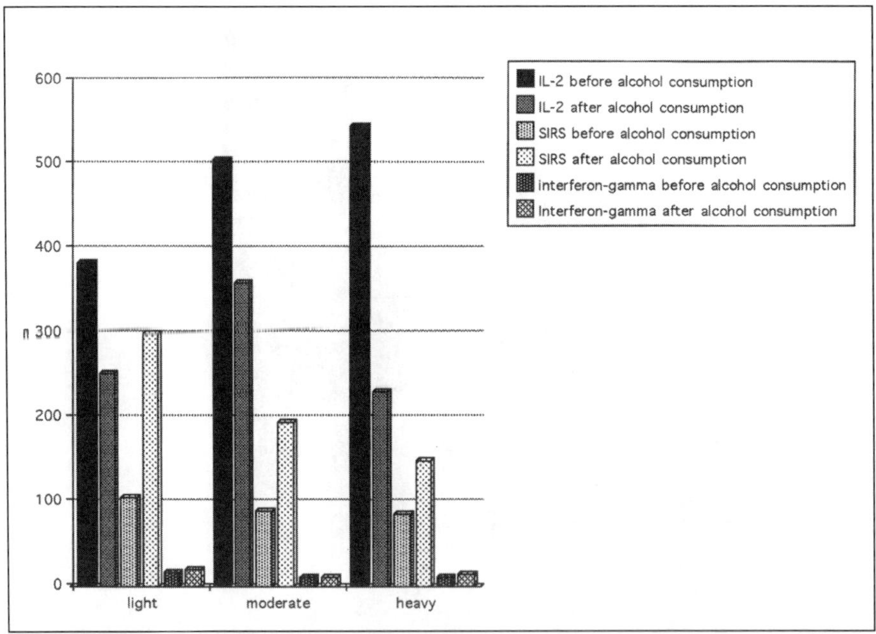

Figure 17. Effect of alcohol ingestion on T-cell functions in absence of HIV-1 infection: both IL-2 and SIRS were measured by functional and ELISA assays. Significantly less IL-2 was secreted after alcohol consumption than before. Similarly, SIRS was significantly less after alcohol ingestion than before.

Table 1. Ethanol Levels (wt/vol) in the Volunteers' Plasma Measured at 30 Min Before and at Various Points After Ethanol Infusion

Time	S1	S2	S3	S4	S5	S6	S7	S8	S9
-0.5	0	0	0	0	0	0	0	0	0
0.5	0.028	0.074	0.097	0.075	0.067	0.091	0.094	0.063	0.050
1	0.012	0.055	0.043	0.057	0.047	0.067	0.066	0.064	0.045
2	0.011	0.030	0.017	0.035	0.038	0.050	0.038	0.029	0.023
24	0.007	0.006	0	0	0	0.007	0.001	0	0
48	0.001	0.001	0	0	0	0	0	0	0

Three control, saline-infused subjects (not shown) demonstrated no detectable ethanol levels in the plasma.

S1–S9: ethanol-infused subjects.

Patients at 72–120 h post-infusion (not shown) demonstrated no detectable ethanol levels in the plasma.

6 weeks, so that assays could be performed in a batch and in a random and blinded manner. All PBMCs were resuspended at a concentration of 10^6 cells/mL in RPMI-1640 medium supplemented with 100 U/mL penicillin, 100 mg/mL streptomycin, 20 mM L-glutamine and 15% heat-inactivated fetal calf serum [tissue culture media (TCM); Life Technologies, Gaithersburg, MD, USA]. Cell viability after thawing was >85%. There were no significant differences in the viabilities of PBMCs from ethanol-infused versus saline-infused individuals. Cultures for HIV-1 replication and for production of IL-1, IL-2, IFN-γ, TNF-α, and GM-CSF were set up within 2–3 h after the cells were thawed. All incubations were performed at 37°C in 5% CO_2 and 95% air. All the HIV-1 replication assays were performed on the same day.

Plasma from each specimen was used to measure plasma ethanol levels, utilizing the Sigma alcohol diagnostic kit (Sigma Chemical, St. Louis, MO, USA). This kit is an alcohol dehydrogenase (ADH)-based color development system. ADH converts ethanol to acetaldehyde in the presence of NADH, which is trapped at pH 9.0. The plasma ethanol concentrations in all 12 individuals were unmeasurable in the specimens obtained 30 min before the infusions of ethanol. In all specimens obtained at each time period after 48 h post-infusion, ethanol concentrations were below detection levels, indicating that none of the controls had any further exposure to ethanol during the course of the studies (see Table 1).

Infusion of ethanol was associated with increased replication of HIV-1 in the PBMCs infected in vitro, as determined by HIV-1 p24 antigen ELISAs of the supernatants of cultures that had been incubated for 13 days post-infection with $TCID_{50}$ of HIV-1. HIV-1 p24 antigen levels were significantly higher in the PBMC cultures of all individuals infused with ethanol compared to controls (Figure 18; *P*<0.001). There were individual variations in the levels of HIV-1 p24 antigen in cultures infected with the same $TCID_{50}$ dose of HIV-1 virions. Our laboratory and others have previously reported these variations (835). Increased levels of HIV-1 p24 antigen expression began to appear in the PBMC cultures 30 min after the infusion of ethanol (152%) and peaked 2 h post-infusion (207%). Nevertheless, the differences in HIV-1 replication between pre- and post-ethanol specimens were highly significant (*P*<0.001) throughout the entire course of the studies (6 days).

Influence of CD8+ T Cells on HIV-1 Replication in PBMCs

PBMCs of one aliquot, from each specimen, were depleted of CD8+ T cells by 2 cycles of panning, as previously described (833). Briefly, PBMCs were incubated with a monoclonal anti-CD8 antibody, then panned on goat anti-mouse immunoglobulin-coated 96-well culture plates at 4°C. The CD8+ lymphocytes remained adherent, and the easily resuspended cells were used as the test population. Control cells for these experiments were the same

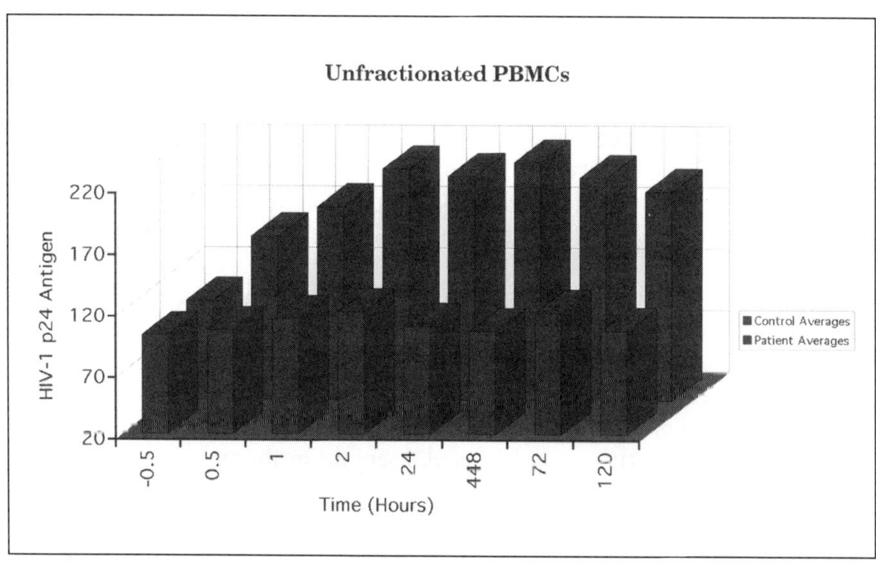

Figure 18. HIV-1 replication in PBMCs isolated from 9 individuals infused with ethanol, compared to 3 controls infused with normal saline. PBMCs were isolated before infusions and then at various time intervals after ethanol or saline infusion, up to 6 days. PBMCs were infected with cell-free HIV-1. On day 13, supernatants were harvested for HIV-1 p24 antigen assays. Mean values of HIV-1 p24 antigen levels of the 3 controls and the 9 ethanol-infused individuals are shown, at various time points of PBMC isolation. The data are expressed as percentages of controls, where HIV-1 p24 antigen levels at baseline (-30 min before infusion) from each individual are compared with the subsequent HIV-1 p24 antigen levels. The following formula was used to express % of control: % of control = mean HIV-1 p24 antigen levels (pg/mL) at a time point post-infusion / mean HIV-1 p24 antigen level (pg/mL) at -30 min (baseline level) × 100. Standard deviations within the replicate wells for each experimental variable were less than 10%.

PBMC populations panned in the above manner, without prior incubation with the anti-CD8 antibody. Adherence of mononuclear phagocytes was minimal at 4°C. The degree of depletion of CD8+ T cells was measured by fluorescence-activated cell sorting (FACS) analysis. After 2 cycles of panning, lymphocyte preparations contained less than 2% CD8+ T cells.

The depleted cell populations were cultured with HIV-1 for 13 days, in parallel with the unfractionated PBMCs, and HIV-1 p24 antigen levels were compared. As shown in Figure 19, the removal of CD8+ T cells from the PBMCs resulted in significant increases in HIV-1 p24 antigen levels ($P<0.001$), in all 12 subjects when compared to unfractionated PBMCs. When HIV-1 p24 antigen levels were compared to saline-infused and ethanol-infused PBMCs after CD8+ T-cell depletion, there was no significant difference in the average increase in the HIV-1 p24 antigen levels between these 2 groups. The percent increase in the HIV-1 p24 antigen levels ranged from 122%–276% compared to unfractionated PBMCs. Nevertheless, at 2 time points (2 h and 48 h), there was a significant difference ($P<0.05$) between the saline-infused and the ethanol-infused subjects (Figure 19). This may be secondary to alterations in cytokine profiles induced by ethanol (see

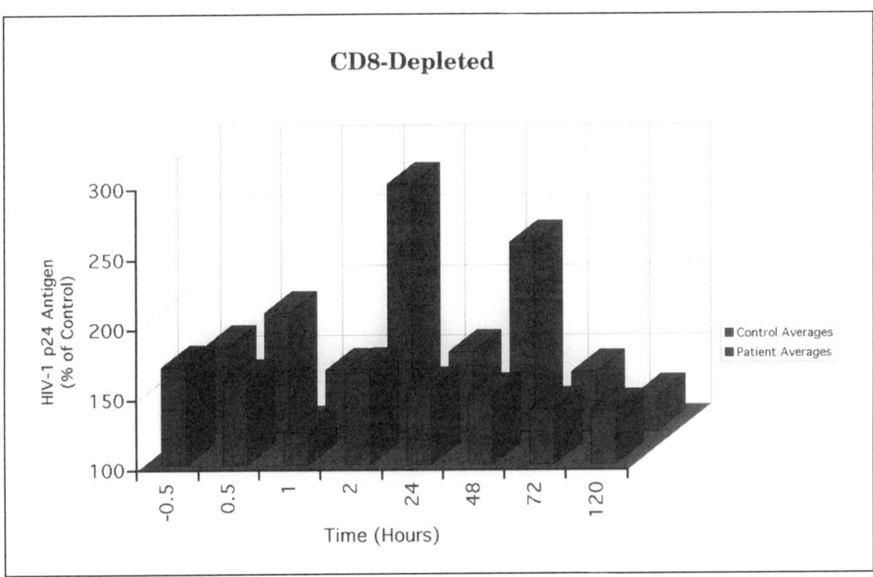

Figure 19. Increased HIV-1 replication after CD8+ T-cell depletion. PBMCs from the 12 HIV-1-seronegative volunteers were cultured for 13 days as described in Figure 18 above, except CD8+ T cells were depleted by panning with an anti-CD8 monoclonal antibody. Supernatants were analyzed for HIV-1 p24 antigen levels. Mean values of HIV-1 p24 antigen levels of 3 saline-infused controls and 9 ethanol-infused individuals, at various times of PBMCs isolation, are illustrated. The data are expressed as % of controls, where HIV-1 p24 antigen levels (pg/mL) at all points were compared to HIV-1 p24 antigen levels at the corresponding baseline HIV-1 p24 antigen levels. The % of control for each time point was calculated according to the formula described in Figure 18 above. Standard deviations within the replicate wells for each experimental variable were less than 10%.

below). These findings may indicate that some portion of the observed increase in HIV-1 replication, after ethanol infusion, may primarily be the result of the effects of ethanol on CD8+ T-cell functions, and part of this effect may be secondary to alterations in the expression of certain cytokines.

Reconstitution with Allogeneic or Autologous CD8+ T Cells Results in Resistance to HIV-1 Replication

In another series of experiments, PBMCs from each of the 12 individuals were depleted of CD8+ T cells 24 h prior to the HIV-1 replication assay, as described below. CD8+ T cells, panned with the anti-CD8 monoclonal antibody in 96-well plates, were harvested by incubating in 2% lidocaine diluted in phosphate-buffered saline for 10 min. These CD8+ T cells were cultured in TCM containing 40 U/mL of IL-2 for 24 h. The CD8+ T cells were divided into 2 equal portions. One portion was used for the reconstitution of corresponding CD8+ T-cell depleted (autologous) cultures, whereas other portions were mixed together and used in the allogeneic reconstitution experiments. Therefore, each CD8+ T-cell depleted PBMC culture was reconstituted with approximately equal numbers (1×10^4) of autologous or allogeneic CD8+ T cells. These cells were then cultured for 13 days, prior to measurement of HIV-1 replication.

To evaluate if CD8+ T-cell-depleted PBMCs could acquire resistance to HIV-1 replication after reconstitution with allogeneic CD8+ T cells, CD8+ T cells were added back to 24 h cultures of these cells. As shown in Figure 20A, the reconstitution with allogeneic CD8+ T cells, 24 h after the CD8+ T-cell-depleted cultures were exposed to HIV-1, resulted in a significant decrease in HIV-1 production (P<0.001) compared to the unfractionated PBMCs. The reduction in HIV-1 replication ranged from 29%–57% of the corresponding unfractionated (control) values. After reconstitution with allogeneic CD8+ T cells, the reduction of HIV-1 production in the PBMCs of saline-infused individuals was significantly greater (P<0.05; ranging from 29%–46% of unfractionated PBMC values), compared to PBMCs from ethanol-infused subjects (ranging from 44%–57%). This reduced capacity of allogeneic CD8+ T cells to reconstitute anti-HIV-1 activity was most probably due to the ethanol exposure of these cells in vivo, but may be at least partly due to confounding factors from mixed lymphocyte reactions resulting from combining lymphocytes from various individuals.

As shown in Figure 20B, the reconstitution with autologous CD8+ T cells of each control individual's cultures resulted in a significant reduction in HIV-1 replication, ranging from 22% to 46%, as compared to unfractionated PBMCs from the corresponding saline-infused subjects (P<0.003), whereas CD8+ T cells reconstituted to the corresponding autologous culture wells from ethanol-infused PBMCs did not exhibit a significant inhibition of HIV-1 replication for up to 2 h (ranging from 75% to 128% of the unfractionated

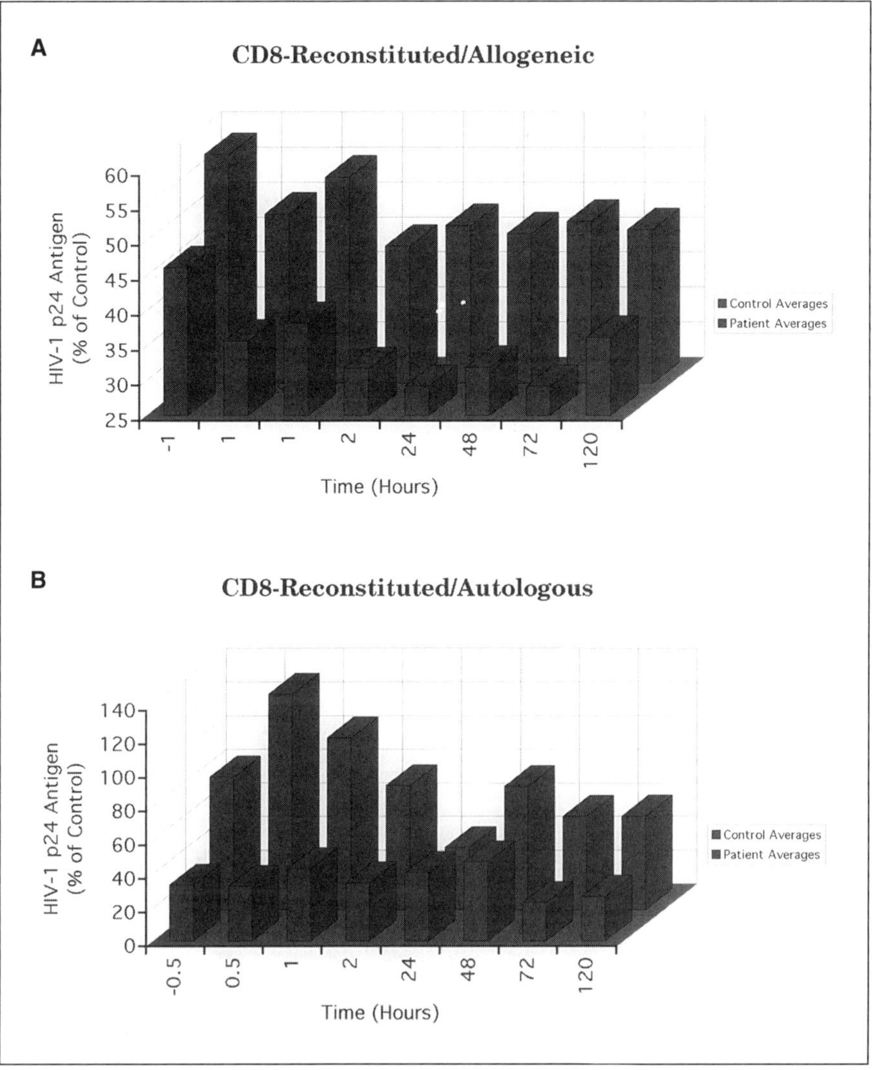

Figure 20. Decreased replication of HIV-1 in cultures reconstituted with allogeneic and autologous CD8+ T cells. PBMCs from 12 HIV-1-seronegative volunteers were cultured for 13 days, as described in Figure 18. CD8+ T cells were cultured in 96-well plates in the presence of tissue culture media containing 40 U/mL of IL-2 for 24 h. One-half of the CD8+ T cells were used for the reconstitution of corresponding CD8+ T cell-depleted (autologous) cultures, whereas the other half was mixed together and used in the allogeneic reconstitution experiments. Therefore, each PBMC CD8+ T-cell-depleted culture was reconstituted with approximately equal numbers of autologous or allogeneic CD8+ T cells (1×10^4 cells/well). These cells were then cultured for 13 days, prior to measurement of HIV-1 replication. Mean values of HIV-1–p24 antigen levels of 3 saline-infused controls and 9 ethanol-infused individuals, at various times of PBMCs isolation, are illustrated. (A) Allogeneic reconstitutions; (B) Autologous reconstitutions. The data are expressed as % of controls. The mean HIV-1 p24 antigen levels at each time point in the saline- or ethanol-infused groups were compared against HIV-1 p24 antigen levels at the corresponding time point in the unfractionated PBMCs, by modification of the formula described in Figure 18. Standard deviations within the replicate wells for each experimental variable were less than 10%.

PBMC control values). In these cultures, HIV-1 p24 antigen levels were somewhat higher than the unfractionated PBMC control levels (128% at 30 min and 102% at 1 h after the ethanol infusion). However, the capacity of CD8+ T cells to reduce HIV-1 p24 antigen levels after autologous CD8+ T-cell reconstitutions appeared to have markedly recovered in samples harvested 24 h after ethanol infusion. These data further support the hypothesis that the ethanol effects on HIV-1 replication are tied to alterations in CD8 cellular function.

The recovery of CD8+ T-cell function 24 h after ethanol infusion may be due to the presence of ethanol or its metabolites in the blood circulation up to 24 h. Ethanol increases intracellular NADH (27). Ethanol-induced membrane perturbations may also influence the optimal functions of various PBMCs, including CD8+ T cells and monocytes. The ability of CD8+ T cells to communicate with other cells, respond to other cells' signals, and exert their influence is mainly dependent on the proper fluidity of the plasma membrane. Ethanol exposure has been reported to change the plasma membrane tolerance to fluidation. It is conceivable that such a change would affect the transmembrane signaling of the CD8+ T cells. This possibility is under investigation in our laboratories. Further evidence for the influence of ethanol or its metabolites comes from the depressed cytokine production in ethanol-infused individuals and the recovery of such cytokines 24 h after the infusion (described below). It is interesting that both autologous and allogeneic CD8+ T cells reconstituted the resistence of PBMCs against HIV-1, suggesting that a common, non-MHC related factor(s) is in operation against HIV-1. As I have suggested, an RNA-based anti-HIV-1 effect can explain such a broad, non-MHC effect.

Effect of Ethanol Infusion on T-Cell and Monocyte Functions in the Absence of HIV-1 Infection

Cytokines play a pivotal role in the regulation and development of the immune system. Both HIV-1 infection and ethanol consumption have been shown to influence cytokine production and immune functions. As such, various arms of the immune system are reported to be affected by retroviral infections and by ethanol exposure. Since CD4+ T cells and monocytes are considered to be the main targets of HIV-1 infection in vivo, it was pertinent to explore the functional parameters of these 2 cell populations, by evaluating their capacity to produce various cytokines after ethanol exposure in vivo. There was a significant (P<0.001) decrease in the in vitro production of IL-2 by PBMCs after infusion with ethanol. The decrease was most pronounced at 1 h after ethanol infusion (27% of pre-ethanol infusion control), but remained below the control levels throughout the course of the studies (6 days). There were similar significant decreases in the production of TNF-α and IL-1 after ethanol infusion, which were approximately one-third that of the control values, for up to 24 h after ethanol infusion. The production of IFN-γ exhibited a significant reduction up to 1 h after the infusion of ethanol, but the levels promptly reached the pre-ethanol infusion levels thereafter. There was no significant difference in the levels of immunoreactive GM-CSF, between pre- and post-ethanol infusion groups (Figure 21).

It appears that the more adverse effects of ethanol, with regard to cytokine production, last about 24 h after ethanol exposure in vivo. The production of 3 cytokines, IL-1, IL-2 and TNF-α, are the most significantly altered. The recovery phase may be a function of intracellular metabolism of ethanol or cellular replacement by the bone marrow. It is instructive to note that the functional capacity of CD8+ T cells in the autologous reconstitution experiments also exhibited recovery 24 h after ethanol exposure.

In conclusion, our studies have suggested that a single episode of alcohol consumption, in amounts that frequently occur during social drinking, influences HIV-1 infection of PBMCs in vitro. A parallel depression in functions attributed to both helper and suppressor T cells was also demonstrated. Beer was the primary beverage consumed, but the fact that the same abnormalities were observed in the many study subjects who ingested most of their ethanol as wine, whiskey, vodka, and other alcoholic beverages made it less likely that the these effects were caused by some component of beer, other than ethanol. However, there was a formal possibility that the effects observed were the result of intestinal factors released during alcohol consumption and absorption. This prompted us to extend the previous studies by utilizing direct intravenous infusions of pure ethanol, which is the subject of the present investigation. In addition, the mechanisms of ethanol-induced increased HIV-1 replication were evaluated, by exploring the effects of ethanol on CD8+ T cells and cytokine expression.

The increased production of HIV-1 p24 antigen after ethanol infusion in the unfractionated PBMCs confirms our previous conclusion that HIV-1 replication in cell cultures can be significantly augmented after exposure to ethanol in vivo. These data demonstrate that ethanol itself, rather than other compounds within alcoholic drinks, led to these alterations in HIV-1 expression. This might be a direct effect on the circulating target cells for HIV-1 or be secondary to an ethanol-altered release of cytokines from those cells. Of note, ethanol does not lead to an acute alteration in absolute levels of CD4+ or CD8+ T cells in vivo. A significant portion of the increased HIV-1 p24 antigen levels, in the cultures of PBMCs isolated from post-ethanol infusion subjects, appears to be due to the effect of ethanol on CD8+ T cells.

It appears that normally functioning CD8+ T cells are very important in resisting an initial HIV-1 infection or maintenance of asymptomatic states in individuals already exposed to HIV-1. In recent years, information has accumulated that suggests an increased viral load in adult HIV-1-seropositive patients correlates with CD4+ T-cell depletion and disease progression (836). The viral and CD4+ T-cell kinetics reported by Wei et al. (462) demonstrated that, a few months after initial exposure to HIV-1 when the early viremic

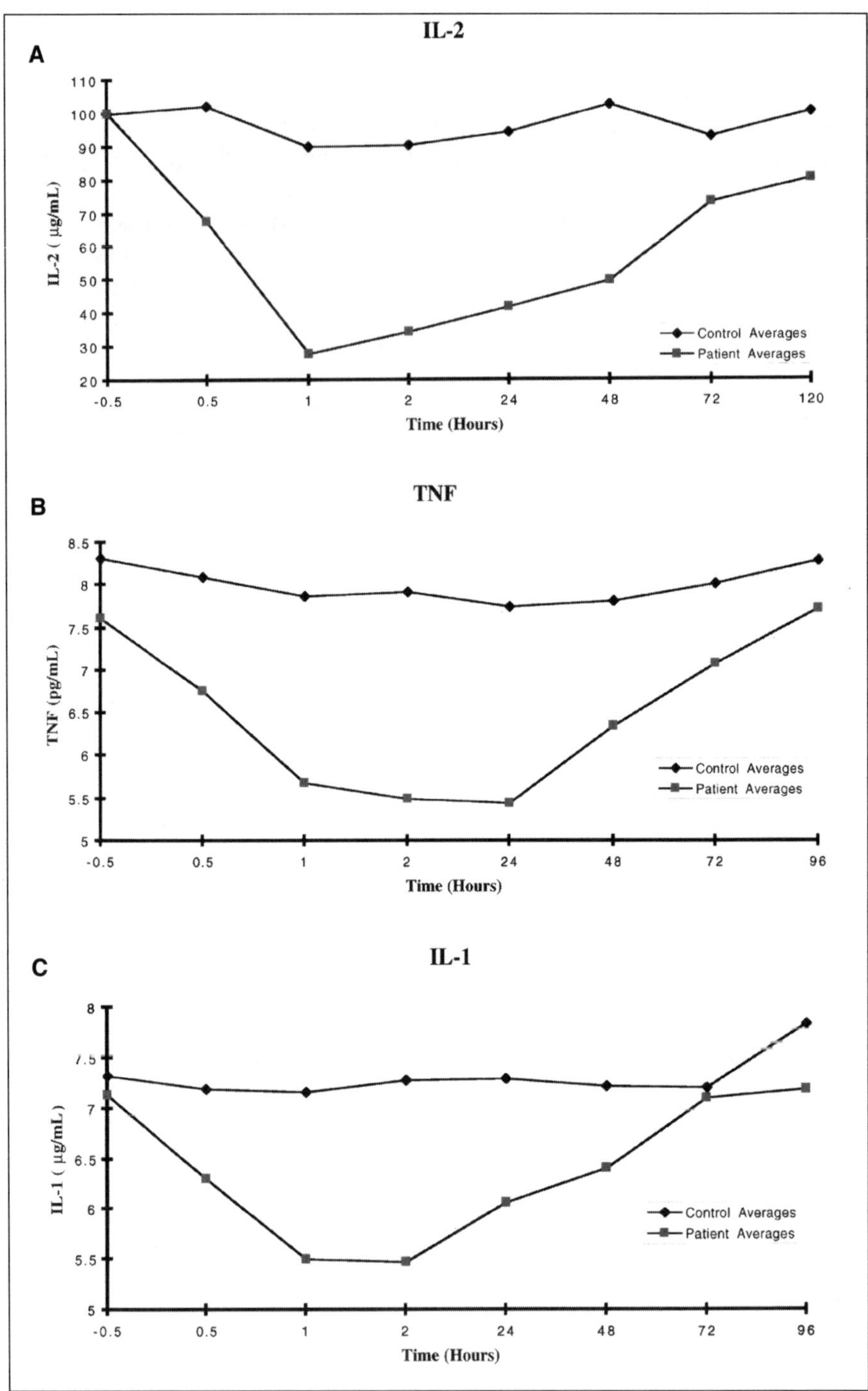

Figure 21. See legend on next page.

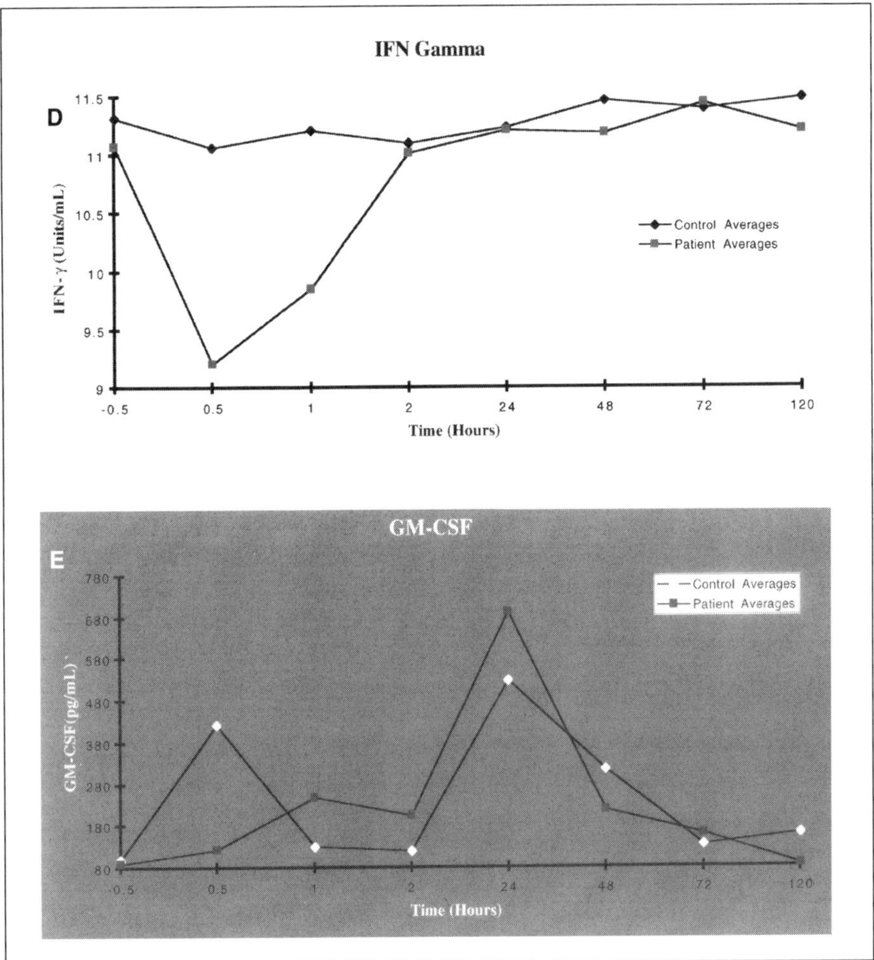

Figure 21. Alterations of cytokine expression by ethanol. (A) IL-2 levels in 48 h supernatants of Con A-stimulated PBMCs. IL-2 levels are illustrated as the concentrations of IL-2 measured by ELISA. The stimulation induced by Con A in the PBMCs was measured in the supernatants obtained from cultures of PBMCs harvested prior to infusion of ethanol and at various time periods thereafter. These were compared to the parallel samples from control subjects (saline-infused). The mean stimulation indices for the ethanol-infused and saline-infused subjects are illustrated. (B) TNF-α and (C) IL-1 levels in 72 h supernatants of PMA-stimulated PBMC. These cytokines levels are shown as the quantity of each cytokine secreted by the PBMC cultures obtained from each experimental variable, as described above. The stimulation induced by supernatants obtained from cultures of PBMCs harvested prior to infusion of ethanol and at various time periods thereafter is compared to the parallel PMA-induced stimulated cultures (saline-infused controls). The mean stimulation indices for the ethanol-infused and saline-infused subjects are illustrated. (D) IFN-γ levels in 72 h supernatants of Con A-stimulated PBMCs. IFN-γ levels are shown as the quantity of cytokine secreted by the PBMC cultures, obtained for each experimental variable. The stimulation induced by supernatants obtained from cultures of PBMC, harvested prior to infusion of ethanol, and various time periods thereafter, is compared to the parallel harvested PBMCs from saline-infused control subjects. The mean stimulation indices for the ethanol-infused and saline-infused subjects are illustrated. (E) GM-CSF levels in 72 h supernatants of Con A-stimulated PBMC. GM-CSF levels are shown as the quantity measured by ELISA. The mean stimulation indices for the ethanol-infused and saline-infused subjects are illustrated. Standard deviations within replicate wells were less than 10%.

phase has passed and a so-called long, clinically latent phase has started, this is not a period of viral inactivity [as was suggested by Baltimore's group (456, 478–479)], but an active process in which significant numbers of CD4+ T cells are being killed by HIV-1 infection, and a measurable number of virions are produced in both progressors and LTNPs. These processes of infection, cell death, and replacement of dead cells lead to an equilibrium. Wei et al. (462) demonstrated that the mean CD4+ T-cell turnover rate in HIV-1-infected individuals was 1.8×10^9 cells per day, whereas the half-life for HIV-1 virions (mean half-life) was 1.3–3.3 days. This study indicated a rapid turnover of CD4+ T cells and plasma virions in adult HIV-1-seropositive individuals with progressive HIV-1 infection, which again points toward the basic hypothesis I have proposed, i.e., if individuals are exposed to high doses of HIV-1 initially, it is difficult for the natural molecular immunity to keep pace with the increasing viral production. However, it appears that if someone has consumed alcohol just before exposure to HIV-1 (by digestive or intravenous route), and the molecular immunity is even transiently compromised, the threshold of virus that can cause disease rather than induce protection is changed in favor of HIV-1. Therefore, in order to prevent the development of AIDS or prolong the asymptomatic phase, all measures should be taken to foster the protective arms of the immune system.

In contrast to patients who are progressive, the LTNPs also show certain levels of HIV-1 viral load but much less (one-tenth) than their progressive counterparts. This supports the hypotheses that in the majority of the cells of LTNPs, HIV-1 is blocked at the preintegration level (451, 455–458), and a minority of their cells are producing virus. In these individuals in whom the amount of virus produced is low, the number of cells being killed is also significantly very low.

In this series of experiments we have demonstrated that the modified susceptibility of PBMCs to infection with HIV-1, observed after ethanol infusion, is associated with concomitant deficiencies in CD8+ T-cell functions, as well as in T-helper and monocyte/macrophage functions. In studies discussed earlier, we analyzed the percentage of PBMC subpopulations, including CD4+, CD8+, and B lymphocytes plus monocytes, which demonstrated significant alterations in ethanol-exposed versus saline-exposed control groups. Although not proven, the data from our studies and other investigations (described earlier) suggest that these associations may be causally related. Keeping in mind the data regarding the anti-HIV-1 effects of CD8+ T cells and the overwhelming evidence that ethanol consumption alters the immune system, our studies stressed the evaluation of the effects of ethanol infusion on T lymphocytes and specifically on CD8+ T cells. Together, these observations suggest that CD8+ T cells in the HIV-1-infected, healthy individual provide protection against further spread of HIV-1 to CD4+ T cells and/or monocytes, and ethanol potentially interferes with one or more of the CD8+ T-cell-mediated protective mechanisms. This might adversely alter the natural protective balance between the host's anti-retroviral capabilities and HIV-1's degree of virulence. These data suggest that exogenous agents may alter HIV-1 replication in vivo. As such, various environmental stimuli may affect the natural history of HIV-1 infections (59–60). In addition, our studies in which we infused ethanol are unique because they eliminate the role of condiments and nonalcoholic components of alcoholic beverages in inducing adverse effects on the immune system.

Between the time of HIV-1 seroconversion and the development of early stages of AIDS, there is a considerable asymptomatic period. As mentioned above (462), this represents an equilibrium phase in which a degree of virally induced CD4+ T-cell destruction is balanced with cell replacement. This equilibrium phase may vary from 3 to 10 years; 10%–25% of HIV-1-infected individuals will develop AIDS-defining illnesses by 4 years, 30%–40% by 8 years, and 35%–50% in 10 years. One of the potential outcomes of ethanol use during HIV-1 infection might be that the so-called clinically silent or latent phase of the disease would be reduced. A large retrospective/prospective study by the Multicenter AIDS Cohort Study followed 1706 homosexual men who were seropositive for HIV-1 and who were free of AIDS-defining illnesses at the time of entry (831). A questionnaire was given to these subjects at the beginning of the study and at monthly intervals regarding their alcohol consumption habits. The study showed that the latent period was not shortened by the use of alcohol: the percentages of HIV-1-seropositive men who developed clinical, symptomatic AIDS during the first 18 months of enrollment into the study were 9.2% for abstainers and 6.7% for those who were heavy drinkers before being admitted into the study (more than 2 drinks per day). Continuing the use of greater amounts of alcohol was not associated with a higher than 18-month risk of AIDS. Actually, among HIV-1-seropositive men, heavier alcohol consumption was associated with a lower prevalence of persistent generalized lymphadenopathy ($P = 0.01$). However, some limitations of this study may detract from the importance of its conclusions. Because it may take up to 10 years for 50% of HIV-1 infected individuals to develop AIDS, a study with an end point of 18 months may not show what would happen if the subjects were followed for a much longer time. The lower prevalence of generalized adenopathy found in heavy drinkers in this study could also be interpreted as a worsening of the prognosis for these patients. It could represent the lymphoid depletion that heralds the onset of symptomatic AIDS (1,567,573–580).

Our studies may provide an explanation for the reported high incidence of HIV-1-seropositive individuals in various alcohol treatment programs, and the rapid progression to AIDS after HIV-1 seroconversion in alcoholics (745-747,829,837). These experiments extend our previous findings that exposure to ethanol may influence the initial stages of HIV-1 infection and possibly alter the delicate balance between the host and the virus (HIV-1 infection, cell death, and replacement) in asymptomatic individuals. Ingestion of ethanol may, as well, increase the likelihood of HIV-1 infection of an individual if it occurs prior to or during exposure to HIV-1, for example, at times of high-risk sexual activity.

LINK BETWEEN COCAINE AND HIV-1 INFECTION

The biological effects of substances of abuse, especially their stimulatory effect on the immune system, may significantly contribute to the outcome of an infection. The prevalence of HIV-1 seropositivity among substance abusers is disturbingly high. As reported by Sterk (756), HIV-1 seropositivity among intravenous cocaine abusers was 46%, and of those who used both cocaine and crack intravenously, 84% were HIV-1 seropositive. Similarly, Chaisson et al. (430) reported that intravenous cocaine use significantly increased the risk of HIV-1 infection, with a HIV-1-seroprevalence rate of 35% in daily cocaine users. There is a suggestion that the high prevalence of HIV-1 infection in cocaine abusers may be due to a disinhibiting effect of the abused substance, resulting in increased willingness to participate in high-risk behaviors. However, a possible direct effect of cocaine on the immune system and thus the potential increased susceptibility of the host to HIV-1 infection was first suggested by Ginzburg et al. (838) and Marmor et al. (839), who reported that ever having used cocaine was associated with KS (risk factor, 20.0) in a dose-response manner, in a survey of HIV-1-seropositive homosexual men. Similarly, Bigger et al. (840) found a significant association between cocaine use and a depression of T-helper to T-suppressor lymphocyte ratios. If an effect of cocaine on the immune system is that it enhances an individual's susceptibility to HIV-1 infection, then the dangers of cocaine use multiply significantly. Despite a profound increase in cocaine abuse in recent years, only a few detailed studies regarding the effects of cocaine on the immune system have been conducted (841–843). A growing body of evidence, though, indicates that various substances of abuse, including cocaine, alcohol, and opiates, exhibit immunomodulatory properties and could serve as cofactors in the potentiation of HIV-1 replication.

My laboratory has been conducting studies on the immunomodulatory effects of cocaine and its potential effect on HIV-1 replication. In order to determine the potential immunomodulatory effect of cocaine, we isolated PBMCs from 8 volunteers with no history of cocaine use. The following is a summary of data from my laboratory as well as from numerous other laboratories that demonstrates the adverse effects of cocaine on lymphocyte functions (750).

Replication of HIV-1 in the Presence of Cocaine in Persistently Infected T-Lymphocytic and Monocytoid Cell Lines

In order to determine if cocaine exerts any HIV-1 stimulation in dormant cells carrying HIV-1 in an integrated form, we decided to utilize cell lines that either carry HIV-1 in a latent form or are chronically infected but produce small amounts of HIV-1 in a steady state (called productively infected cell lines). Therefore, we exposed several CD4+ T-lymphocytic cell lines, ACH-2 (latently infected), H9/IIIB and SUP-T_1 (chronically but productively infected with HIV-1 or the monocytoid cell lines), U1 (latently infected), and U937/HIV-1 (chronically productively infected with HIV-1) to 25 mg/mL and 50 mg/mL of cocaine. Such an exposure did not result in significantly higher levels of HIV-1 at 72 h after treatment or up to 10 days post-treatment, as compared to control cultures (Figure 22). Presence of one of the active metabolites of cocaine, benzoylecgonine, at 25 mg/mL and 50 mg/mL, did not lead to increased levels of HIV-1 p24 antigen in the supernatants of these cell lines either. In addition, exposure of these productively and latently HIV-1-infected cell lines to a combination of cocaine (25 mg/mL) and benzoylecgonine (25 mg/mL) did not stimulate HIV-1 replication (data not shown). In our pilot studies conducted in advance of these experiments, we had determined that cell lines used in these experiments were relatively more sensitive to the toxic effects of cocaine than were PBMCs. Therefore, we have shown only the results from the lower concentrations of cocaine for comparative analysis in Figure 23. In the presence of PMA (another mitogen, which ap-

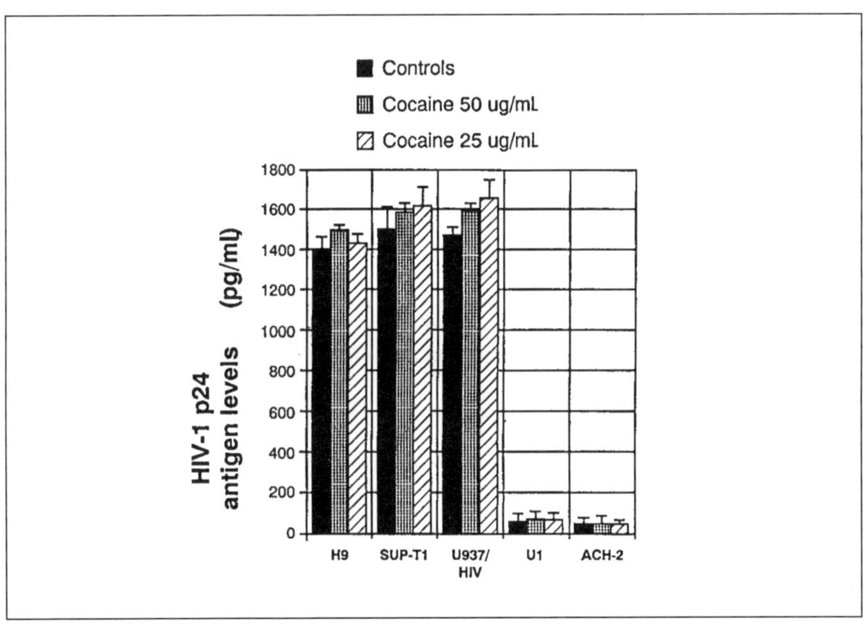

Figure 22. Effect of cocaine on HIV-1 replication in chronically infected cell lines. HIV-1 p24 antigen levels in the supernatants of freshly cultured H9/IIIB, SUP-T1, ACH-2, U1 and U937/HIV-1 cells, harvested after 72 h in the presence of 50 mg/mL and 25 mg/mL of cocaine, are illustrated. HIV-1 p24 antigen levels were assayed by antigen capture ELISA. Mean values for 6 wells per experimental variable are illustrated. Cocaine (50 mg/mL) did not affect viability or proliferation of any cell line evaluated (data not shown). Standard deviations were all less than 10%.

pears to break down molecular immunity; 50 ng/mL), the U1 and ACH-2 cell lines produced significant amounts of HIV-1 p24 antigen. However, the addition of cocaine to PMA-treated cultures did not result in significantly higher levels of HIV-1 p24 antigen. Therefore cells that already have a blocked HIV-1 replication appear nonsensitive to the effect of cocaine (Figure 22).

Susceptibility of PBMCs to Infection with HIV-1 in the Presence of Cocaine

PBMCs from 8 healthy volunteers were exposed to either 50 mg/mL of cocaine, 50 mg/mL of benzoylecgonine, or a combination of cocaine plus benzoylecgonine, in vitro. Twenty-four hours after infection with HIV-1, the PBMCs were washed 3 times with media to remove unbound HIV-1, cocaine, and/or benzoylecgonine. Supernatants from these cultures were collected on the 4th, 7th, and 10th day post-infection, and HIV-1 p24 antigen levels were measured by the ELISA method. As shown in Figure 23, the cumulative data from all 8 individuals indicated that the exposure to cocaine resulted in significantly ($P<0.05$) higher levels of HIV-1 replication in the PBMC cultures by the 10th day post-infection. In 6 out of 8 individuals, levels of HIV-1 p24 antigen after exposure to 50 mg/mL cocaine were augmented from 128% to 280%. The effect of cocaine on HIV-1 replication was significant in subjects A, B, C, and D, with less of an effect in subjects E and F. The cumulative mean HIV-1 p24 antigen levels from the 8 subjects indicated that exposure to

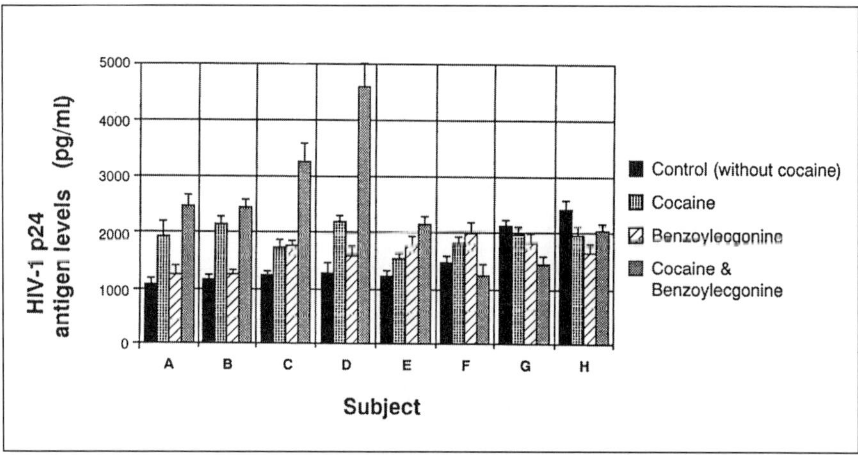

Figure 23. Effect of cocaine and its major metabolite on HIV-1 replication in PBMC, in vitro. HIV-1 p24 antigen levels in the supernatants of PBMC cultures, harvested after 10 days of culture in tissue culture media containing 6 U/mL of rIL-2, were measured as in Figure 22. Mean HIV-1 p24 antigen levels in supernatants of each individual's PBMCs are illustrated. Control PBMCs (black bars) were not exposed to cocaine or its by-product. Striped bars represent PBMCs exposed to cocaine. Diagonal gray bars represent PBMCs exposed to benzoylecgonine and checkered bars represent PBMCs exposed to both cocaine and benzoylecgonine. Standard deviations were all less than 10%.

50 mg/mL of benzoylecgonine led to no significantly increased levels of HIV-1 p24 antigen in the PBMC cultures. However, benzoylecgonine significantly increased HIV-1 p24 antigen production in subjects C, E, and F ($P<0.04$). Also, for individuals C and D, there was a strong synergism noted between cocaine and benzoylecgonine. However, the cumulative mean HIV-1 p24 antigen levels from the 8 individuals indicated that exposure to cocaine and benzoylecgonine led to no significant synergistic activity. These data indicate that exposure to cocaine at the time of HIV-1 infection (early stages) may result in severe consequences as opposed to during the stages in which the individual is already infected. However, since these are in vitro data, the immunostimulatory effect of cocaine and its consequences for later stages of infection cannot be completely ruled out (see below).

As shown in Figure 24, exposure to cocaine also resulted in increased syncytia formation, as compared to untreated cells from the same individual, in the PBMCs of all 8 subjects tested. Thus, a second sensitive measurement of HIV-1 replication documents that cocaine can significantly ($P<0.001$) increase HIV-1 production from unstimulated PBMCs.

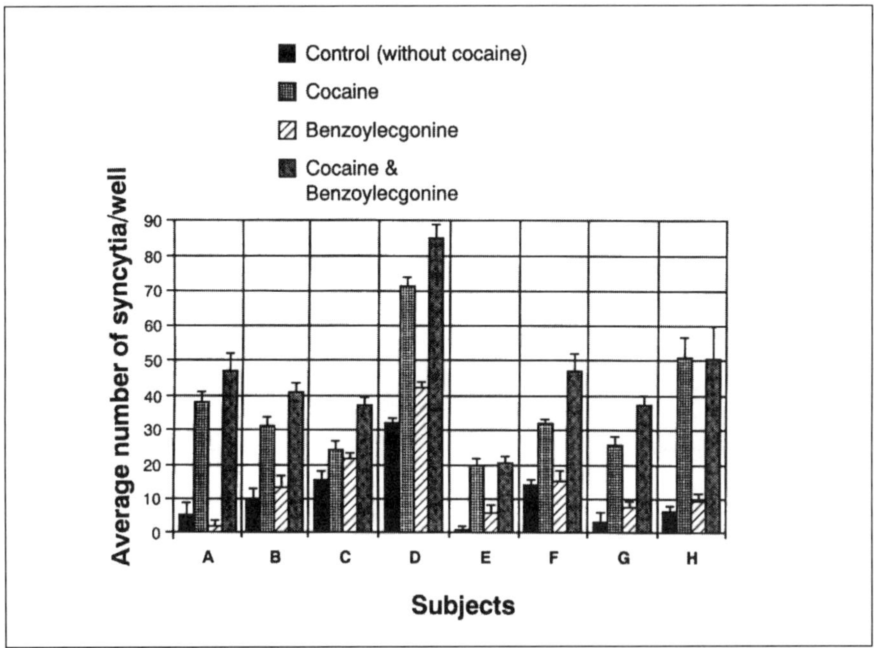

Figure 24. Effect of cocaine and one of its metabolites, benzoylecgonine, on HIV-1-induced syncytia formation in PBMCs in vitro. Overnight syncytia formation, between SUP-T_1 indicator cells and PBMCs, which were exposed to cocaine, benzoylecgonine or their combination and infected with HIV-1 for 10 days, are illustrated. They key to the legend is the same as in Figure 22. Cocaine, benzoylecgonine, or a combination of these agents did not affect PBMC viability (data not shown). Standard deviations were all less than 10%.

Determination of Active HIV-1 Replication by In Situ Hybridization

In order to evaluate the status of HIV-1 replication at a molecular level, we performed in situ hybridization of cultured cells utilizing an HIV-1 *gag* probe. Unstimulated PBMCs, infected with $TCID_{50}$ of HIV-1, exhibited the presence of HIV-1-specific RNA only in 1%–2% of cells. When PBMCs were exposed to cocaine (50 mg/mL) and infected with HIV-1, significantly higher ($P<0.001$) percentages of PBMCs (7%–9%) exhibited evidence of active HIV-1 replication.

In these studies, conducted with PBMCs isolated from 8 healthy HIV-1-seronegative individuals, we demonstrated that exposure to cocaine or its metabolite, at levels usually associated with social cocaine/crack abuse, markedly influences the level of HIV-1 production in PBMCs infected with HIV-1 in vitro (Figures 23 and 24). In all 8 individuals, syncytia formation was significantly increased, and levels of HIV-1 p24 antigen in 6 out of 8 individuals' PBMC culture supernatants indicated significantly higher degrees of HIV-1 replication. The analysis of the PBMCs by in situ hybridization also revealed that a significantly higher percentage of cells in cocaine-exposed PBMC cultures were expressing HIV-1-specific RNA. The maximum augmentation of HIV-1 replication by cocaine, as measured by syncytia formation, was 7-fold higher than that in control PBMC cultures and up to 280% higher by HIV-1 p24 antigen assay. In vitro exposure to the major active by-product of cocaine, benzoylecgonine, resulted in increased levels of HIV-1 production, but cumulative data indicated that it was statistically not significant, even though in 3 out of 8 individuals the HIV-1 p24 antigen levels were markedly increased.

Syncytia formation, the fusion of cells into multinucleated giant cells, is commonly observed in cultures of retroviruses as a cytopathic effect of the infection. In the case of HIV-1, this fusion involves the CD4 molecules of the indicator cells and the gp41/gp120 glycoproteins of HIV-1. Optimal viral replication and syncytia formation, even in the presence of rIL-2, requires other mitogenic or antigenic stimulation of the T lymphocytes, but some HIV-1 replication and transient syncytia formation can occur in normal lymphocytes in the absence of such stimulation. It was under the latter conditions that the assay system was applied in this study. We reasoned that the low levels of baseline cellular activity might allow the assay to be more sensitive to any increased surface expression of gp120/gp41 on infected cells that might be induced by cocaine. In addition, PBMCs not stimulated with PHA might more closely resemble the state of the majority of lymphocytes in vivo. Use of the SUP-T_1 cell line, which expresses a very high density of CD4 molecules on its cell surface and forms large syncytia, is a sensitive assay for measuring cells expressing low densities of HIV-1 gp120/gp41 antigens. Therefore, the syncytia formation assay may represent the precise state of HIV-1-infected PBMCs. The in situ hybridization assay also measures unspliced viral RNA expression and not viral protein expression or virion release.

The molecular mechanism(s) leading to this cocaine-induced effect on HIV-1 replication remains an active area of current investigation in my laboratory (see Figure 25). The increased HIV-1 p24 antigen levels, syncytia formation, and cells actively transcribing viral RNA in the PBMC cultures might be the result of a combination of factors including: *(i)* a direct or co-stimulatory effect of cocaine on the CD4+ lymphocytes, the primary site of HIV-1 replication in this system, or *(ii)* the effect of cocaine on CD8+ T cells, which have been demonstrated to control the replication of HIV-1 in vitro in

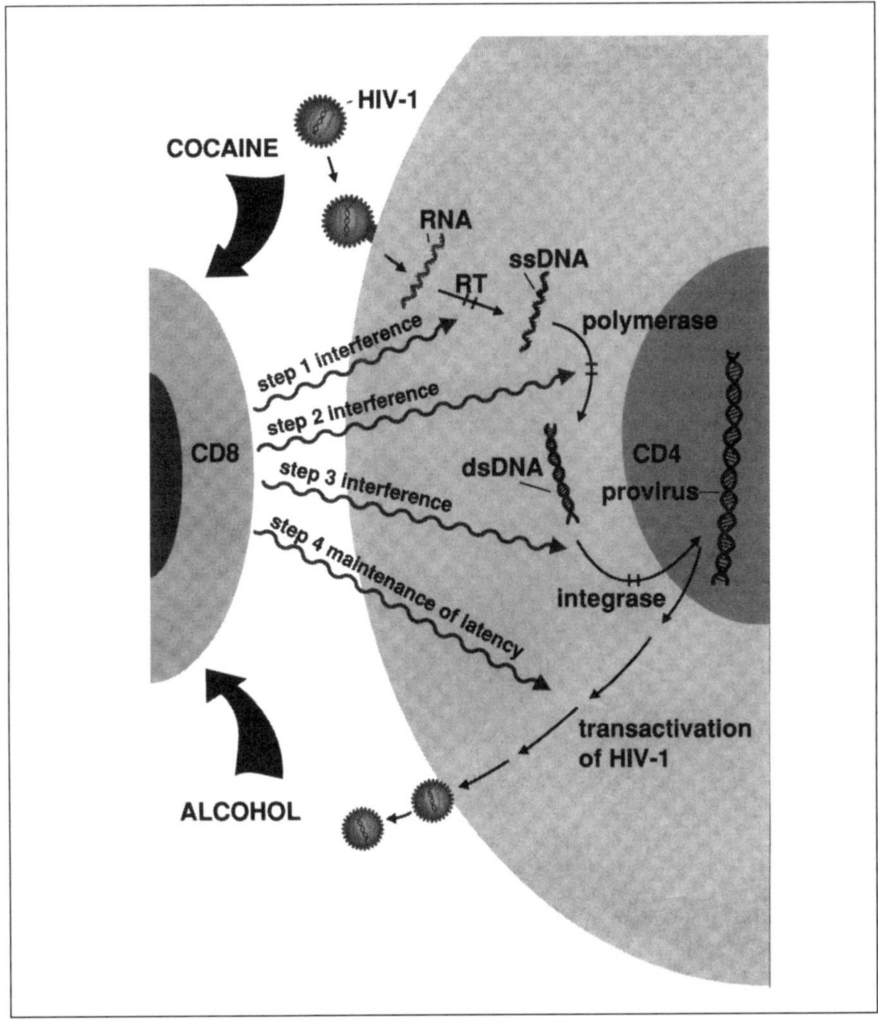

Figure 25. Molecular anti-retroviral immunity. Multistep, anti-retroviral molecular immune mechanisms and their potential interactions with CD8+ T cells are illustrated.

PBMCs isolated from HIV-1-seropositive individuals (36–38).

It is of note that cocaine had no effect on HIV-1 replication in persistently HIV-1-infected CD4+ lymphocytic and monocytoid cell lines. Numerous mechanisms might account for these findings. The cocaine-induced augmentation of HIV-1 replication in PBMCs may be CD8+ T-cell mediated. It is also possible that these cell lines lack receptors for cocaine. However, it is very unlikely that all 6 cell lines have lost receptors for cocaine. We believe that the observed wide range of differences in the ability of PBMCs to produce HIV-1 p24 antigen, after exposure to cocaine or its metabolite, represents a natural variation among different individuals, which may be dependent on many factors (835). It is also possible that certain individuals are genetically less susceptible to the adverse effects of cocaine on their immune system than others (835). Exposure to cocaine plus benzoylecgonine also resulted in a significant increase in the HIV-1 p24 antigen levels ($P<0.05$), in the same 6 out of 8 individuals. Exposure to the 2 agents, in combination, appeared to produce a small but statistically insignificant additive effect. It is possible that each agent is affecting PBMCs through an independent mechanism.

Previously, Peterson et al. (757,844) reported that cocaine potentiates HIV-1 replication in human PBMCs in vitro, possibly by a modulation of transforming growth factor beta (TGF-β). Recently, Shapshak et al. (845) demonstrated that cocaine and cocaethylene (another by-product of cocaine and ethanol co-ingestion) accelerate AIDS progression in African-American women, in vivo, and HIV-1 replication in their PBMCs, in vitro. They evaluated 86 HIV-1-seropositive and 44 HIV-1-seronegative African-American women at 6-month intervals. Immunology, epidemiology, toxicology (hair and urine), and virological studies were performed using standard procedures. Logistic regression analysis showed that progression was associated with RNA virus load and self-reported use of both crack/cocaine and alcohol, and was inversely related to the percentage of CD8+ CD38- T cells. Kaplan-Meier survival plots indicated increased deaths with increased virus load, self-reported cocaine use frequency, and decreased CD4+ T-cell counts. Hair cocaine-metabolite toxicology by gas chromatography/mass spectroscopy correlated with self-reported crack/cocaine and alcohol use during the 30 days before testing. Cocaine (cocaethylene) abuse stimulated HIV-1 replication in cultures, in vitro. These studies, as well as our own, may have implications for cocaine's direct biological effect on T lymphocytes. Cocaine and metabolites appear to accelerate HIV-1 infection, and cocaine-dependent behavior must be treated to reduce the spread of AIDS. Importantly, cocaine is one of many substances of abuse, including alcohol and opioids, which affect replication of HIV-1 (48,49). Alcohol is a frequent cofactor used with cocaine, and these substances may interact in their effects on HIV-1 expression in vivo.

In vitro studies, various epidemiological studies, and some recent studies conducted in animal models (430,750–757,822,837,846–849) indicate that the immunomodulations caused by cocaine may support an environment in which HIV-1 replication is more efficient than in the intact immune system. These experiments indicate, however, that a modified susceptibility of PBMCs to infection with HIV-1, observed after exposure to cocaine, is associated with increased HIV-1 replication in these target cells, in vitro. Recent data have suggested that HIV-1 mainly exists in vivo in an unintegrated state in quiescent lymphocytes, and this may be the predominant form in mainly HIV-1-infected individuals treated with reverse transcriptase inhibitors (559,717,770–774); therefore, I suggest that the evaluation of cocaine and other biological modifiers of HIV-1 replication should be performed in systems that more closely mimic the unstimulated T lymphocyte in vivo.

LINK BETWEEN AMYL NITRITE AND HIV-1 INFECTION

Amyl nitrite has been used medically since 1867 in the management of coronary insufficiency. However, it currently has a very limited role in medicine. Beginning in the late 1960s and into the early 1970s, reports began to surface that nitrite inhalants were being abused predominantly by homosexual men to augment the physical pleasure of sexual intercourse. Soon nitrite inhalants became known as poppers, and abuse patterns widened. As a street drug, poppers were frequently used on social occasions, often in night clubs, parties, and other social occasions to enhance euphoric effects and as a stimulant. A more widespread pattern of use was associated with overt sexual activities. Although awareness of the adverse health effects of nitrite abuse was raised in the 1970s, real concerns surfaced with the rise of the AIDS epidemic and the growing body of data suggesting that the volatile nitrites may induce immunomodulations or might otherwise be a cofactor in the pathogenesis of HIV-1 infection and certain AIDS-related syndromes (e.g., KS). For example, of the first 5 homosexual men with AIDS reported to the CDC, all had used nitrite inhalants, but only 1 had abused intravenous drugs and only 2 were reported to be promiscuous (183).

Various clinical and epidemiological studies and some recent studies conducted in animal models indicate that the immunomodulations induced by the nitrites may act as cofactors in the development of KS in AIDS patients (reviewed in References 2 and 850). Most importantly, there is evidence that nitrites may compromise the immune cell activity and the in vitro polyclonal induction of IgG and IgM synthesis. In one study (reviewed in Reference 850) the mice were exposed to amyl nitrite and analyses of various immune-related parameters were carried out. The results showed that exposure to amyl nitrite can induce changes in immune function even after short exposure to moderate doses. The results demonstrate that exposure to sublethal doses of amyl nitrite can cause a significant decrease in helper cells, thus resulting in an inverted T-cell helper (CD4+) to suppressor (CD8+) cell ratio. Mean body weight was also shown to be decreased after 8 weeks, and the decrease became statistically significant by the end of 21 weeks of exposure. The gross pathological observation of selected organs also showed statistically significant damage to the lungs in the exposed group. Another parameter tested was the resistance of exposed mice to pathogenic intracellular *Listeria monocytogenes*, used to assess the competence of T lymphocytes and macrophages. Peak resistance was reached on day 6 for the control group (40% survival) but was delayed until day 14 (20% survival) in the exposed group. These studies demonstrated that chronic inhalation of amyl nitrite can lead to a decrease in helper cells, thus altering the T-cell helper (CD4+) to suppressor (CD8+) cell ratio, which is the same phenomenon that occurs in AIDS victims. This suggests a link between amyl nitrite inhalation and cellular immunity depression. However, it is important to remember that the doses used to test the hypothesis were much higher than those a nitrite abuser would normally use.

ARE SUBSTANCES OF ABUSE THE CAUSE OF AIDS?

The Drug–AIDS Hypothesis

According to Dr. Peter Duesberg (2), "All AIDS diseases in America and Europe that exceed their long-established, normal background are caused by the long-term consumption of recreational drugs and by AZT and its analogs. Hemophilia–AIDS, transfusion–AIDS, and extremely rare AIDS cases of the general population reflect the normal incidence of AIDS-defining diseases in these groups plus the AZT-induced incidence of these diseases under a new name." The key to this so-called drug–AIDS hypothesis is that only long-term consumption causes irreversible AIDS-defining diseases, and that there is no HIV-1.

Many people would like to know the answers to the questions raised by the proponents of this drug–AIDS dogma. In my opinion, believing that AIDS is caused only by the long-term use of drugs is like hiding one's head in the sand.

It is true that in Western countries, a high level of substance abuse generally is associated with an increased risk of AIDS (429–431,742,745–747). However, such a correlation is inevitable since individuals who abuse drugs also stand a good chance of being exposed to relatively high doses of HIV-1. In addition, as outlined by well-documented scientific data, exposure to certain drugs (i.e., alcohol and cocaine) weakens the arm of the immune system that protects against retroviruses, and exposure to HIV-1 at that specific time makes individuals much more susceptible to infection (though transiently). Therefore, there is no doubt that individuals who abuse drugs are more exposed to high doses of HIV-1 and also stand a better chance of widespread HIV-1 dissemination as a result of the weakened state of their molecular immunity. However, with the exception of alcohol and cocaine, there is no drug(s), to the best of my knowledge, that has been documented to adversely affect the normal functions of CD8+ T cells; therefore, it is my belief that a direct correlation observed in the incidence of AIDS and the abuse of drugs other than alcohol and cocaine is due largely to the increased exposure of abusers to high doses of HIV-1 (due to increased high-risk sexual activities and intravenous drug injections).

It is true that HIV-1 infection is more common among intravenous drug users, in babies born to mothers who abuse drugs, and in male drug users. Obviously, if one group has a greater chance of being exposed to HIV-1, through substance abuse or sexual activity, then the incidence of HIV-1 would be higher in this group. In this group, many other infections are also more common, like hepatitis B and HHV-8 (which is associated with KS). Also, immunity against HIV-1 is reduced due to the use of certain drugs like alcohol and cocaine, as described above.

Low Percentage of PBMCs are Infected with HIV-1

Dr. Duesberg was probably baffled, and reasonably so, by the observations made in earlier reports from Dr. Robert Gallo's laboratory that the PBMCs from individuals dying from AIDS exhibited only 1 in 5000 to 1 in 100 000 T cells infected with HIV-1 (188). This information was based on a relatively insensitive technique called in situ hybridization. With the introduction of more sensitive methods like PCR, quantitative PCR, and ISPCR, old concepts based on less sensitive methods were revised.

Since the introduction of thermostable DNA polymerase, *Taq*, which brought automation and convenience to PCR, many scientists, including myself, have been paying special attention to the development of PCR in situ (189,191–195). I started working on ISPCR techniques in the beginning of 1987, and it took me almost 4 years before I felt comfortable about the validity of this method (189). As I mentioned, the actual percentage of HIV-1-infected cells in the PBMCs has been a subject of controversy (188). Various modifications of the PCR method have been used to quantitatively or semiquantitatively assess the relative frequencies of HIV-1-infected cells in PBMCs, lymph nodes, and other cell types (reviewed in Reference 578). One of the major drawbacks of the standard PCR method (which is performed in microtubes with nucleic acid isolated from cells in tissues) has been that the procedure does not allow the association of amplified signals of a specific genetic segment with the histological cell types(s). The ability to identify individual cells carrying a specific gene(s) or a portion of a genetic fragment under the microscope is extremely useful in delineating various aspects of normal and pathological conditions. For example, this technique could be used in various leukemias and lymphomas, where specific aberrant gene sequences are associated with malignancy. The HIV-1 virus has been demonstrated to infect CD4+ lymphocytes, monocytes, B lymphocytes, fibroblasts, sperm, oral mucosal epithelial cells, and various cells of the central nervous system (106,189,191,578,957,810). Although the CD4+ cells may be the primary reservoir for HIV-1 in the bloodstream, and the monocyte/macrophage may be the major reservoir in solid tissues (191), it is highly desirable to identify all cell types that carry HIV-1 in vivo, as well as which cell types are actively producing HIV-1. My laboratory was the first to report the actual percentage of PBMCs infected with HIV-1 by using an ISPCR technique (189).

Initially, we evaluated 56 patients infected with HIV-1; the percentage of PBMCs with HIV-1 ranged from 0.1% to 13.5%. CD4+ cells infected with HIV-1 ranged from 0.2% to 69% in the 42 HIV-1-infected patients who were evaluated. We used the ISPCR technique to determine the proportion of PBMCs in unfractionated PBMCs, and also separated CD4+ cells from PBMCs by immunomagnetic beads from HIV-1-infected patients in different stages of disease. Studies using this technique demonstrated higher levels of HIV-1 provirus in unfractionated PBMCs of infected persons than had been demonstrated in many previous studies. None of the PBMCs from 11 HIV-1-seronegative patients were found to be positive for HIV-1 provirus by the ISPCR method. The percentages of HIV-1-infected CD4+ cells increased significantly with advancing stages of disease. These procedures demonstrated that, in HIV-1 infection, the proportion of PBMCs that are infected appears to be at least 10 times higher than previously described, and these data also suggest that in certain infected individuals, high levels of infected PBMCs may harbor the HIV-1 provirus. This has been confirmed and extended by several groups, using a related ISPCR technique (191–195).

AIDS in Central Africa Defies the Drug–AIDS Hypothesis

As described earlier, AIDS might be the result of accidental exposure to pre-HIV viruses in a form of vaccine in Central Africa. If this proposal is true, then one would expect that regardless of drug use or abuse, this population would be predominantly infected. Therefore, from the estimated 23 million individuals who are infected with HIV-1 worldwide, over 14 million individuals are in sub-Sahara Africa. Out of these 14 million, 820 000 have been diagnosed with AIDS. In parts of the world where drug abuse is relatively uncommon, such a high number of HIV-1-infected individuals defies the drug–AIDS hypothesis. In addition, in parts of the world where substance abuse is rare (e.g., Pakistan and Saudi Arabia), many HIV-1 cases have been reported. (In Pakistan an estimated 80 000 individuals are infected with HIV-1.) If AIDS is solely the result of substance abuse, then the highest number of cases should be from the countries where substance abuse and alcohol abuse are most common. However, if one looks at the number of cases around the globe, this drug–AIDS hypothesis does not pan out. For example, from the total estimated 23 million HIV-1-infected people around the globe, 570 000 HIV-1-infected individuals reside in Europe, 1.3 million in Latin America, 750 000 in North America, 270 000 in the Caribbean, 200 000 in North Africa and the Middle East, 5.2 million in Southeast Asia, 50 000 in Eastern Europe and only 13 000 in Australia. Obviously, this distribution does not coincide with drug-abusing populations. Australia and Sweden are the top consumers of substances of abuse and alcohol in the world but are relatively very low on the HIV-1 infection list. In Australia there were a total of 5737 reported AIDS cases until 1995 (total population over 23 million) and in Sweden there were a total of 1170 reported AIDS cases until 1995 (total population around 8 million): both of these countries are top consumers of alcohol. Clearly this pattern of infection does not fit into the drug–AIDS hypothesis but rather appears to fit into a "seed-and-spread" pattern. If more seeds of HIV-1 are planted from the beginning, more individuals are going to be infected from each of these seeds. And if many of these individuals engage in behavior that allows them to spead the virus effectively to others, then the disease could be disseminated into the population. In sub-Sahara Africa, where presumably a quarter of a million to half a million individuals were inoculated with HIV-1-like viruses, then the initial seed stock would have been quite large (in Kenya, which has a population of 28 million, over 60 000 individuals have died from AIDS). On the other hand, if the Australian population initially received a limited amount of seed (from a few HIV-1-infected individuals who brought the disease from other countries) then the cases of HIV-1 would be expected to be very low. Over 90% of HIV-1-infected individuals are in developed countries and migration to Australia from the developing countries is much lower compared to the United States and Europe, where migration from developing countries is relatively high (more seed). On the African continent, a significant immigration to South Africa from the sub-Sahara has taken place since the end of Apartheid. And, in this country, the incidence of HIV-1 infections has also skyrocketed.

We need to be clear on the fact that substance abuse itself does not cause AIDS. However, consumption of certain chemical substances makes the immune system more vulnerable to HIV-1 if the body is exposed to the virus during a transient immunocompromised state. Unfortunately, the most commonly used substances known to compromise CD8+ T-cell function (i.e., alcohol and cocaine, though transiently) also induce a transient disinhibiting effect, making the act of unsafe sex more possible, and hence increasing the risk of HIV-1 infection. However, there is no evidence that substances of abuse cause AIDS. Use and consumption of chemical substances are not new in human history. If AIDS were solely caused by drugs, then AIDS would have been rampant in Europe and the United States, not in the poorest areas of the world, where people barely have enough money to buy food and millions die each year from starvation. There is little doubt that substances of abuse are cofactors in the development and progression of AIDS but they are not the direct cause. The introduction of an infectious virus into naive human societies allows that virus to be pathogenic. The positive correlation observed among drug abusers and HIV-1 infection is due to high exposure rates of these groups to HIV-1 (as well as a secondary effect of these drugs on CD8+ T cells). This group is not only exposed to HIV-1 but also is exposed to syphilis, herpes, CMV, HHV-8, and many other venereal diseases (which also enhance the replication of HIV-1). It is estimated that 8500 individuals are infected with HIV-1 every day; 90% of these are in developing countries and most are not drug abusers. Out of these 8500 individuals, 1000 children infected are under 15 years of age and 3000 are women. Thus, the majority of the individuals who become infected are not hard-core drug abusers (and many have never used drugs even once in their lives) but are heterosexual men and women, who most likely get infected through sexual contact.

Epilogue

"Of course, it is sure as the sun following the dawn of tomorrow that the high deeds of the microbe hunters have not come to end; there will be others to fashion magic bullets. And they will be waggish men and original ... for it is not from a mere combination of incessant work and magnificent laboratories that such marvelous cures are to be got."

Paul de Kruif
Microbe Hunters

The most serious hurdle in the development of an effective vaccine against HIV-1 has been the lack of convincing evidence regarding the true nature of immunity that correlates with protection. The critical analyses of the experimental studies in various animal models of AIDS, especially in rhesus macaques, individuals with an apparent resistance to HIV-1 infection, and individuals who are LTNPs, have provided very important information regarding the true nature of protection. There is growing evidence that neither HI responses nor the traditionally understood viral-specific CTLs play any important role in the inhibition of HIV-1 replication in vivo. The majority of the HIV-1 vaccine strategies that have received the greatest attention to date, including the use of recombinant HIV-1 envelope glycoprotein immunogens, live vaccinia virus subunits, and many vaccine approaches to elicit virus-specific CTLs, have given disappointing results. I believe it is futile to attempt to develop vaccines against HIV-1 by eliciting HIV-1-specific HI or CMI responses, since successful vaccines can only be made by mimicking the host's natural defenses. In this book, I have presented a description of and preliminary evidence for the existence of a new form of immunity, molecular immunity, which appears to provide the real protection against the retroviral–lentiviral invasion. I have presented data from my laboratory which indicates that this newly described immunity works by repertoires of small RNAs, present in CD8+/NK+ cells. These RNA repertoires are the result of our long evolutionary symbiotic relationship with retroviruses. Upon encountering a retrovirus, these small RNAs probably form a triple helix with the invading virus and block entry to the nucleus. This inhibition takes place predominantly at the preintegration step of retroviral replication. Upon blocking a particular retrovirus at the preintegration phase, multiple copies (millions) of the specific blocker RNAs are reproduced by the protective machinery of the host and are sent to distant locations. These RNAs provide the specific immunity against that retrovirus to the cells receiving the specific protective RNAs. HIV-1 is a rather new lentivirus for which human populations are a naive host. Some of its genes are highly pathogenic to various cells in our body, including our immune, nervous, and vascular systems. In the case of HIV-1 infection, I have proposed that there is a race between HIV-1, which tries to infect as many cells as possible to reach a threshold number of infected cells at the initial stage of infection, and CD8+/NK+ cells, which produce protective RNAs against HIV-1 and protect as many cells as possible. If initially a majority of the cells are protected by the protective RNAs, the HIV-1 viral load will remain relatively low, and the individual will remain asymptomatic (a LTNP or, in some cases, HIV-1 seronegative). However, if HIV-1 reaches a significant number of cells before molecular immunity can send enough protective RNAs, the individual will produce too many virions that reach too many cells and overcome the protective machinery, and will thus develop AIDS. The outcome of the race between HIV-1 infection and the anti-HIV-1-specific RNA-based immunity depends on the initial viral dose, as well as percentages of cells stimulated at the time of HIV-1 exposure. If the initial viral dose is low, the HIV-1-specific molecular immunity can reach a significant number of cells and protect the host. An optimal protective response depends on intact molecular immunity. However, certain naturally occurring physiological conditions [i.e., stress, depression (827–828), infancy, old age (72–75)] or exposure to certain immunomodulatory agents [i.e., cocaine, alcohol, steroids, exposure to UV light or radiation, etc. (455–458, 745–758,760–764, 827–849)] can allow even small doses of HIV-1 to cause damage to the infected host.

I have provided numerous examples, including experimental data in macaques and chimpanzees, as well as natural evidence in humans, which strongly suggest that a live attenuated virus or a replication-defective virus could serve as a vaccine. An understanding of the molecular mechanisms involved in protection against retroviruses can help us design a suitable vaccine against HIV-1 and other lentiviruses.

I believe that the real natural defense against HIV-1 lies inside the CD8+/NK+ cells, and fostering this intracellular molecular immunity would bring us closer to the development of a vaccine against HIV-1. I also believe that the most practical form of vaccine would be an attenuated lentiviral agent, genetically related to HIV-1.

I have expressed serious concerns regarding the use of a retroviral vaccine for human or even animal gene therapy. Currently, many types of retroviral- and lentiviral-based gene therapies are in progress. These forms of gene therapy have been shown to create new types of retroviruses, which probably have never existed in nature, and experimental animals or humans are naive hosts for these newly emerging retroviruses or lentiviruses (111–112, 787,789–791). These newly formed viruses may cause new and potentially even more destructive epidemics than AIDS. Recently, Patience et al. (791) reported that a pig endogenous retrovirus is capable of infecting human cells in vitro. In another study, a replication-defective MuLV vector was used to transduce bone marrow cells from the macaque with a marker gene. Instead, recombination took place, a replication-competent virus arose, and lymphomas developed in 3 out of 10 monkeys within a year (178). I am issuing a strong warning to the scientific community that widespread use of retroviral- or lentiviral-based gene therapy is extremely dangerous. Such forms of gene therapy should be evaluated carefully and moved forward very slowly.

Recently, several US health agencies, including the Food and Drug Administration, the National Institutes of Health, and the CDC, have agreed to allow limited clinical trials of animal-to-human transplantation. From even the limited knowledge we have about retroviruses, we should all have serious concerns regarding xenotransplantation. Pigs (the proposed donor animals for xenotransplantation) carry many retroviruses. Human and animal retroviruses also carry an enormous potential for recombination, and xenotransplantation has been shown to create new types of retroviruses—which would be novel for the human immune system. The transplanted tissue would be a veritable breeding ground for replication of high doses of newly recombined retroviruses (178,451,787,791). The pig endogenous retrovirus (PERV-PK) is capable of infecting human cells in vitro. I believe that a reasonable observation period (3–5 years) should be allowed to decipher the adverse effects of this type of experimentation.

Currently there is great interest in the utilization of SHIV, a chimera virus containing the internal genes of SIV and the external HIV protein (Env). Although the study of retroviral recombination has been extensive and we have been able to obtain a great deal of information from SHIV, naturally occurring genetic recombination between SIVs and HIV-1 has not been studied extensively. Chimeric viruses have been artificially created using molecular cloning techniques in order to study their biological properties (131,186). HIV-1/SIV_{mac} recombinants and HIV-1/SIV_{agm} recombinants have been made and used to infect primates and humans (851,852). These viruses replicate well inside monkeys and humans, and actively infect the host's PBMCs (853–855). They also show that the recombinant nature of these viruses increased their host range to include both primates and humans, and can also alter their pathogenicity. These chimeric lentiviruses were artificially created, but we need to know if they recombine naturally in vivo.

I believe that the live attenuated vaccine against HIV-1 already exists in the bloodstreams of those individuals who received CHAT-1 live polio vaccine in the Ruzizi Valley, near Lake Tanganyika. These individuals carry the sort of viral particles that we can utilize for future AIDS vaccines. If these individuals have survived for over 50 years with a kind of attenuated lentivirus related to HIV-1, we should explore the possibility of using these lentiviruses for mass vaccination.

References

1.**Pantaleo, G. et al.** 1993. HIV infection is active and progressive in lymphoid tissue during the clinically latent stage of disease. Nature 362:355.

2.**Duesberg, P.H.** 1997. Inventing the AIDS Virus. Regnery Publishing, Washington, DC.

3.**Orgel, L.E. et al.** 1980. Selfish DNA: the ultimate parasite. Nature 284:604.

4.**Temin, H.M.** 1970. Malignant transformation of cells by viruses. Perspect. Biol. Med. 4:26.

5.**Coffin, J.M.** 1996. Retroviridae: the viruses and their replication, p. 1767. In B.N. Fields et al. (Eds), Fields Virology. Lippincott-Raven, Philadelphia.

6.**Villareal, L.P.** 1997. On virus, sex, and motherhood. J. Virol. 71:859.

7.**Coffin, J.M.** 1992. Retrovirus variation and evolution, p. 221. In J. Levy (Ed.), The Retroviridae. Plenum Press, New York.

8.**Doolittle, R.F. and C. Sapienza.** 1980. Selfish genes, the phenotypic paradigm, and genome evolution. Nature 284:601.

9.**Phillips, A.N.** 1996. Reduction of HIV concentration during acute infection: independence from a specific immune response. Science 271:497.

10.**Siegel, F. et al.** 1995. Neither whole inactivated virus immunogen nor passive immunoglobulin transfer protects against SIVagm infection in the African green monkey natural host. J. Acquir. Immune Defic. Syndr. 8:217.

11.**Mitchell, W.M. et al.** 1995. Antibodies to the putative SIV infection-enhancing domain diminish beneficial effects of an SIV gp160 vaccine in rhesus macaques. AIDS 9:27.

12.**Girard, M.P.** 1990. Progress in the development of SIV vaccines. AIDS (Suppl.) 4:143.

13.**Karzon, D.T. et al.** 1992. Development of a vaccine for the prevention of AIDS, a critical appraisal. Vaccine 10:1039.

14.**Kent, K.A. et al.** 1994. Passive immunization of cynomolgus macaque with immune sera or a pool of neutralizing monoclonal antibodies failed to protect against challenge with SIV_{mac251}. AIDS Res. Hum. Retroviruses 10:189.

15.**Orentas, R.I. et al.** 1990. Induction of CD4+ human cytolytic T cell-specific for HIV-infected cell by a gpl60 subunit vaccine. Science 248:1234.

16.**Ruprecht, R.M. et al.** 1990. Vaccination with a live retrovirus: the nature of the protective immune response. Proc. Natl. Acad. Sci. USA 87:5558.

17.**Heeney, J. et al.** 1993. The resistance of HIV-infected chimpanzees to progression to AIDS correlates with absence of HIV-related T-cell dysfunction. J. Med. Primatol. 22:194.

18.**Eichberg, J.W. et al.** 1987. T-cell responses to human immunodeficiency virus (HIV) and its recombinant antigens in HIV- infected chimpanzees. J. Virol. 61:3804.

19.**Montelaro, R.C. et al.** 1995. Vaccines against retroviruses, p. 605. In J.A. Levy (Ed.), The Retroviridae. Plenum Press, New York.

20.**Hoth, D.F. et al.** 1994. HIV vaccine development: a progress report. Ann. Int. Med. 8:603.

21.**Girard, M. et al.** 1996. Failure of a human immunodeficiency virus type 1 (HIV-1) subtype B-derived vaccine to prevent infection of chimpanzees by an HIV-1 subtype E strain. J. Virol. 70:8229.

22.**Mascola, J.R. et al.** 1993. Summary report: workshop on potential risks of antibody-dependent enhancement in human HIV vaccine trails. AIDS Res. Hum. Retroviruses 9:1175.

23.**Clerici, M. et al.** 1992. Cell mediated immune response to HIV-1 in seronegative homosexuals with recent sexual exposure to HIV-1. J. Infect. Dis. 165:1012.

24.**Rowland-Jones, S. et al.** 1995. HIV-specific cytotoxic T-cell in HIV-exposed but uninfected Gambian women. Nat. Med. 1:59.

25.**Langlade-Demoyen, P. et al.** 1994. Human immunodeficiency virus (HIV) -specific cytotoxic T lymphocytes in noninfected heterosexual contact of HIV-1 infected patients. J. Clin. Invest. 93:1293.

26.**Paxton, W.A. et al.** 1996. Relative resistance to HIV-1 infection of CD4 lymphocytes from persons who remain uninfected despite multiple high-risk sexual exposure. Nat. Med. 2:412.

27.**Hirsch, V.M. et al.** 1993. A distinct African lentivirus from Sykes' monkeys. J. Virol. 67:1517.

28.**Muller, M.C. et al.** 1993. Simian immunodeficiency viruses from Central and Western Africa: evidence for a new species-specific lentivirus in tantalus monkeys. J. Virol. 67:1227.

29.**Allan, J.S. et al.** 1990. Isolation and characterization of simian immuno-deficiency viruses from two subspecies of African green monkeys. AIDS Res. Hum. Retroviruses 6:275.

30.**Ohta, Y. et al.** 1988. Isolation of simian immunodeficiency virus from African green monkeys and seroepidemiologic survey of the virus in various non human primates. Int. J. Cancer 41:115.

31.**Fultz, P.N. et al.** 1989. Isolation of a T-lymphocyte retrovirus from naturally infected sooty mangabey monkeys. Proc. Natl. Acad. Sci. USA 83:5286.

32.**Gao, F. et al.** 1992. Human infection by genetically diverse SIVsm-related HIV-2 in West Africa. Nature 358:495.

33.**Huet, T. et al.** 1994. Genetic organization of a chimpanzee lentivirus related to HIV-I. Nature 345:356.

34.Peeters, M. et al. 1989. Isolation and partial characterization of an HIV-related virus occurring naturally in chimpanzees in Gabon. AIDS 3:625.
35.Francis, D. et al. 1984. Infection of chimpanzees with lymphadenopathy-associated virus. Lancet ii: 1270.
36.Peeters, M. et al. 1992. Isolation and characterization of a new chimpanzee lentivirus (simian immunodeficiency virus isolate cpz-ant) from a wild-capture chimpanzee. AIDS 6:447.
37.Nara, P. et al. 1987. Persistent infection of chimpanzees with human immunodeficiency virus: serological responses and properties of reisolated viruses. J. Virol. 61:3173.
38.Kanki, P.J. et al. 1985. Serologic identification and characterization of a macaque T-lymphotropic retrovirus closely related to HTLV-III. Science 230:1199.
39.Krugner-Higby, L. et al. 1990. Serological survey for two simian retroviruses in macaques and African green monkeys. Lab. Animal Sci. 40:24.
40.Lowenstine, L.J. and N.W. Lerche. 1986. Retrovirus infections of nonhuman primates: a review. J. Zoo Animal Med. 19:16872.
41.Lowenstine, L.J. et al. 1986. Seroepidemiologic survey of captive Old-World primates for antibodies to human and simian retroviruses, and isolation of a lentivirus from sooty mangabeys (Cercocebus atys). Int. J. Cancer 38:563.
42.Schneider, J. et al. 1987. Serological and structural comparison of HIV, SIVmac, SIVagm and SIVsm, four primate lentiviruses. Ann. Inst. Pasteur Virol. 138:93.
43.Honjo, S. and M. Hayaml. 1988. Isolation of simian immunodeficiency virus from African green monkeys and seroepidemiologic survey of the virus in various non-human primates. Int. J. Cancer 41:115.
44.McNulty, W.P. et al. 1985. Isolation of a new serotype of simian acquired immune deficiency syndrome type D retrovirus from Celebes black macaques (*Macaca nigra*) with immune deficiency and retroperitoneal fibromatosis. J. Virol. 56:571.
45.Villinger, F. et al. 1991. Detection of occult simian immunodeficiency virus SIVsmm infection in asymptomatic seronegative nonhuman primates and evidence for variation in SIV gag sequence between in vivo- and in vitro-propagated virus. J. Virol. 65:1855.
46.Muller, M.C. et al. 1993. Simian immunodeficiency viruses from central and western Africa: evidence for a new species-specific lentivirus in tantalus monkeys. J. Virol. 67:1227.
47.Grankvist, O. et al. 1992. Improved detection of HIV-2 DNA in clinical samples using a nested primer-based polymerase chain reaction. AIDS 5:286.
48.Dietrich, U. et al. 1989. A highly divergent HIV-2 related isolate. Nature 342:948.
49.Hirsh, V. et al. 1989. An African primate lentivirus (SIVsm) closely related to HIV-2. Nature 339:389.
50.Alter, H.J. et al. 1984. Transmission of HTLV-III infection from human plasma to chimpanzees: an animal model of AID. Science 226:549.
51.Girard, M. et al. 1991. Immunization of chimpanzees confers protection against challenge with human immunodeficiency virus. Proc. Natl. Acad. Sci. USA 88:542.
52.Zarling, J. et al. 1987. Proliferative and cytotoxic T cells to AIDS virus glycoproteins in chimpanzees immunized with a recombinant vaccinia virus expressing AIDS virus envelope glycoproteins. J. Immunol. 139:988.
53.Kestens, L. et al. 1995. Phenotypic and functional parameters of cellular immunity in chimpanzee with a naturally acquired simian immunodeficiency virus infection. J. Infect. Dis. 172:957.
54.Sakuragi, J. et al. 1992. Functional classification of simian immuno-deficiency virus isolated from a chimpanzee by transactivators. Virology 189:354.
55.Ferrari, G. et al. 1993. The impact of HIV-l infection on phenotypic and functional parameters of cellular immunity in chimpanzees. AIDS Res. Hum. Retroviruses 9:647.
56.Warren, J.T. and M. Dolatshahi. 1992. Worldwide survey of AIDS vaccine challenge studies in nonhuman primates: vaccines associated with active and passive immune protection from live virus challenge. J. Med. Primatol. 21:139.
57.Warren, J.T. and M. Dolatshahi. 1993. First updated and revised survey of worldwide HIV and SIV vaccine challenge studies in nonhuman primates: progress in first and second order studies. J. Med. Primatol. 22:203.
58.Sutjipto, S. et al. 1990. Inactivated simian immunodeficiency virus vaccine failed to protect rhesus macaques from intravenous or genital mucosal infection but delayed disease in intravenously exposed animals. J. Viro. 64:2290.
59.Johnson, P.R. et al. 1992. Inactivated whole SIV vaccine in macaques: evaluation of protective efficacy against challenge with cell-free virus or infected cells. AIDS Res. Hum. Retroviruses 8:1501.
60.Almond, N. et al. 1992. Population sequence analysis of a simian immunodeficiency virus (32H reisolate of SIVmac251): a virus stock used for international vaccine studies. AIDS Res. Hum. Retroviruses

8:77.
61.**Murphey-Corb, M.** 1997. Live-attenuated HIV vaccines: how safe is safe enough? Nat. Med. 3:17.
62.**Hoover, E.A.** 1994. Incomplete protection, but suppression of virus burden, elicited by subunit simian immunodeficiency virus vaccines. J. Virol. 68:1843.
63.**Hu, S.-L. et al.** 1992. Protection of macaques against SIV infection by subunit vaccines of SIV envelope glycoprotein gpl60. Science 255:456.
64.**Baskerville, A. et al.** 1993. Studies on the specificity of the vaccine effect elicited by inactivated simian immunodeficiency virus. AIDS Res. Hum. Retroviruses 9:13.
65.**Putkonen, P. et al.** 1993. Whole inactivated SIV vaccine grown on human cells fails to protect against homologous SIV grown on simian cells. J. Med. Primatol. 22:100.
66.**Daniel, M.D. et al.** 1992. Protective effects of a live attenuated SIV vaccine with a deletion in the nef gene. Science 258:1938.
67.**Putkonen, P. et al.** 1995. Long-term protection against SIV-induced disease in macaque vaccinated with a live attenuated HIV-2 vaccine. Nat. Med. 1:914.
68.**Travers, K. et al.** 1995. Natural protection against HIV-1 infection provided by HIV-2. Science 268:1612.
69.**Bonhoeffer, S. and M. Nowak.** 1995. Can live attenuated virus work as post-exposure treatment. Immunol. Today 16:131.
70.**Baba, T.W. et al.** 1995. Pathogenicity of live attenuated SIV after mucosal infection of neonatal macaques. Science 267:1820.
71.**Shibata, R. et al.** 1996. Resistance of previously infected chimpanzees to successive challenges with a heterologous intraclade B strain of HIV-1. J. Virol. 70:4361.
72.**Putkonen, P. et al.** 1990. Infection of cynomolgus monkey with HIV-2 protects against pathogenic consequences of a subsequent simian immunodeficiency virus infection. AIDS 4:783.
73.**Wyand, M.S. et al.** 1997. Resistance of neonatal monkeys to live attenuated vaccine strains of simian immunodeficiency virus. Nat. Med. 3:32.
74.**Desrosiers, R.C.** 1992. HIV with multiple gene deletions as a live attenuated vaccine for AIDS. AIDS Res. Hum. Retroviruses 8:1457.
75.**Black, K.P. et al.** 1997. IgA immunity in HIV type 1-infected chimpanzees. II. Mucosal immunity. AIDS Res. Hum. Retroviruses 13:1273.
76.**Marthas, M.L. et al.** 1992. Efficacy of live attenuated and whole-inactivated simian immunodeficiency virus vaccines against vaginal challenge with virulent SIV. J. Med. Primatol. 21:99.
77.**Marthas, M. et al.** 1993. Viral determinants of simian immuno-deficiency virus (SIV) virulence in rhesus macaques assessed using attenuated and pathogenic molecular clones of SIVmac. J. Virol. 67:6047.
78.**Weiss, R.A.** 1988. Foamy retroviruses: a virus in search of a disease. Nature 333:497.
79.**Mergia, A. and P.A. Luciw.** 1991. Replication and regulation of primate foamy viruses. Virology 184:475.
80.**Aguzzi, A.** 1994. Neurotoxicity of human foamy virus in transgenic mice. Verh. Dtsch. Ges. Pathol. 78:180.
81.**McCune, J.M.** 1997. Animal models of HIV-1 diseases. Science 278: 2141.
82.**Tinkle, B.T. et al.** 1997. Transgenic dissection of HIV genes involved in lymphoid depletion. J. Clin. Invest. 100:32.
83.**Vellutini, C. et al.** 1995. Development of lymphoid hyperplasia in transgenic mice expressing the HIV tat gene. AIDS Res. Hum. Retroviruses 11:21.
84.**Sugamura, K. and Y. Hinuma.** 1992. Human retroviruses: HTLV-I and HTLV-II, p. 399. In J.A. Levy (Ed.), The Retroviridae. Plenum Press, New York.
85.**Chen, C.-H. et al.** 1993. CD8+ lymphocyte-mediated inhibition of HIV-l long terminal repeat transcription: a novel antiviral mechanism. AIDS Res. Hum. Retroviruses 9:1079.
86.**Cao, Y. et al.** 1995.Virologic and immunologic characterization of long-term survivors of human immunodeficiency virus type 1 infection. N. Engl. J. Med. 332:201.
87.**Liu, R. et al.** 1996. Homozygous defect in HIV-1 coreceptor accounts for resistance of some multiply-exposed individuals to HIV-1 infection. Cell 86:367.
88.**Fauci, A.S.** 1988. The human immunodeficiency virus: infectivity and mechanisms of pathogenesis. Science 239:617.
89.**Pantaleo, G. et al.** 1993. New concepts in the immuno-pathogenesis of human immunodeficiency virus infection. N. Engl. J. Med. 328:327.
90.**Fauci, A.S.** 1992. Multifactorial nature of human immunodeficiency virus disease: implications for therapy. Science 262:1011.
91.**Auger, I. et al.** 1988. Incubation periods for paediatric AIDS patients. Nature 336:575.
92.**Blanche, S. et al.** 1994. Relation of the course of HIV infection in children to the severity of the dis-

ease in their mothers at delivery [see comments]. N. Engl. J. Med. 330:308.
93.**Duliege, A.M. et al.** 1992. Natural history of human immunodeficiency virus type 1 infection in children: prognostic value of laboratory tests on the bimodal progression of the disease. Pediatr. Infect. Dis. J. 11:630.
94.**Galli, L. et al.** 1995. Onset of clinical signs in children with HIV-1 perinatal infection. Italian Register for HIV Infection in Children. AIDS 9:455.
95.**Dickover, R.E. et al.** 1995. Rapid increases in load of human immunodeficiency virus correlate with early disease progression and loss of CD4 cells in vertically infected infants. J. Infect. Dis. 170:1279.
96.**Shrager, L.K. et al.** 1994. Long-term survivors of HIV-1 infection:definitions and research challenges. AIDS Suppl. 8:S95.
97.**Scott, G.B. et al.** 1989. Survival in children with perinatally acquired human immunodeficiency virus type 1 infection. N. Engl. J. Med. 321:1791.
98.**Wade, A.M. et al.** 1992. Age-related standards for T-lymphocyte subsets based on uninfected children born to human immunodeficiency virus 1-infected women. Pediatr. Infect. Dis. J. 11:1018.
99.**CDC Report.** 1996. Persistent lack of detectable HIV-1 antibody in a person with HIV infection. MMWR Morb. Mortal. Wkly. Rep. 45:181.
100.**Alastair, J. and J. Wood.** 1995. Management of occupational exposure to blood-borne viruses. N. Engl. J. Med. 332:443.
101.**Marcus, R.** 1988. Surveillance of health care workers exposed to blood from patients infected with the human immunodeficiency virus. N. Engl. J. Med. 319:1118.
102.**Detels, R. et al.** 1994. Resistance to HIV-1 infection. J. Acquir. Immune Defic. Syndr. 7:1263.
103.**DeGruttola, V. et al.** 1989. Infectiousness of HIV between male homosexual partners. J. Clin. Epidemiol. 42:849.
104.**Prevots, D.R. et al.** 1994. The epidemiology of heterosexually acquired HIV infection and AIDS in Western industrialized countries. AIDS 8:S109.
105.**Taylor, R.** 1994. Quiet clues to HIV-1 immunity: do some people resist infection? J. NIH Res. 6:29.
106.**Bagasra, O. et al.** 1994. Detection of HIV-1 proviral DNA in sperm from HIV-1-infected men. AIDS 8:1669.
107.**Borzy, MS. et al.** 1988. Detection of human immunodeficiency virus in cell-free seminal fluid. J. Acquir. Immune Defic. Syndr. 1:419.
108.**Boeke, I.D. and P. I Stoye.** 1998. Retrotransposons, endogenous retroviruses, and the evolution of retroelements. In J.M. Coffin et al. (Eds.), Retroviruses. Cold Spring Harbor Laboratory Press, Plainview.
109.**Marshall, E.** 1995. Gene therapy's growing pains. Science 269:1050.
110.**Crystal, R.G.** 1995. Transfer of genes to humans: early lessons and obstacles to success. Science 270:404.
111.**Bordignon, C. et al.** 1995. Gene therapy in peripheral blood lymphocytes and bone marrow for ADA-immunodeficient patients. Science 270:470.
112.**Blaese, R.M. et al.** 1995. T lymphocyte-directed gene therapy for ADA- SCID: initial trial results after 4 years. Science 270:475.
113.**Robinson, H.L.** 1978. Inheritance and expression of chicken genes that are related to avian leukosis sarcoma virus genes. Curr. Top. Microbiol. Immunol. 83:1.
114.**Nikiforov, M.A. and A.V. Gudkov.** 1994. ART-CH: a VL30 in chickens? J. Virol. 68:846.
115.**DesGroseillers, L., and P. Jolicoeur.** 1983. Physical mapping of the Fv-1 tropism host range determinant of BALB/c murine leukemia viruses. J. Virol. 48:685.
116.**Ou, C.Y. et al.** 1983. Nucleotide sequences of gag-pol regions that determine the Fv-1 host range property of BALB/c N-tropic and B-tropic murine leukemia viruses. J. Virol. 48:779.
117.**Gardner, M. et al.** 1986. Molecular mechanism of an ecotropic MuLB restriction gene Akvr-1/Fv-4 in Califonia wild mice. Curr. Top. Microbiol. Immunol. 127:338.
118.**Nisini, R. et al.** 1994. Lack of evidence for a superantigen in lymphocytes from HIV-discordant monozygotic twins. AIDS 8:443.
119.**Chang, J. et al.** 1996. Twin studies demonstrate a host cell genetic effect on productive human immunodeficiency virus infection of human monocytes and macrophages in vitro. J. Virol. 70:7792.
120.**Park, C.L. et al.** 1987. Transmission of human immunodeficiency virus from parents to only one dizygotic twin. J. Clin. Microbiol. 25:1119.
121.**Benveniste, R. et al.** 1993. Prior exposure to subinfectious doses of SIV protects macaques from subsequent virus challenge [abstr 81]. 11th Annual Nonhuman Primate Models for AIDS, Madison, WI, September 11–14.
122.**Ho, D.D. and Y. Cao.** 1995. Long-term survivors of human immunodeficiency virus type I infection. N. Engl. J. Med. 332:1647.

123.Deacon, N.J. et al. 1995. Genomic structure of an attenuated quasispecies of HIV-1 from a blood transfusion donor and recipients. Science 270:988.

124.Fultz, P.N. et al. 1990. Humoral response to SIV/SMM infection in macaque and mangabey monkeys. J. Acquir. Immune Defic. Syndr. 3:319.

125.Chakrabarti, L. et al. 1987. Sequence of simian immunodeficiency virus from macaque and its relationship to other human and simian retroviruses. Nature 328:543.

126.Cocchi, F. et al. 1995. Identification of RANTES, MIP-1α and MIP-1β as the major HIV suppressive factors produced by CD8+ T cells. Science 270:1811.

127.Choe, H. et al. 1996. The β-chemokine receptors CCR3 and CCR5 facilitate infection by primary HIV-1 isolates. Cell 85:1135.

128.Alkhatib, G. et al. 1996. CC CKR5: a Rantes, MIP-1α, MIP 1β receptor as a fusion cofactor for macrophage-tropic HIV-1. Science 272:1955.

129.Samson, M. et al. 1996. Resistance to HIV-1 infection in caucasian individuals bearing mutant alleles of CCR-5 chemokine receptor gene. Nature 382:722.

130.Dean, M. et al. 1996. Genetic restriction of HIV-1 infection and progression to AIDS by a deletion allele of the CKR5 structural gene. Science 273:1856.

131.Heilman, C.A. and D. Baltimore. 1998. HIV vaccines—where are we going? Nat. Med. 4:532.

132.Walker, C.M. et al. 1989. CD8-positive T lymphocytes control of HIV replication in cultured CD4-positive cells varies among infected individuals. Cell Immunol. 199:470.

133.Walker, C.M. et al. 1991. Inhibition of human immunodeficiency virus replication in acutely infected CD4+ cells involves a non-cytotoxic mechanism. J. Virol. 65:5921.

134.Bagasra, O. et al. 1993.The role of CD8+ lymphocytes on unstimulated peripheral blood lymphocytes to infection with HIV-1. Immunol. Lett. 35:83.

135.Kannagi, M. et al. 1988. Suppression of simian immuno-deficiency virus replication in vitro by CD8-positive lymphocytes. J. Immunol. 140:2237.

136.Kannagi, M. et al. 1990. Interference with human immunodeficiency virus (HIV) replication by CD8+ T cells in peripheral blood leukocytes of asymptomatic HIV carriers in vitro. J. Virol. 64:3799.

137.Brinchmann, J.E. et al. 1990. CD8+ T cells inhibit HIV-1 replication in naturally infected CD4+ T cells: evidence for a soluble inhibitor. J. Immunol. 144:2961.

138.Walker, C.M. and J.A. Levy. 1989. A diffusible lymphokine produced by CD8-positive T lymphocytes suppresses HIV replication. Immunology 66:628.

139.Walker, C.M. et al. 1991. CD8+ T cells from HIV-1-infected individuals inhibit acute infection by human and primate immunodeficiency viruses. Cell Immunol. 137:420.

140.Lingner, J. et al. 1997. Reverse transcription motifs in the catalutic subunit of telomerase. Science 276:561.

141.San Miguel, P. et al. 1996. Nested retrotransposons in the intergenic regions of the maize genome. Science 274:765.

142.Martin, M.A. et al. 1981. Identification and cloning of endogenous retroviral sequences present in human DNA. Proc. Natl. Acad. Sci. USA 78:4892.

143.Horwitz, M.S. et al. 1992. Novel human endogenous sequences related to human immunodeficiency virus type 1. J. Virol. 66:2170.

144.Curcio, M.J. and M. Belfort. 1996. Retrohoming: cDNA-mediated mobility of group II introns requires a catalytic RNA. Cell 84:9.

145.Moloney, J.B. 1995. The history of retroviruses, p. 237. In G.M. Cooper et al. (Eds.), The DNA Provirus: Howard Temin's Scientific Legacy. ASM Press, Washington, DC.

146.Temin, H.M. 1980. Origin of retroviruses from cellular moveable genetic elements. Cell 121:599.

147.Doolittle, R.F. et al. 1989. Origins and evolutionary relationships of retroviruses. Q. Rev. Biol. 64:1.

148.Xiong, Y. and T.H. Eickbush. 1990. Origin and evolution of retroelements based upon their reverse transcriptase sequences. EMBO J. 9:3353.

149.Eickbush, T.H. 1992. Transposing without ends: the non-LTR retrotransposable elements. New Biologist 4:430.

150.McClure, M.A. 1991. Evolution of retroposons by acquisition or deletion of retrovirus-like genes. J. Biol. Evol. 8:835.

151.McClure, M.A. 1993. Evolutionary history of reverse transcriptase, p. 425. In A.M. Skalka and S.P. Goff (Eds.), Reverse Transcriptase. CSH Laboratory Press, Cold Spring Harbor.

152.McDonald, J.F. 1993. Evolution and consequences of transposable elements. Curr. Opin. Genet. Dev. 3:855.

153.Samuelson, L. et al. 1990. Retroviral and pseudogene insertion sites reveal the lineage of human salivary and pancreatic amylase genes from a single gene during primate evolution. Mol. Cell Biol. 10:2513.

154.Toh, H. et al. 1985. Retroviral gag and DNA endonuclease coding sequences in IgE-binding factor. Nature 318:388.

155.Stavenhagen, J. and D. Robins. 1988. An ancient provirus has imposed androgen regulation on the adjacent mouse sex-limited protein gene. Cell 55:247.

156.Banville, D. and Y. Boie. 1989. Retroviral long terminal repeat is the promoter of the gene encoding the tumor-associated calcium-binding protein oncomodulin in the rat. J. Mol. Biol. 207:481.

157.Bultman, S.J. et al. 1994. Molecular analysis of reverse mutations from nonagouti (a) to black and tan (a′) and white-bellied agouti (AW) reveals alternative forms of agouti transcripts. Genes Dev. 8:481.

158.McClintock, B. 1952. Chromosome organization and genic expression. Cold Spring Harbor Symp. Quant. Biol. 16:13.

159.McClintock, B. 1957. Controlling elements and the gene. Cold Spring Harbor Symp. Quant. Biol. 21:197.

160.Lampson, B.C. et al. 1989. Reverse transcriptase with concomitant ribonuclease H activity in a cell-free system of branched RNA-linked msDNA of Myxococcus xanthus. Cell 56:701.

161.Gessain, A. et al. 1995. Isolation and molecular characterization of a human T-cell lymphotropic virus type II (HTLV-II), subtype B, from a healthy Pygmy living in a remote area of Cameron: an ancient origin for HTLV-II in Africa. Proc. Natl. Acad. Sci. USA 92:4041-4045.

162.Shippen-Lentz, D. and E.H. Blackburn. 1990. Functional evidence for an RNA template in telomerase. Science 247:546.

163.Danilevskaya, O. et al. 1994. Structure of Drosophila HeT-A transposon: a retrotransposon-like element forming telomeres. Chromosoma 103:215.

164.Kennell, J.C. et al. 1993. Reverse transcriptase activity associated with maturase-encoding group II introns in yeast mitochondria. Cell 73:133.

165.Hickey, D.A. et al. 1989. A general model for the evolution of nuclear pre-mRNA introns. J. Theor. Biol. 137:41.

166.Gilbert, W. 1978. Why genes in pieces? Nature 271:501.

167.Mizrokhi, L.J. et al. 1988. Jockey, a mobile Drosophila element similar to mammalian LINEs, is transcribed from the internal promoter by RNA polymerase II. Cell 54:685.

168.Wu, J. et al. 1990. Negative regulation of the human E-globin gene by transcriptional interference: role of an Alu repetitive element. Mol. Cell Biol. 10:1209.

169.Jass, D.H. et al. 1995. Gene conversion as a secondary mechanism of short interspersed element (SINE) evolution. Mol. Cell. Biol. 15:19.

170.Weiner, A.M. and N. Maizels. 1987. tRNA-like structures tag the 3′-ends of genomic RNA molecules for replication: implications for the origin of protein synthesis. Proc. Natl. Acad. Sci. USA 84:7383.

171.Coffin, J.M. 1993. Reverse transcription and evolution, p. 445. In A.M. Skalka and S.P. Goff (Eds.), Reverse Transcriptase. CSH Laboratory Press, Cold Spring Harbor.

172.Hodgson, C.P. 1996. The Retroelements, p. 1. In C.P. Hodgson (Ed.), Retro-Vector for Human Gene Therapy. R.G. Landes Co, New York.

173.Sommerfeld, H.J. et al. 1996. Telomerase activity: a prevalent marker of malignant human prostate tissue. Cancer Res. 56:218.

174.Hiyama, E. et al. 1996. Telomerase activity in human breast tumors. J. Natl. Cancer Inst. 88:116.

175.Kim, N.W. et al. 1994. Specific association of human telomerase activity with immortal cells and cancer. Science 266:2011.

176.Courtney, M.G. et al. 1982. Evidence for an early evolutionary origin and locus polymorphism of mouse VL30 DNA sequences. J. Virol. 43:511.

177.Giri, C.P. et al. 1982. Discrete regions of sequence homology between cloned rodent VL30 genetic elements and AKV-related MuLV provirus genomes. Nucleic Acids Res. 11:305.

178.Vanin, E.F. et al. 1994. Characterization of replication-competent retroviruses from nonhuman primates with virus-induced T-cell lymphomas and observations regarding the mechanisms of oncogenesis. J. Virol. 68:4241.

179.Martin, M.A. et al. 1981. Identification and cloning of endogenous retroviral sequences present in human DNA. Proc. Natl. Acad. Sci. USA 78:4892.

180.Callahan, R. et al. 1985. A new class of endogenous human retroviral genomes. Science 229:1208.

181.Mager, D.L. and J.D. Freeman. 1987. Human endogenous retrovirus-like genome with type C pol sequences and gag sequences related to human T-cell lymphotropic viruses. J. Virol. 61:4060.

182.Hoffenbach, A. et al. 1989. Unusually high frequencies of HIV-1-specific cytotoxic T lymphocytes in humans. J. Immunol. 142:452.

183.Gottlieb, M.S. et al. 1981. Pneumocystis carinii pneumonia and mucosal candidiasis in previously

healthy homosexual men. N. Engl. J. Med. 305:1425.
184.Coffin, J.M. et al. 1986. Human immunodeficiency virus. Science 232:697.
185.Desrosiers, R.C. and N.L. Letvin. 1987. Animal models for acquired immunodeficiency syndrome. Rev. Infect. Dis. 9:438.
186.Hayami, M. and T. Igarashi. 1997. SIV/HIV-1 chimeric viruses having HIV-1 env gene: a new animal model and a candidate for attenuated live vaccine. Leukemia (Suppl. 3) 11:95.
187.Desrosiers, R.C. et al. 1989. Vaccine protection against simian immunodeficiency virus infection. Proc. Natl. Acad. Sci. USA 86:6353.
188.Harper, M.F. et al. 1986. Detection of lymphocytes expressing human T-lymphotropic virus type III in the lymph nodes and peripheral blood from infected individuals by in situ hybridization. Proc. Natl. Acad. Sci. USA 83:772.
189.Bagasra, O. et al. 1992. Detection of human immunodeficiency virus type 1 in mononuclear cells by in situ polymerase chain reaction. N. Engl. J. Med. 326:1385.
190.Wei, X. et al. 1995. Viral dynamics in human immunodeficiency virus type 1 infection. Nature 373:117.
191.Bagasra, O. and R.J. Pomerantz. 1993. HIV-1 provirus is demonstrated in peripheral blood monocytes in vivo: a study utilizing an in situ PCR. AIDS Res. Hum. Retroviruses 9:69.
192.Patterson, B.K. et al. 1993. Detection of HIV-1 DNA and messenger RNA in individual cells by PCR-driven in situ hybridization and flow cytometry. Science 260:976.
193.Embretson, J. et al. 1993. Analysis of human immunodeficiency virus-infected tissues by amplification and in situ hybridization reveals latent and permissive infections at single-cell resolution. Proc. Natl. Acad. Sci. USA 90:357.
194.Embretson, J. et al. 1993. Massive covert infection of helper T lymphocytes and macrophages by HIV during the incubation period of AIDS. Nature 362:359.
195.Patterson, B.K. et al. 1995. Detection of CD4+ T cells harboring human immunodeficiency virus type 1 DNA by flow cytometry using simultaneous immunophenotyping and PCR-driven in situ hybridization: evidence of epitope masking of the CD4 cell surface molecule in vivo. J. Virol. 69:4316.
196.Broder, S. 1988. Pathogenic human retroviruses. N. Engl. J. Med. 318:243.
197.Desrosiers, R.C. et al. 1989. HIV-related lentiviruses of nonhuman primates. AIDS Res. Hum. Retroviruses 5:465.
198.Doolittle, R.F. et al. 1989. Origins and evolutionary relationships of retroviruses. Q. Rev. Biol. 64:1.
199.McClure, M.A. et al. 1988. Sequence comparisons of retroviral proteins: relative rates of change and general phylogeny. Proc. Natl. Acad. Sci. USA 85:2469.
200.Shih, A. et al. 1991. Evolutionary implications of primate endogenous retroviruses. Virology 182:495.
201.Bryant, M.L. et al. 1985. Molecular comparison of retroviruses associated with human and simian AIDS. Hematol. Oncol. 3:187.
202.Callahan, R., D. et al. 1986. Endogenous MMTV proviral genomes in feral Mus musculus domesticus. Curr. Top. Microbiol. Immunol. 1 27:362.
203.Sculte, A.M. et al. 1996. Human trophoblast and choriocarinoma expression of the growth factor pleiotropin attributable to germ-line insertion of an endogenous retrovirus. Proc. Natl. Acad. Sci. USA 93:14759.
204.Herst, H. et al. 1996. Expression of human endogenous retrovirus K elements in germ cell and trophoblastic tumors. Am. J. Pathol. 149:1727.
205.Cohen, J.C. and H.E. Varmus. 1979. Endogenous mammary tumour virus DNA varies among wild mice and segregates during inbreeding. Nature 278:418.
206.Coppola, M.A. and W.R. Green. 1994. Cytotoxic T lymphocyte responses to the envelope proteins of endogenous ecotropic and mink cytopathic focus-forming murine leukemia viruses in H-2B mice. Virology 202:500.
207.Djaffar, I. et al. 1990. Detection of IAP related transcripts in normal and transformed rat cells. Biochem. Biophys. Res. Commun. 169:222.
208.Frisby, D.P. et al. 1979. The distribution of endogenous chicken retrovirus sequences in the DNA of galliform birds does not coincide with avian phylogenetic relationships. Cell 17:623.
209.Ha Lee, Y.M. and J.M. Coffin. 1991. Relationship of avian retrovirus DNA synthesis to integration in vitro. Mol. Cell. Biol. 11:1419.
210.Kukolj, G. et al. 1997. Subcellular localization of avian sarcoma viruses and human immunodeficiency virus type 1 integrases. J. Virol. 71:843.
211.Hardy, W.J., Jr. 1980. Feline leukemia virus disease, p. 3. In W.D. Hardy, Jr. et al. (Eds.), Feline Leukemia Virus. Elsevier/North-Holland, New York.
212.Mathes, L.E. et al. 1978. Abrogation of lymphocyte blastogenesis by a feline leukaemia virus pro-

tein. Nature 274:687.

213.**Hardy, W.J., Jr.** 1980. The virology, immunology and epidemiology of the feline leukemia virus, p. 33. In W.D. Hardy, Jr. et al. (Eds.), Feline Leukemia Virus. Elsevier/North-Holland, New York.

214.**Wooley D.P. et al.** Direct demonstration of retroviral recombination in rhesus monkey. J. Virol. 71:9650.

215.**D'Souza, M.P. et al.** 1993. International collaboration comparing neutralization and binding assays for monoclonal antibodies to simian immunodeficiency virus. AIDS Res. Hum. Retroviruses 9:415.

216.**Bohannon, R.C. et al.** 1991. Isolation of a type D retrovirus from B-cell lymphomas of a patient with AIDS. J. Virol. 65:5663.

217.**Daniel, M.D. et al.** 1984. A new type D retrovirus isolated from macaques with an immunodeficiency syndrome. Science 223:602.

218.**Gardner, M.B. and P.A. Marx.** 1987. Induction of simian acquired immune deficiency syndrome (SAIDS) with a molecular clone of a type D SAIDS retrovirus. J. Virol. 61:3066.

219.**Ilyinskii, P. et al.** 1991. Antibodies to type D retrovirus in talapoin monkeys. J. Gen. Virol. 72:453.

220.**Koo, H.M. et al.** 1992. Reticuloendotheliosis type C and primate type D oncoretroviruses are members of the same receptor interference group. J. Virol. 66:3448.

221.**Krause, H. et al.** 1989. Molecular cloning of a type D retrovirus from human cells (PMFV) and its homology to simian acquired immunodeficiency type D retroviruses. Virology 173:214.

222.**Gravell, M. et al.** 1984. Transmission of simian AIDS with type D retrovirus isolate. Lancet 1:334.

223.**Benveniste, R.E. et al.** 1993. Detection of serum antibodies in Ethiopian baboons that cross-react with SIV, HTLV-I, and type D retroviral antigens. J. Med. Primatol. 22:124.

224.**Benveniste, R.E. et al.** 1993. Long-term protection of macaques against high-dose type D retrovirus challenge after immunization with recombinant vaccinia virus expressing envelope glycoproteins. J. Med. Primatol. 22:74.

225.**Berman, P.W. et al.** 1990. Protection of chimpanzees from infection by HIV-1 after vaccination with recombinant glycoprotein gpl20 but not gpl60. Nature 345:622.

226.**Salk, J. et al.** 1992. A strategy for prophylactic vaccination against HIV. Science 260:1270.

227.**Brody, B.A. et al.** 1992. Protection of macaques against infection with simian type D retrovirus (SRV-1) by immunization with recombinant vaccinia virus expressing the envelope glycoproteins of either SRV-1 or Mason-Pfizer monkey virus (SRV-3). J. Virol. 66:3950.

228.**Maier, D.L. and J.D. Freernan.** 1987. Human endogenous retrovirus like genome with type C pol sequences and gag sequences related to human T-cell lymphotropic viruses. J. Virol. 61:4060.

229.**Ueno, H. et al.** 1983. Frequency and antigenicity of type C retrovirus-like particles in human placentas. Virchows Arch. A Pathol. Anat. Histopathol. 400:31.

230.**Rhee, S.S. and E. Hunter.** 1990. A single amino acid substitution within the matrix protein of a type D retrovirus converts its morphogenesis to that of a type C retrovirus. Cell 63:77.

231.**Stephenson, J.R. et al.** 1976. Immunological cross reactivity of Mason-Pfizer monkey virus with type C RNA viruses endogenous to primates. Nature 261:609.

232.**Todaro, G.J. et al.** 1978. MAC-l, a new genetically transmitted type C virus of primates: "low frequency" activation from stumptail monkey cell cultures. Cell 13:775.

233.**Todaro, G.J. et al.** 1978. Endogenous New World primate type C viruses isolated from owl monkey (Aotus trivirgatus) kidney cell line. Proc. Natl. Acad. Sci. USA 75:1004.

234.**Jerabek, L.B. et al.** 1984. Detection and immunochemical characterization of a primate type C retrovirus-related p30 protein in normal human placentas. Proc. Natl. Acad. Sci. USA 81:6501.

235.**Vencables, J.W. et al.** 1995. Abundance of an endogenous retroviral envelope protein in placental trophoblasts suggests a biological function. Virology 211:589.

236.**Boyd, M.T. et al.** 1993. The human endogenous retrovirus ERV-3 is upregulated in differentiating placental trophoblast cells. Virology 196:905.

237.**Larsson, E. et al.** 1994. Expression of an endogenous retrovirus (ERV3 HERV-R) in human reproductive and embryonic tissues—evidence for a function for envelope gene products. Ups. J. Med. Sci. 99:113.

238.**Lower, R. et al.** 1991. Identification of a rev-related protein by analysis of spliced transcripts of the human endogenous retroviruses HTDV/HERV-K. J. Virol. 69:141.

239.**Benit, L. et al.** 1997. Cloning of a new murine endogenous retrovirus, MuERV-L with strong similarity to the human HERV-L element and with a gag coding sequence closely related to the Fv1. J. Virol. 71:5652.

240.**Goodchild, N.L. et al.** 1993. Recent evolutionary expansion of a subfamily of RTVL-H human endogenous retrovirus-like elements. Virology 96:778.

241.**Guilbert, L. et al.** 1993. The trophoblast as an integral component of a macrophage-cytokine network. Immunol. Cell Biol. 71:49.

242.Wilkinson, D.A. et al. 1993. Autonomous expression of HERV-H endogenous retrovirus-like elements in human cells. J. Virol. 64:2157.
243.Wilkinson, D.A. et al. 1991. Analysis of the DNA-binding and activation properties of human transcription factor AP-2. Genes Dev. 5:670.
244.Johnson, P.M. 1993. Immunobiology of the human placental trophoblast. Exp. Clin. Immunogenet. 10:118.
245.Hirose, Y. et al. 1993. Presence of env genes in members of HERV-H family of human endogenous retrovirus-like elements. Virology 192:52.
246.Johansen, T. et al. 1989. Members of HERV-H family of human endogenous retrovirus-like elements are expressed in placenta. Gene 79:259.
247.Lavine, M.D. and N.E. Beckage. 1995. Polydnaviruses: potent mediators of host insect immune dysfunction. Parasitol. Today 11:368.
248.Frankel, W.N. et al. 1990. A linkage map of endogenous murine leukemia proviruses. Genetics 124:221.
249.Storye, J.P. et al. 1991. Virological events leading to spontaneous AR thymomas. J. Virol. 65:1273.
250.Calarco, P.G. 1979. Intracisternal A particles in preimplantation embryos of feral mice (Mus musculus). Intervirology 11:321.
251.Head, J.R. 1991. Rodent maternal-fetal immune interactions. Curr. Opin. Immunol. 3:767.
252.Lyden, T.W. et al. 1995. Expression of endogenous HIV-1 crossreactive antigens within normal human extravillous trophoblast cells. J. Reprod. Immunol. 28:233.
253.Mwenda, J.M. et al. 1994. A murine monoclonal antibody (RV3-27) raised against isolated human placental endogenous retroviral particles and reactive with syncytiotrophoblast. J. Reprod. Immunol. 26:75.
254.Nilsson, B.O. et al. 1992. Human oocytes express murine retroviral equivalents. Virus Genes 6:221.
255.Ober, C. 1992. The maternal-fetal relationship in human pregnancy: an immunogenetic perspective. Exp. Clin. Immunogenet. 9:1.
256.Prachar, J.A. et al. 1994. Retrovirus like particles produced by human embryonal cells and cell lines derived from human malignancies. Il. Protein structure. Neoplasma 34:129.
257.Sinier, M.F. et al. 1993. LINE-1: a human transposable element. Gene 135:183.
258.Sionov, R.V. et al. 1993. Trophoblasts protect the inner cell mass from macrophage destruction. Biol. Reprod. 49:588.
259.Stewart, C.L. et al. 1992. Blastocyst implantation depends on maternal expression of leukaemia inhibitory factor. Nature 359:76.
260.Branciforte, D. and S.L. Martin. 1994. Developmental and cell type specificity of LINE-1 expression in mouse testis: implications for transposition. Mol. Cell Biol. 14:2584.
261.Huani, T.T.J. and P.G. Calarco. 1981. Immunoprecipitation of intracisternal A-particle-associated antigens from preimplantation mouse embryos. J. Natl. Cancer Inst. 67:1129.
262.Golovkina, T.V. et al. 1990. Distribution of mouse mammary tumor virus-related sequences does not correlate with the taxonomic position of their hosts. Virus Genes 4:85.
263.Imai, S.M. et al. 1994. Distribution of mouse mammary tumor virus in Asian wild mice. J. Virol. 68:3437.
264.Jurka, J. et al. 1995. Ubiquitous mammalian-wide interspersed repeats (MIRs) are molecular fossils from the mesozoic era. Nucleic Acids Res. 23:170.
265.Mietz, J.A. et al. 1987. Nucleotide sequence of a complete mouse intracisternal A- particle genome: relationship to known aspects of particle assembly and function. J. Virol. 61:3020.
266.Papaioannou, V. and R.L. Gardner. 1979. Investigation of the lethal yellow Ay/Ay embryo using mouse chimaeras. J. Embryol. Exp. Morphol. 52:153.
267.Piko, L. et al. 1984. Amounts, synthesis, and some properties of intracisternal A particle-related RNA in early mouse embryos. Proc. Natl. Acad. Sci. USA 81:488.
268.Sorhaui, H. and B. Grinde. 1993. Evolution of mouse mammary tumor virus-related sequences in the human genome. Virus Res. 30:53.
269.Franklin, G.C. et al. 1988. Expression of human sequences related to those of mouse mammary tumor virus. J. Virol. 62:1203.
270.Gardner, M.B. et al. 1994. The simian retroviruses: SIV and SRV, p. 133. In J.A. Levy (Ed.), The Retroviridae, vol 3. Plenum Press, New York.
271.Cichutek, K. and S. Norley. 1993. Lack of immune suppression in SIV-infected natural hosts. AIDS (Suppl) 1:S25.
272.Kestler, H.W. et al. 1988. Comparison of simian immunodeficiency virus isolates. Nature 331:619.
273.Franchini, G. et al. 1987. Sequence of simian immunodeficiency virus and its relationship to the human immunodeficiency viruses. Nature 328:539.

274.Gardner, M.B. and P.A. Luciw. 1992. Simian retroviruses, p. 127. In G.P. Wormser (Ed.), AIDS and Other Manifestations of HIV Infection. Raven Press, New York.
275.Gardner, M.B. et al. 1988. Non-human primate retrovirus isolates and AIDS, p. 171. In I.K. Perk (Ed.), Immunodeficiency Disorders and Retroviruses. Academic Press, New York.
276.Fultz, P.N. et al. 1990. SIVsmm infection of macaque and mangabey monkeys: correlation between in vivo and in vitro properties of different isolates. Dev. Biol. Stand. 72:253.
277.Koralnik, I.J. et al. 1994. Phylogenetic associations of human and simian T-cell leukemia/lymphotropic virus type I strains: evidence for interspecies transmission. J. Virol. 68:2693.
278.Larsson, E. et al. 1989. Human endogenous proviruses. Curr. Top. Microbiol. Immunol. 148:115.
279.Neel, J.V. et al. 1994. Virologic and genetic studies relate Amerind origins to the indigenous people of the Mongolia/Manchuria/southeastern Siberia region. Proc. Natl. Acad. Sci. USA 91:10737.
280.Shaw, G.M. and B.H. Hahn. 1988. Identification of a novel retroviral gene unique to human immunodeficiency virus type 2 and simian immunodeficiency virus SIVmac. J. Virol. 62:3501.
281.Khan, A.S. et al. 1991. SIV of stump-tailed macaque (SIVstm) is a divergent Asian isolate. J. Med. Primatol. 20:167.
282.Shadan, F.F. and L.P. Villarreal. 1996. The evolution of small DNA viruses of eukaryotes: past and present considerations. Virus Genes 11:239.
283.Vandamme, A.M. et al. 1994. Primate T-lymphotropic virus type I LTR sequence variation and its phylogenetic analysis: compatibility with an African origin of PTLV-I. Virology 202:212.
284.Wilkinson, D.A. et al. 1993. Evidence for a functional subclass of the RTVL-H family of human endogenous retrovirus-like sequences. J. Virol. 67:2981.
285.Adachi, A. et al. 1986. Production of acquired immunodeficiency syndrome-associated retrovirus in human and nonhuman cells transfected with an infectious molecular clone, 7. Virology 59:284.
286.Allan, J.S. 1992. Viral evolution and AIDS. J. NIH Res. 4:51.
287.Emau, P. et al. 1991. Isolation from African Sykes' monkeys (Cercopithecus mitis) of a lentivirus related to human and simian immunodeficiency viruses. J. Virol. 65:2135.
288.Norley, S.G. 1996. SIVagm infection of its natural African green monkey host. Immunol. Lett. 51:53.
289.Benjamini, E. et al. 1991. Isolation and characterization of the neutralizable epitope of simian retrovirus-l (SRV-I) and of the cell receptor for the virus. Adv. Exp. Med. Biol. 303:71.
290.Blackbourn, D.J. et al. 1992. Detection of simian immunodeficiency virus RNA from infected rhesus macaques by the polymerase chain reaction. J. Virol. Methods 37:109.
291.Bohm, R.P. Jr. et al. 1993. Neonatal disease induced by SIV infection of the rhesus monkey (Macaca mulatta). AIDS Res. Hum. Retroviruses 9:1131.
292.Daniel, M.D. et al. 1987. Long-term persistent infection of macaque monkeys with the simian immunodeficiency virus. J. Gen. Virol. 68:3183.
293.Daniel, M.D. et al. 1988. Prevalence of antibodies to 3 retroviruses in a captive colony of macaque monkeys. Int. J. Cancer 41:601.
294.Bottinger, D. et al. 1991. Simian immunodeficiency virus (SIVsm) isolation from blood and brain of experimentally infected macaques. AIDS 5:445.
295.Brinkmann, R. et al. 1993. In vitro and in vivo infection of rhesus monkey microglial cells by simian immunodeficiency virus. Virology 195:561.
296.Bryant, M.L. et al. 1986. Immunodeficiency in rhesus monkeys associated with the original Mason-Pfizer monkey virus. J. Natl. Cancer Inst. 77:957.
297.Desrosiers, R.C. 1990. The simian immunodeficiency viruses. Annu. Rev. Immunol. 8:557.
298.Burns, D.P. and R.C. Desrosiers. 1990. Sequence variability of simian immunodeficiency virus in a persistently infected rhesus monkey. J. Med. Primatol. 19:317.
299.Burns, D.P. and R.C. Desrosiers. 1991. Selection of genetic variants of simian immunodeficiency virus in persistently infected rhesus monkeys. J. Virol. 65:1843.
300.Chalifoux, L.V. et al. 1987. Lymphadenopathy in macaques experimentally infected with the simian immunodeficiency virus (SIV). Am. J. Pathol. 128:104.
301.Chen, Z.W. et al. 1992. Predominant use of a T-cell receptor V beta gene family in simian immunodeficiency virus Gag-specific cytotoxic T lymphocytes in a rhesus monkey. J. Virol. 66:3913.
302.Doms, R.W. et al. 1990. Human immunodeficiency virus types 1 and 2 and simian immunodeficiency virus env proteins possess a functionally conserved assembly domain. J. Virol. 64:3537.
303.Grant, S.K. et al. 1991. Purification and biochemical characterization of recombinant simian immunodeficiency virus protease and comparison to human immunodeficiency virus type 1 protease. Biochemistry 30:8424.
304.Grief, C. et al. 1989. The morphology of simian immunodeficiency virus as shown by negative staining electron microscopy. J. Gen. Virol. 70:2215.
305.Colombini, S. et al. 1989. Structure of simian immunodeficiency virus regulatory genes. Proc. Natl.

Acad. Sci. USA 86:4813.

306.Courgnaud, V. et al. 1992. Genetic differences accounting for evolution and pathogenicity of simian immunodeficiency virus from a sooty mangabey monkey after cross-species transmission to a pig-tailed macaque. J. Virol. 66:414.

307.Debouck, C. 1991. Substrate specificity of the human immunodeficiency virus type 1 and simian immunodeficiency virus proteases. Adv. Exp. Med. Biol. 306:407.

308.Henrickson, R.V. et al. 1984. Clinical features of simian acquired immunodeficiency syndrome (SAIDS) in rhesus monkeys. Lab. Anim. Sci. 34:146.

309.McClure, H.M. et al. 1989. Spectrum of disease in macaque monkeys chronically infected with SIV/SMM. Vet. Immunol. Immunopathol. 21:13.

310.Miura, T. et al. 1989. Genetic analysis and infection of SIV_{AGM} and SIV_{MND}. J. Med. Primatol. 18:255.

311.Naidu, Y.M. et al. 1988. Characterization of infectious molecular clones of simian immuno-deficiency virus (SIVmac) and human immunodeficiency virus type 2: persistent infection of rhesus monkeys with molecularly cloned SIVmac. J. Virol. 62:4691.

312.Tristem, M. et. al. 1990. Origin of vpx in lentiviruses [letter]. Nature 347:341.

313.Tristem, M. et al. 1992. Evolution of the primate lentiviruses: evidence from vpx and vpr. EMBO J. 11:3405.

314.Hirsch, V.M. and P.R. Johnson. 1992. Pathogenesis of experimental SIV infection of macaques. Semin. Virol. 3:175.

315.Ciochon, R.L. and A.B. Chiarelli. 1980. Evolutionary Biology of the New World Monkeys and Continental Drift. Plenum Press, New York.

316.Daniel, M.D. et al. 1988. Simian immunodeficiency virus from African green monkeys. J Virol. 62:4123.

317.Henderson, L.E. et al. 1988. Molecular characterization of gag proteins from simian immunodeficiency virus (SIVmne). J. Virol. 62:2587.

318.Henderson, L.E. et al. 1988. Isolation and characterization of a novel protein (x-orf product) from SIV and HIV-2. Science 241:199.

319.Henderson, L.E. et al. 1990. Gag precursors of HIV and SIV are cleaved into six proteins found in the mature virions. J. Med. Primatol. 19:411.

320.Khan, A.S. et al. 1991. A highly divergent simian immunodeficiency virus (SIVstm) recovered from stored stump-tailed macaque tissues. J. Virol. 65:7061.

321.Lerche, N.W. et al. 1986. Inapparent carriers of simian acquired immune deficiency syndrome type D retrovirus and disease transmission with saliva. J. Natl. Cancer Inst. 77:489.

322.Lerche, N.W. et al. 1987. Natural history of endemic type D retrovirus infection and acquired immune deficiency syndrome in group-housed rhesus monkeys. J. Natl. Cancer Inst. 79:847.

323.Lowenstine, L.J. et al. 1992. Evidence for a lentiviral etiology in an epizootic of immune deficiency and lymphoma in stump-tailed macaques (Macaca arctoides). J. Med. Primatol. 21:1.

324.Allan, J.S. et al. 1991. Species-specific diversity among simian immunodeficiency viruses from African green monkeys, J. Virol. 65:2816.

325.Fomsgaard, A. et al. 1991. A highly divergent proviral DNA clone of SIV from a distinct species of African green monkey. Virology 182:397.

326.Johnson, P.R. et al. 1990. Simian immunodeficiency viruses from African green monkeys display unusual genetic diversity. J. Virol. 64:1086.

327.Kanki, P.J. et al. 1986. New human T-lymphotropic retrovirus related to simian T-lymphotropic virus type 111 (STLV-lllagm). Science 232:238.

328.Baier, M. et al. 1989. Molecularly cloned simian immunodeficiency virus SIVagm3 is highly divergent from other SIVagm isolates and is biologically active in vitro and in vivo. J.Virol. 63:5119.

329.Kraus, G. et al. 1989. Isolation of human immunodeficiency virus-related immunodeficiency viruses from African green monkeys. Proc. Natl. Acad. Sci. USA 868:2892.

330.Krohn, K. et al. 1993. Transcomplementation of simian immunodeficiency virus rev with human T-cell leukemia virus type 1 rex. J. Virol. 67:5681.

331.Norley, S.G. et al. 1990. Immunological studies of the basis for the apathogenicity of simian immunodeficiency virus from African green monkeys. Proc. Natl. Acad. Sci. USA 87:9067.

332.Tomonaga, K. et al. 1993. Isolation and characterization of simian immunodeficiency virus from African white-crowned mangabey monkeys (Cercocebus torquatus lunulatus). Arch. Virol. 129:77.

333.Almond, N. et al. 1995. Protection by attennuated simian immunodeficiency virus in macaques against challenge with virus-infected cells. Lancet 345:1342.

334.Tsujimoto, H. et al. 1988. Isolation and characterization of simian immunodeficiency virus from mandrills in Africa and its relationship to other human and simian immunodeficiency viruses. J. Virol.

62:4044.
335.**Henrickson, R.V. et al.** 1984. Simian AIDS: isolation of a type D retrovirus and transmission of the disease. Science 223:1083.
336.**MacKenzie, M.R. et al.** 1986. Pathogenesis of simian AIDS in rhesus macaques inoculated with type D retroviruses. Am. J. Vet. Res. 47:863.
337.**Goldstein, S. et al.** 1990. Detection of SIV antigens by HIV-l antigen capture immunoassays. J. Acquir. Immune Defic. Syndr. 3:98.
338.**Pan, L.Z. et al.** 1991. Lack of detection of human immunodeficiency virus in persistently seronegative homosexual men with high or medium risks for infection. J. Infect. Dis. 164:962.
339.**Soniano, V. et al.** 1990. Silent HIV infection in heterosexual partners of seropositive drug abusers in Spain. Lancet 335:860.
340.**Rowland-Jones, S. et al.** 1993. HIV-1-specific cytotoxic T-cell in an HIV-exposed but uninfected infant. Lancet 341:860.
341.**Higgins, J.R. et al.** 1992. Shared antigenic epitopes of the major core proteins of human and simian immunodeficiency virus isolates. J. Med. Primatol. 21:65.
342.**Jolly, C.J. et al.** 1996. SIVagm incidence over two decades in a natural population of Ethiopian grivet monkeys (Ceropithecs aethiops). J. Med. Primatol. 25:78.
343.**Fine, D.L. and L.O. Arthur.** 1981. Expression of natural antibodies against endogenous and horizontally transmitted macaque retroviruses in captive primates. Virology 112:49.
344.**Haigwood, N.L. et al.** 1992. Characterization of group specific antibodies in primates: studies with SIV envelope in macaques. J. Med. Primatol. 21:82.
345.**Hartung, S. et al.** 1992. Quantitation of a lentivirus in its natural host: simian immunodeficiency virus in African green monkeys. J. Virol. 66:2143.
346.**Kodama, T. et al.** 1989. Prevalence of antibodies to SIV in baboons in their native habitat. AIDS Res. Hum. Retroviruses 5:337.
347.**Kwang, H.S. et al.** 1987. Viremia, antigenemia, and serum antibodies in rhesus macaques infected with simian retrovirus type 1 and their relationship to disease course. Lab. Invest. 56:591.
348.**Lairmore, M.D.** 1990. SIV, STLV-I and type D retrovirus antibodies in captive rhesus macaques and immunoblot reactivity to SIV p27 in human and rhesus monkey sera. AIDS Res. Hum. Retroviruses 6:1233.
349.**Taylor, J.F. et al.** 1972. Kaposi's sarcoma in Uganda: geographic and ethnic distribution. Br. J. Cancer 26:483.
350.**Taylor, J.F. et al.** 1971. Kaposi's sarcoma in Uganda: a clinico-pathological study. Int. J. Cancer 122.
351.**Hutt, M.S.R.** 1984. Kaposi's sarcoma. Br. Med. Bull. 40:355.
352.**Oettle, A.G. et al.** 1962. Geographical and racial differences in the frequency of Kaposi's sarcoma as evidence of environmental or genetic causes. Ann. Acta Int. Contra. Cancer 18:330.
353.**Beral, V.** 1991. Epidemiology of Kaposi's sarcoma. Cancer Surv. 10:5.
354.**Weber, J.** 1984. Is AIDS an epidemic form of African Kaposi's sarcoma? J. R. Soc. Med. 77:572.
355.**Courtois, G. et al.** Preliminary report on mass vaccination of man with live attenuated poliomevlitis virus in the Belgian Congo and Ruanda-Urundi. Br. Med. J. 1958:187..
356.**Zhu, et al.** 1998. An African HIV-1 sequence from 1959 and implications for the origin of the epidemic. Nature 391:594.
357.**Chang, Y. et al.** Sequences in AIDS-associated Kaposi's sarcoma. Science 266:1869.
358.**Said, J.W. et al.** 1997. Kaposi's sarcoma-associated herpesvirus/human herpesvirus type 8 encephalitis in HIV-positive and -negative individuals. AIDS 11:1119.
359.**Broitman, S.L. et al.** 1987. Formation of the triple-stranded polynucleotide helix, poly(A.A.U). Proc. Natl. Acad. Sci. USA 84:5120.
360.**Protozanova, E. and R.B. Macgregor.** 1996. Kinetic footprinting of DNA triplex formation. Anal. Biochem. 243:92.
361.**Doranz, B.J. et al.** 1996. A dual tropic primary HIV-1 isolate that uses Fusin and β-chemokine receptors CKR-5, CKR-3 and CKR-2β as fusion cofactors. Cell 85:1149.
362.**Dragic, T. et al.** 1996. HIV-1 entry into CD4 cells is mediated by the chemokine receptor CC-CKR-5. Nature 381:667.
363.**Feng, Y. et al.** 1996. HIV-1 entry cofactor: functional cDNA cloning of a seven-transmembrane G protein-coupled receptor. Science 272:872.
364.**Cairns, J.S. and M.P. D'Souza.** 1998. Chemokines and HIV-1 second receptors: the therapeutic connection. Nat. Med. 4:563.
365.**Kantor, A.B. and L.A. Herzenberg.** 1993. Origin of murine B cell lineages. Annu. Rev. Immunol. 11:501.
366.**Black, F.L.** 1975. Infectious diseases in primitive societies. Science 187:515.

367.Paulson, H.J. 1987. Tuberculosis in native Americans: indigenous or introduced. Rev. Infect. Dis. 9:1180.

368.Grigg, E.R.N. 1958. The arcana of tuberculosis, III. Epidemiologic history of tuberculosis in the United States. Am. Rev. Tuberc. Pulm. Dis. 78:426.

369.Sharp, W.D. 1983. Prehistoric tuberculosis in the Americas: essay review. Trans. Stud. Coll. Physicians Phila. 5:278.

370.Lerche, N.W. et al. 1984. Epidemiologic aspects of an outbreak of acquired immunodeficiency in rhesus monkeys (Macaca mulatta). Lab. Anim. Sci. 34:146.

371.Sharp, P.M. et al. 1995.Cross-species transmission and recombination of viruses. Philos. Trans. Soc. Lond. Biol. Scil. 349:41.

372.Hirsch, V.M. et al. 1995. Induction of AIDS by simian immunodeficiency virus from an African green monkey: species-specific variation in pathogenicity correlates with the extent of in vivo replication. J. Virol. 69:955.

373.Weigler, B.J. et al. 1990. A cross sectional survey for B virus antibody in a colony of group housed rhesus macaques. Lab. Anim. Sci. 40:257.

374.Kannagi, M. et al. 1986. Humoral immune responses to T cell tropic retrovirus simian T lymphotropic virus type 111 in monkeys with experimentally induced acquired immune deficiency-like syndrome. J. Clin. Invest. 78:1229.

375.Kestler, H. et al. 1989. Use of infectious molecular clones of simian immunodeficiency virus for pathogenesis studies. J. Med. Primatol. 18:305.

376.King, N.W. et al. 1990. Comparative biology of natural and experimental SIVmac infection in macaque monkeys: a review. J. Med. Primatol. 19:109.

377.Letvin, N.L. et al. 1985. Induction of AIDS-like disease in macaque monkeys with T-cell tropic retrovirus STLV-III. Science 230:71.

378.Morton, W.R. et al. 1989. Transmission of the simian immunodeficiency virus SIVmne in macaques and baboons. J. Med. Primatol. 18:237.

379.Fukasawa, M. et al. 1988. Sequence of simian immunodeficiency virus from African green monkey, a new member of the HIV/SIV group. Nature 333:457.

380.Fultz, P.N. 1991. Replication of an acutely lethal simian immunodeficiency virus activates and induces proliferation of lymphocytes. J. Virol. 65:4902.

381.Fultz, P.N. et al. 1986. Isolation of a T-lymphotropic retrovirus from naturally infected sooty mangabey monkeys (Cercocebus atys). Proc. Natl. Acad. Sci. USA 83:5286.

382.Fultz, P.N. et al. 1989. Identification and biologic characterization of an acutely lethal variant of simian immunodeficiency virus from sooty mangabeys (SIV/SMM). AIDS Res. Hum. Retroviruses 5:397.

383.Shibata, R. et al. 1990. Construction and characterization of an infectious DNA clone and of mutants of simian immunodeficiency virus isolated from the African green monkey. J. Virol. 64:307.

384.Vogel, P. 1993. Evidence of horizontal transmission of Pneumocystis carnii pneumonia in simian immunodeficiency virus-infected rhesus macaques. J. Infect. Dis. 168:836..

385.Miller, C.J. et al. 1989. Genital mucosal transmission of simian immunodeficiency virus: animal model for heterosexual transmission of human immunodeficiency virus. J.Virol. 63:4277.

386.Cooper, R. et al. 1989. A lack of evidence of sexual transmission of a simian immunodeficiency agent in a semifree-ranging group of mandrills [letter]. AIDS 3:764.

387.Novembre, F.J. et al. 1991. Molecular diversity of SIVsmm/PBj and a cognate variant, SIVsmm/PGg. J. Med. Primatol. 20:188.

388.Novembre, F.J. et al. 1992. SIV from stump-tailed macaques: molecular characterization of a highly transmissible primate lentivirus. Virology 186:783.

389.Ochs, H.D. 1991. Maternal-fetal transmission of SIV in macaques: disseminated adenovirus infection in an offspring with congenital SIV infection. J. Med. Primatol. 20:193.

390.Otsyula, M. 1996. Prevalence of antibodies against simian immunodeficiency virus (SIV) and simian T-lymphotropic virus (STLV) in a colony of non-human primates in Kenya, East Africa. Ann. Trop. Med. Parasitol. 96:65.

391.Peeters, M. et al. 1989. Isolation and partial characterization of an HIV-related virus occurring naturally in chimpanzees in Gabon. AIDS 3:625.

392.Colebunders, R.L. et al. 1988. Breast feeding and transmission of HIV. Lancet 2:1487.

393.Weinbreck, P. et al. 1988. Postnatal transmission of HIV infection. Lancet 2:482.

394.Stiehm, E.R. and P. Vink. 1991. Transmission of human immunodeficiency virus by breast feeding. J. Pediatr. 118:410.

395.Miller, C.J. et al. 1990. Effect of virus dose and nonoxynol-9 on the genital transmission of SIV in rhesus macaques. J. Med. Primatol. 19:401.

396.Bottiger, D. et al. 1992. Influence of the infectious dose of simian immunodeficiency virus on the acute infection in cynomologus monkeys and on the effect of treatment with 3′-fluorothymidine. Antiviral Chem. Chemother. 3:267.
397.Myers, G. and G.N. Pavlakis. 1992. Evolutionary potential of complex retroviruses, p. 51. In J.A. Levy (Ed.), The Retroviridae, Vol. I. Plenum Press, New York.
398.Myers, G. et al. 1992. The emergence of simian/human immunodeficiency viruses. AIDS Res. Hum. Retroviruses 8:373.
399.Napier, J.R. and P.H. Napier. 1986. The Natural History of the Primates. MIT Press, Cambridge.
400.Baier, M. et al. 1990. Complete nucleotide sequence of a simian immunodeficiency virus from African green monkeys: a novel type of intragroup divergence. Virology 176:216.
401.Baier, M. et al. 1991. Development in vivo of genetic variability of simian immunodeficiency virus. Proc. Natl. Acad. Sci. USA 88:8126.
402.I i, Y. et al. 1989. Genetic diversity of simian immunodeficiency virus. J. Med. Primatol. 18:261.
403.Li, Y. et al. 1989. Extensive genetic variability of simian immunodeficieny virus from African green monkeys. J. Virol. 63:1800.
404.Castro, B.A. et al. 1991. Persistent infection of baboons and rhesus monkeys with different strains of HIV-2. Virology 184:219.
405.Fomsgaard, A. et al. 1993. Genetic variation of the SIVagm transmembrane glycoprotein in naturally and experimentally infected primates. AIDS 7:1041.
406.Johnson, P.R. and V.M. Hirsch. 1992. Genetic variation of simian immunodeficiency viruses in nonhuman primates. AIDS Res. Hum. Retroviruses 8:367.
407. Centers for Disease Control. 1992. Anonymous survey for simian immunodeficiency virus (SIV) seropositivity in SIV-laboratory researchers—United States. MMWR Morb. Mortal. Wkly. Rep. 41:814.
408.Khabbaz, R. et al. 1992. Seroconversion to simian immunodeficiency virus(SIV) in two laboratory workers [abstr 91]. Tenth Annual Symposium on Nonhuman Primate Models for AIDS, Puerto Rico.
409.Pau, C.P. et al. 1992. Simian immunodeficiency virus needlestick accident in a laboratory worker. Lancet 340:271.
410.Khabbaz, R.F. et al. 1994. Brief report: infection of a laboratory worker with simian immunodeficiency virus. N. Engl. J. Med. 330:172.
411.Horowitz, L.G. 1996. Emerging Viruses. Pub. Tetrahedan, Rockport, p. 180.
412.Agy, M.B. et al. 1991. Viral and cellular gene expression in CD4+ human lymphoid cell lines infected by the simian immunodeficiency virus, SIV/Mne. Virology 183:170.
413.Clapham, P.R. et al. 1991. Specific cell surface requirements for the infection of CD4-positive cells by human immunodeficiency virus types 1 and 2 and by simian immunodeficiency virus. Virology 181:703.
414.Firpo, P.P. et al. 1992. Macaque CD4+ T-cell subsets: influence of activation on infection by simian immuno-deficiency viruses (SIV). AIDS Res. Hum. Retroviruses 8:357.
415.Fomsgaard, A. et al. 1992. Cloning and sequences of primate CD4 molecules: diversity of the cellular receptor for simian immunodeficiency virus/human immunodeficiency virus. Eur. J. Immunol. 22:2973.
416.Koenig, S. et al. 1989. Selective infection of human CD4+ cells by simian immuno-deficiency virus: productive infection associated with envelope glycoprotein-induced fusion. Proc. Natl. Acad. Sci. USA 86:2443.
417.Jones, W.C. et al. 1992. Heterogeneity in the recognition of the simian immunodeficiency virus envelope glycoprotein by CD4+ T cell clones from immunized macaques. J. Immunol. 149:3120.
418.McEntee, M.F. et al. 1991. Rhesus monkey macrophages infected with simian immunodeficiency virus cause rapid lysis of CD4-bearing lymphocytes. J. Gen. Virol. 72:317.
419.Watanabe, M. et al. 1989. Effect of recombinant soluble CD4 in rhesus monkeys infected with simian immunodeficiency virus of macaques. Nature 337:267.
420.Werner, A. et al. 1990. Soluble CD4 enhances simian immuno-deficiency virus SIVagm infection. J. Virol. 64:6252.
421.Reinhhardt, V. and A. Roberts. 1997. The African polio vaccine—acquired immune deficiency syndrome connnection. Med. Hypotheses 48:367.
422.Willerford, D.M. et al. 1990. Simian immunodeficiency virus is restricted to a subset of blood CD4+ lymphocytes which includes memory cells. J. Immunol. 144:3779.
423.Zuckerman, A.J. and R.A. Weiss. 1987. HIV infection of primate lymphocytes and conservation of the CD4 receptor. Nature 330:487.
424.Horwitz, M.S. et al. 1992. Novel human endogenous sequences related to human immunodeficiency virus type 1. J. Virol. 66:2170.

425.Hirsch, V.M. et al. 1989. An African primate lentivirus (SIVsm) closely related to HIV-I. Nature 339:389.

426.Cook, S.F. 1946. The incidence and significance of disease among the Aztec and related tribes. Hispanic Am. Historical Rev. 36:320.

427.Piot, P. 1996. A global response. Science 272:1855.

428.Simon, F. et al. 1998. Identification of a new human immunodeficiency virus type 1 distinct from group M and O. Nat. Med. 4:1032.

429.Lohrenz, L.J. et al. 1978. Alcohol problems in several Midwestern homosexual communities. J. Stud. Alcohol 39:1959.

430.Chaisson, R.E. et al. 1989. Cocaine use and HIV infection in intravenous drug users in San Francisco. JAMA 261:561.

431.Stall, R. et al. 1988. A comparison of alcohol and drug use patterns of homosexual and heterosexual men: The San Francisco Men's Health Study. Drug Alcohol Depend. 22:63.

432.Heise, C. et al. 1993. Simian immunodeficiency virus infection of the gastrointestinal tract of rhesus macaques: functional, pathological, and morphological changes. Am. J. Pathol. 142:1759.

433.Heise, C. et al. 1993. Distribution of SIV infection in the gastrointestinal tract of rhesus macaques at early and terminal stages of AIDS. J. Med. Primatol. 22:187.

434.Essex, M. and P.J. Kanki. 1988. The origins of the AIDS virus. Sci. Am. 259:6446.

435.Desrosiers, R.C. 1986. Origin of the human AIDS virus. Nature 319:728.

436.Essex, M. 1994. Simian immunodeficiency virus in people. N. Engl. J. Med. 330:209.

437.Gotch, F. et al. 1993. Cytotoxic T lymphocyte epitopes shared between HIV-l, HIV-2 and SIV. J. Med. Primatol. 22:119.

438.Baba, T.M. et al. 1996. Infection and AIDS in adult macaques after nontraumatic oral exposure to cell-free SIV. Science 272:1486.

439.Curtis, T. 1992. Origin of the AIDS virus. RollingStone Magazine, March 19, p. 55.

440.Lukashov, V.L. et al. 1995. Intrahost human immunodeficiency virus type 1 evolution is related to length of the immunocompetent period. J. Virol. 69:6911.

441.Huminer, D. et al. 1987. AIDS in the preAIDS era. Rev. Infect. Dis. 9:1102.

442.Saxinger, W.C. et al. 1985. Evidence of exposure to HTLV-III in Uganda before 1973. Science *227*:1036.

443.Serwadda, D. et al. 1985. Slim disease: a new disease in Uganda and its association with HTLV-III infection. Lancet *2*:849.

444.Chintu, C. et al. 1995. Childhood cancers in Zambia before and after the HIV epidemic. Arch. Dis. Child. 73:100.

445.Ganeshan, S. et al. 1997. Human immunodeficiency virus type 1 genetic evolution in children with different rates of development of disease. J. Virol. 71:663.

446.Wolinsky, S.M. et al. 1996. Adaptive evolution of human immunodeficiency virus-type 1 during the natural course of infection. Science 272:537.

447.Hirsch, V.M. et al. 1989. SIV adaption to human cells. Nature 341:573.

448.Varmus, H.E. and R. Swanstrom. 1985. Replication of retroviruses, p. 74. In R.Weiss et al. (Eds.), RNA Tumor Viruses, 2nd edition. Cold Spring Harbor Laboratory, Cold Spring Harbor.

449.Luciw, P. and N.J. Leung. 1992. Viral DNA synthesis, p. 51. In J. Levy (Ed.), The Retroviridae. Plenum Press, New York.

450.Gilboa, E. et al. 1979. A detailed model of reverse transcription and tests of crucial aspects. Cell 18:93.

451.Miller, M.D. et al. 1997. Human immunodeficiency virus type 1 preintegration complexes: studies of organization and composition. J. Virol. 71:5382.

452.Dalgleish, A.G. et al. 1984. The CD4 +(T4) antigen is an essential component of the receptor for the AIDS retrovirus. Nature 312:763.

453.Maddon, P.J. et al. 1988. HIV infection does not require endocytosis of its receptor, CD4. Cell 54:865.

454.Bknjouad, A. et al. 1993. N-linked oligosaccharides of simian immunodeficiency virus envelope glycoproteins are dispensable for the interaction with the CD4 receptor. Biochem. Biophys. Res. Commun. 190:311.

455.Zack, J.A. et al. 1990. HIV-1 entry into quiescent primary lymphocytes: molecular analysis reveals a labile, latent viral structure. Cell. 61:213.

456.Stevenson, M. 1997. Molecular mechanisms for the regulation of HIV replication, persistence and latency. AIDS (Suppl. A) 11:25.

457.Bagasra, O. et al. 1993. High percentage of CD4-positive lymphocytes harbor the HIV-1 provirus in the blood of certain infected individuals. AIDS 7:1419.

458.Bukrinsky, M.I. et al. 1991. Quiescent T-lymphocytes as an inducible virus reservoir in HIV-1 infection. Science 254:423.
459.Reyes, R.A. and G.L. Cockerell. 1996. Unintegrated bovine leukemia virus DNA: association with viral expression and disease. J. Virol. 70:4961.
460.Pang, S. et al. 1990. High levels of unintegrated HIV-1 DNA in brain tissue of AIDS dementia patients. Nature 343:85.
461.Pauza, C.D. et al. 1994. 2-LTR circular viral DNA as a marker for human immunodeficiency virus type 1 in vivo. Virology 205:470.
462.Wei, X. et al. 1995. Viral dynamics in human immunodeficiency virus type 1 infection. Nature 373:117.
463.Temin, H.M. and S. Mizutani. 1970. RNA-dependent DNA polymerase in virions of Rous sarcoma virus. Nature 226:1211.
464.Luo, G. and J. Taylor. 1990.Template switching by RT during DNA synthesis. J.Virol. 64:4321.
465.Omer, C.A. et al. 1984. Evidence for involvement of an RNA primer in initiation of strong-stop plus strand DNA synthesis during reverse transcriptase in vitro. J. Virol. 50:465.
466.Ramsey, C.A. and A.T. Panganiban. 1993. Replication of the retroviral terminal repeat sequence during in vivo reverse transcription. J. Virol. 67:4114.
467.Jones, J.S. et al. 1994. One retroviral RNA is sufficient for synthesis of viral DNA. J.Virol. 68:207.
468.Aldovini, H. and B.D. Walker (Eds.). 1990. Techniques in HIV Research. Stockton Press, New York.
469.Whiting, S.H. and J.J. Champoux. 1994. Strand displacement synthesis capability of moloney murine leukemia virus reverse transcriptase. J. Virol. 68:4747.
470.Collin, M. and S. Gordon. 1994. The kinetics of HIV reverse transcription are slower in primary human macrophages than in a lymphoid cell line. Virology 200:114.
471.Bukrinsky, M.I. et al. 1992. Active nuclear import of HIV-1 preintegration complexes. Proc. Natl. Acad. Sci. USA 89:6580.
472.Bukrinsky, M.I. et al. 1993. A nuclear localization signal within HIV-1 matrix protein that governs infection of non-dividing cells. Nature 365:666.
473.Kubo, I. 1997. Abrogation of in vitro suppression of human immunodeficiency virus type 1 (HIV-1) replication mediated by CD8+ T-lymphocytes of asymptomatic HIV-1 carriers by Staphylococcal Enterotoxin B and phorbol ester through induction of tumor necrosis factor alpha. J. Virol. 71:7560.
474.Del Llano, A.M. et al. 1993. The combined assessment of cellular apoptosis, mitochondrial function and proliferative response to pokeweed mitogen has prognostic value in SIV infection. J. Med. Primatol. 22:1.
475.Cullen, B.R. and W.C. Greene. 1989. Regulatory pathways governing HIV-1 replication. Cell 58:423.
476.Sharp, P.A. and R.A. Marciniak. 1989. HIV Tar: an RNA enhancer? Cell 59:229.
477.Jones, K.A. et al. 1986. Activation of the AIDS retrovirus promoter by the cellular transcription factor, Sp1. Science 232:755.
478.Lenardo, M.J. and D. Baltimore. 1989. NF-kB: a pleiotropic mediator of inducible and tissue-specific gene control. Cell 58:227.
479.Nabel, G. and Baltimore, D. 1987. An inducible transcription factor activates expression of human immunodeficiency virus in T cells. Nature 326:712.
480.Gosh, S. et al. 1990. Cloning of the p50 DNA binding subunit of NF-kB: homolog to rel and dorsal. Cell 62:1019.
481.Duh, E.J. et al. 1989. Tumor necrosis factor α activates HIV type 1 through induction of nuclear factor binding to NF-kB sites in the long terminal repeat. Proc. Natl. Acad. Sci. USA 86:5974.
482.Osborn, L. 1989. Tumor necrosis factor α and interleukin 1 stimulate the human immunodeficiency virus enhancer by the activation of the nuclear factor kB. Proc. Natl. Acad. Sci. USA 86:2336.
483.Kieran, M. et al. 1990. The DNA binding subunit of NF-kB is identical to factor KBF1 and homologous to the rel oncogene product. Cell 62:1007.
484.Ghosh, S. and D. Baltimore. 1990. Activation of in vitro of NF-kB by phosphorylation of its inhibitor, IkB. Nature 344:678.
485.Leonard, J.C. et al. 1989. The NF-kB binding sites in the HIV-1 LTR are not required for viral infectivity. J. Virol. 63:4919.
486.Folks, T. et al. 1987. Cytokine induced expression of HIV-1 in a chronically-infected promonocyte cell line. Science 238:800.
487.Gimble, J.M. et al. 1988. Activation of the HIV LTR by herpes simplex virus type 1 is associated with induction of a nuclear factor that binds to the NF-kB/core enhancer sequence. J. Virol. 62:4104.
488.Kim, Y-S. and R. Risser. 1993. TAR-independent transactivation of the murine virus major immediate-early promoter by the Tat protein. J. Virol. 67:239.

489.Barry, P.A. 1990. Molecular interactions between human immunodeficiency virus type 1 and human cytomegalovirus. Ann. N.Y. Acad. Sci. 616:54.

490.Zeichner, S.L. et al. 1991. Linker-scanning mutational analysis of the transcriptional activity of the human immunodeficiency virus type 1 long terminal repeat. J. Virol. 65:2436.

491.Garcia, J.A. et al. 1987. Interactions of cellular proteins involved in the transcriptional regulation of the human immunodeficiency virus. EMBO J. 12:3761.

492.Foon, W. et al. 1988. Alterations in binding characteristics of the human immunodeficiency virus enhancer factor. J. Virol. 62:218.

493.Parrott, C. et al. 1991. Variable role of the long terminal repeat Sp1-binding sites in human immunodeficiency virus replication in T lymphocytes. J. Virol. 65:1414.

494.Ross, E.K. et al. 1991. Contribution of NF-kB and Sp1 binding motifs to the replicative capacity of human immunodeficiency virus type 1: distinct patterns of viral growth are determined by T-cell types. J. Virol. 65:4350.

495.Cullen, B.R. 1990. The HIV-1 Tat protein: an RNA sequence-specific processivity factor? Cell 63:655.

496.Feinberg, M.B. et al. 1991. The role of tat in the human immunodeficiency virus life cycle indicates a primary effect in transcriptional elongation. Proc. Natl. Acad. Sci. USA 88:4045.

497.Braddock, M. et al. 1991. Blocking of tat-dependent HIV-1 RNA modification by an inhibitor of RNA polymerase II processivity. Nature 350:439.

498.Bagasra, O. et al. 1994. CD14 is involved in the control of HIV-1 expression in latently-infected cells by LPS. Proc. Natl. Acad. Sci. USA 89:6285.

499.Taylor, J.P. et al. 1992. Tar-independent transactivation by Tat in cells derived from the CNS: a novel mechanism of HIV-1 gene regulation. EMBO J. *11*:3395.

500.Bagasra, O. et al. 1992. Tar-independent replication of HIV-1 in glial cells. J. Virol. 66:7522.

501.Southgate, C. et al. 1990. Activation of transcriptional by HIV-1 Tat protein tethered to nascent RNA through another protein. Nature 345:640.

502.Berkhout, B. et al. 1989. Tat transactivates the human immunodeficiency virus through a nascent RNA target. Cell 59:273.

503.Roy, S. et al. 1990. A bulge structure in HIV-1 TAR RNA is required for Tat binding and Tat-mediated transactivation. Genes Dev. 4:1365.

504.Dingwall, C. et al. 1990. HIV-1 tat protein stimulated transcription by binding to a U-rich bulge in the stem of the TAR RNA structure. EMBO J. 9:4145.

505.Selby, M.J. and B.M. Peterlin. 1990. Transactivation by HIV-1 TAT via a heterologous RNA binding protein. Cell 62:769.

506.Berkhout, B. and K.-T. Jeang. 1992. Functional roles for the TATA promoter and enhancers in basal and Tat-induced expression of the human immunodeficiency virus type 1 long terminal repeat. J. Virol. 66:139.

507.Gatignol, A. et al. 1991. Characterization of a human TAR RNA-binding protein that activates the HIV-1 LTR. Science 251:1597.

508.Gaynor, B. et al. 1989. Specific binding of a Hela cell nuclear protein to RNA sequences in the human immunodeficiency virus transactivating region. Proc. Natl. Acad. Sci. USA 86:4858.

509.Sheline, C.T. et al. 1991. Two distinct nuclear transcription factors recognize loop and bulge residues of the HIV-1 TAR RNA hairpin. Genes Dev. 5:2508.

510.Marciniak, R.A. et al. 1990. HIV-1 Tat protein transactivates transcription in vivo. Cell 63:791.

511.Marciniak, R.A. et al. 1990. Identification and characterization of a Hela nuclear protein that specifically binds to the transactivation-response (TAR) element of human immuno-deficiency virus. Proc. Natl. Acad. Sci. USA 87:3624.

512.Newstein, M. et al. 1990. Human chromosome 12 encodes a species-specific factor which increases human immunodeficiency virus type 1 tat-mediated transactivation in rodent cells. J. Virol. 64:4565.

513.Harrich, D. et al. 1990. TAR independent activation of the human immunodeficiency virus in phorbol ester stimulated T lymphocytes. EMBO J. 9:4417.

514.Malim, M.H. et al. 1988. Immunodeficiency virus Rev modulates expression of virus regulatory genes. Nature 355:181.

515.Ilyinskii, P.O. et al. 1997. Induction of AIDS by simian immunodeficiency virus lacking NF-kB and SP1 binding elements. J. Virol. 71:1880.

516.Amjad M. and O. Bagasra. 1997. Nature of putative soluble HIV-1 suppressive factors [abstr 100]. 4th Conference on Retroviruses and Related Infections. January 22-26, Washington, DC.

517.Hirsch, M.S. and J.W. Curran. 1996. Human immunodeficiency virus, p. 1953. In B.N. Fields et al. (Eds.), Fields Virology, Lippincott-Raven, Philadelphia.

518.Benveniste, R.E. et al. 1989. Molecular characterization and comparison of simian immunodeficiency virus isolates from macaques, mangabeys, and African green monkeys. J. Med. Primatol. 18:287.

519.Gravell, M. et al. 1989. Infection of macaque monkeys with simian immunodeficiency virus from African green monkeys: virulence and activation of latent infection. J. Med. Primatol. 18:247.

520.Hendry, R.M. et al. 1986. Antibodies to simian immunodeficiency virus in African green monkeys in Africa in 1957-62. Lancet 2:455.

521.Sakakibara, L. et al. 1990. Experimental infection of African green monkeys and cynomolgus monkeys with a SIV_{AGM} strain isolated from a healthy African green monkey. J. Med. Primatol. 19:9.

522.Johnson, P.R. et al. 1990. Molecular clones of SIVsm and SIVagm: experimental infection of macaques and African green monkeys. J. Med. Primatol. 19:279.

523.Shibata, R. et al. 1990. Mutational analysis of simian immunodeficiency virus from African green monkeys and human immunodeficiency virus type 2. J. Med. Primatol. 19:217.

524.Shibata, R. et al. 1990. Generation and characterization of infectious chimeric clones between human immunodeficiency virus type 1 and simian immunodeficiency virus from an African green monkey. J. Virol. 64:5861.

525.Fukasawa, M. et al. 1988. Sequence of simian immunodeficiency virus from African green monkeys, a new member of the HIV/SIV group. Nature 333:457.

526.McKeating, J.A. et al. 1989. Evaluation of human and simian immunodeficiency virus plaque and neutralization assays. J. Gen. Virol. 70:3327.

527.Kent, K.A. et al. 1991. Production of monoclonal antibodies to simian immunodeficiency virus envelope glycoproteins. AIDS 5:829.

528.Kent, K.A. et al. 1992. Identification of two neutralizing and 8 non-neutralizing epitopes on simian immunodeficiency virus envelope using monoclonal antibodies. AIDS Res. Hum. Retroviruses 8:1147.

529.Kirchhoff, F. et al. 1991. Antibody response to the negative regulatory factor (nef) in experimentally infected macaques: correlation with viremia, disease progression, and seroconversion to structural viral proteins. Virology 183:267.

530.Kitagawa, M. et al. 1991. Simian immunodeficiency virus infection of macaque bone marrow macrophages correlates with disease progression in vivo. Am. J. Pathol. 138:921.

531.Ljungdahl-Stahle, E. et al. 1992. Early appearance of simian immunodeficiency virus (SIV) antigen and antibodies as variables in evaluating antiviral drugs in macaques. J. Virol. Methods 37:43.

532.McBride, B. et al. 1993. Comparison of serum antibody reactivities to a conformational and to linear antigenic sites in the external envelope glycoprotein of simian immunodeficiency virus (SIVmac) induced by infection and vaccination. J. Gen. Virol. 74:1033.

533.McEntee, M.F. et al. 1991. Neutralizing antibodies modulate replication of simian immunodeficiency virus SIVmac in primary macaque macrophages. J. Virol. 66:6200.

534.MacKenzie, M. et al. 1986. The hematologic abnormalities in simian acquired immune deficiency syndrome (SAIDS): peripheral blood and bone marrow findings. Lab. Anim. Sci. 36:14.

535.Makoschey, B. et al. 1993. Neutralizing antibodies in SIVmac infected macaques in relation to the course of disease [abstr]. IXth International Conference on AIDS, Berlin.

536.Otteken, A. et al. 1992. Identification of a gag protein epitope conserved among all four groups of primate immunodeficiency vlruses by using monoclonal antibodies. J. Gen. Virol. 73:2721.

537.Samuelsson, A. et al. 1993. Identification of four antibody-binding sites in the envelope proteins of simian immunodeficiency virus SIVsm. AIDS 7:159.

538.Shafferman, A. et al. 1989. Antibody recognition of SIVmac envelope peptides in plasma from macaques experimentally infected with SIV/Mne. AIDS Res. Hum. Retroviruses 5:327.

539.Torres, J.V. et al. 1993. SIV envelope glycoprotein epitopes recognized by antibodies from infected or vaccinated rhesus macaques. J. Med. Primatol. 22:129.

540.Watanabe, M. et al. 1991. Soluble human CD4 elicits an antibody response in rhesus monkeys that inhibits simian immunodeficiency virus replication. Proc. Natl. Acad. Sci. USA 88:120.

541.Zamarchi, R. et al. 1993. In vitro spontaneous production of anti-SIV antibodies is a reliable tool in the follow-up of protection of SIV-vaccinated monkeys. AIDS Res. Hum. Retroviruses 9:1139.

542.Zhang, J.Y. et al. 1988. Simian immunodeficiency virus/delta-induced immunodeficiency disease in rhesus monkeys: relation of antibody response and antigenemia. J. Infect. Dis. 158:1277.

543.Zhang, Y.-J. et al. 1993. Autologous neutralizing antibodies to SIVsm in cynomolgus monkeys correlate to prognosis. Virology 197:609.

544.Liew, F.Y. 1991. Protection in simian immunodeficiency virus-vaccinated monkeys correlates with anti-HLA class I antibody response. J. Exp. Med. 176:1203.

545.Jehuda-Cohen, T. et al. 1991. Transmission of retroviral infection by transfusion of seronegative blood in nonhuman primates. J. Infect. Dis. 163:1223.

546.**Jehuda-Cohen, T. et al.** 1991. Presence of SIV antibodies in the sera of infants born to SIV-seronegative monkeys [letter]. J. Acquir. Immune Defic. Syndr. 4:204.

547.**Anderson, M.G. et al.** 1993. Analysis of envelope changes acquired by SIVmac239 during neuroadaption in rhesus macaques. Virology 195:616.

548.**Joag, S.V. et al.** 1993. Pathogenesis of SIVmac infection in Chinese and Indian rhesus macaques: effects of splenectomy on virus burden. Virology 200:436.

549.**Joag, S.V. et al.** 1993. Antigenic variation of molecularly cloned SIVmac239 during persistent infection in a rhesus macaque. Virology 195:406.

550.**McGraw, T.P. et al.** 1990. Cellular immune response of SIV-infected rhesus macaques. J. Med. Primatol. 19:177.

551.**Popov, J. et al.** 1992. Acute lymphoid changes and ongoing immune activation in SIV infection. AIDS 5:391.

552.**Vowels, B.R. et al.** 1989. Characterization of simian immuno-deficiency virus-specific-mediated cytotoxic response of infected rhesus macaques. AIDS 3:785.

553.**Yamamoto, N.** 1986. Differential susceptibility to the acquired immunodeficiency syndrome retrovirus in cloned cells of human leukemic T-cell line Molt-4. J. Virol. 57:1159.

554.**Polacino, P.S. et al.** 1993. T-cell activation influences initial DNA synthesis of simian immunodeficiency virus in resting T lymphocytes from macaques. J.Virol. 67:7008.

555.**McClure, H.M. et al.** 1990. Nonhuman primate models for evaluation of AIDS therapy. Ann. N. Y. Acad. Sci. 616:287.

556.**McGraw, T.P. et al.** 1990. Simian immunodeficiency virus-specific T-cell-mediated proliferative response of infected rhesus macaques. AIDS 4:191.

557.**Gotch, F.M. et al.** 1991. Cytotoxic T-cell response to simian immunodeficiency virus by cynomolgus macaque monkeys immunized with recombinant vaccinia virus. AIDS 5:317.

558.**Salvato, M.S. et al.** 1994. Cellular immune responses in rhesus macaques infected rectally with low dose simian immunodeficiency virus. J. Med. Primatol.

559.**Kaur, S. et al.** 1997. Cytotoxic T lymphocyte (CTL) immunity to simian immunodeficiency virus (SIV) in sooty mangabeys with natural SIV infection and following experimental infection with SIVmac239 [abstr 731]. 4th Conference on Retroviruses and Related Infections. January 22-26, Washington, DC.

560.**Fultz, P.N. et al.** 1990. Humoral response to SIVsmm infection in macaque and mangabeys. J. Acquir Immune Dedic. Syndr. 3:319.

561.**Beer, B. et al.** 1996. Lack of dichotomy between virus load of peripheral blood and lymph nodes during long-term simian immunodeficiency virus infection in African green monkeys. Virology 219:367.

562.**Hirsch, V.M. et al.** 1995. Induction of AIDS by simian immunodeficiency virus from an African green monkey: species-specific variation in pathogenicity correlates with the extent of in vivo replication. J. Viro. 69:955.

563.**Ochs, H.D. et al.** 1993. Intra-ammiotic inoculation of pigtailed macaque (Macaca nemestrina) fetuses with SIV and HIV-1. J. Med. Primatol. 22:162.

564.**Villinger, F. et al.** 1995. Immunological and virological studies of natural SIV infection of disease-resistant nonhuman primates. Immunol. Lett. 51:59.

565.**Traina-Dorge, V. et al.** 1992. Immunodeficiency and lympho-proliferative disease in an African green monkey dually infected with SIV and STLV-I. AIDS Res. Hum. Retroviruses 8:97.

566.**Ho, D.D. et al.** 1995. Rapid turnover of plasma virions and CD4 lymphocytes in HIV-1 infection. Nature 373:123.

567.**Joag, S.V. et al.** 1997. Animal model of mucosally transmitted human immunodeficiency virus type 1 disease: intravaginal and oral deposition of simian/human immunodeficiency virus in macaques results in systemic infection, elimination of CD4 + T cells, and AIDS. J. Virol. 71:4016.

568.**Marthas, M.L. et al.** 1995. Viral factors determine progression to AIDS in simian immunodeficiency virus-infected newborn rhesus macaques. J. Virol. 69:4198.

569.**Meyer, P.R. et al.** 1985. An immunopathologic evaluation of lymph nodes from monkey and man with acquired immune deficiency syndrome and related conditions. Hematol. Oncol. 3:199.

570.**Racz, P. et al.** 1986. Spectrum of morphologic changes of lymph nodes from patients with AIDS or AIDS-related complexes. Prog. Allergy 37:81.

571.**Wyand, M.S. et al.** 1989. Detection of simian immunodeficiency virus in macaque lymph nodes with a SIVmac envelope probe. J. Med. Primatol. 18:209.

572.**Bagasra, O. et al.** 1993. High percentage of CD4-positive lymphocytes harbor the HIV-1 provirus in the blood of certain infected individuals. AIDS 7:1419.

573.**Miller, C.J. et al.** 1994. Pathology and localization of SIV in the reproductive tract of chronically infected male rhesus macaques. Lab. Invest. 70:255.

574.Bryant, M.L. et al. 1991. Incorporation of 12-methoxydodecanoate into the human immunodeficiency virus 1 gag polyprotein precursor inhibits its proteolytic processing and virus production in a chronically infected human lymphoid cell line. Proc. Natl. Acad. Sci. USA 88:2055.
575.Blackbourn, D.J. et al. 1996. Suppression of HIV replication by lymphoid tissue CD8+ cells correlates with the clinical state of HIV-infected individuals. Proc. Natl. Acad. Sci. USA 93:13123.
576.Nuovo, G.J. et al. 1992. Rapid in situ detection of PCR-amplified-HIV-1 DNA. Diagn. Mol. Pathol. 1:98.
577.Seshamma, T. et al. 1992. A quantitative reverse transcriptase-polymerase chain reaction for HIV-I-specific RNA species. J. Virol. Methods 40:331.
578.Bagasra, O. et al. 1993. Polymerase chain reaction in situ: intracellular amplification and detection of HIV-1 proviral DNA and other specific genes. J. Immunol. Methods 158:131.
579.Haase, A.T. 1986. Pathogenesis of lentivirus infections. Nature 322:130.
580.Embretson, J. et al. 1993. Massive covert infection of helper T lymphocytes and macrophages by HIV during the incubation period of AIDS. Nature 362:359.
581.Mackewicz, C.E. et al. 1995. CD8+ T cells suppress human immuno-deficiency virus replication by inhibiting viral transcription. Proc. Natl. Acad. Sci. USA 92:2308.
582.Powell, J.D. et al. 1993. Inhibition of cellular activation of retroviral replication by CD8+ T cells derived from non-human primates. Clin. Exp. Immunol. 91:473.
583.Chen, C.H. et al. 1993. CD8+ T lymphocyte-mediated inhibition of HIV-1 long terminal repeat transcription: a novel antiviral mechanism. AIDS Res. Hum. Retroviruses 9:1079.
584.Wiviott, L.D. et al. 1990. CD8+ lymphocytes suppress HIV production by autologous CD4+ cells without eliminating the infected cells from culture. Cell. Immunol. 128:628.
585.Jeng, C.R. et al. 1996. Evidence for CD8+ antiviral activity in cats infected with feline immunodeficiency virus. J. Virol. 70:2474.
586.Paliard, X. et al. 1996. RANTES, MIP-1α and MIP-1β are not involved in the inhibition of HIV-1SF33 replication mediated by CD8+ T-cell clones. AIDS 10:1317.
587.Margolick, J.B. et al. 1989. Development of antibodies to HIV-1 is associated with an increase in circulating CD3+ CD4- CD8- lymphocytes. Clin. Immunol. Immunopathol. 51:348.
588.Brinchmann, J.E. et al. 1991. In vitro replication of HIV-1 in naturally infected CD4+ T cells is inhibited by rIFNa2 and by a soluble factor secreted by activated CD8+ T cells, but not by rIFNb, rIFN, or recombinant tumor necrosis factor-a. J. Acquir. Immune Defic. Syndr. 4:480.
589.Agostini, C. et al. 1989. Increased levels of soluble CD8 molecule in the serum of patients with acquired immunodeficiency syndrome (AIDS) and AIDS-related disorders. Clin. Immunol. Immunopathol. 50:146.
590.Reddy, M.M. et al. 1989. Elevated soluble CD8 levels in sera of human immunodeficiency virus-infected populations. J. Clin. Microbiol. 27:257.
591.Pascal, J. et al. 1989. Cell mediated suppression of HIV-specific cytotoxic T lymphocytes. J. Immunol. 143:2193.
592.Pantaleo, G. et al. 1990. Defective clonogenic potential of CD8+ T lymphocytes in patients with AIDS. J. Immunol. 144:1696.
593.Tong, S. et al. 1989. Signaling through T lymphocytes surface proteins, TCR/CD8+ and CD28, activates the HIV-1 long terminal repeat. J. Immunol. 142:702.
594.Henderson, L.A. et al. 1988. Human immunodeficiency virus-induced cytotoxicity for CD8 cells from some normal donors and virus-specific induction of a supressor factor. Clin. Immunol. Immunopathol. 48:174.
595.De Maria, A. et al. 1991. Infection of CD8+ lymphocytes with HIV: requirements for interaction with infected CD4+ cells and induction of infectious virus from chronically infected CD8+ cells. J. Immunol. 146:2220.
596.Kent, S.J. et al. 1996. Detection of simian immunodeficiency virus (SIV)-specific CD8+ T cells in macaques protected from SIV challanged by prior SIV subunits vaccination. J. Virol. 70:4941.
597.Dean, G.A. et al. 1996. Simian immunodeficiency virus infection of CD8+ lymphocytes in vivo. J. Virol. 70:5646.
598.Livingstone, W.J. et al. 1996. Frequent infection of peripheral blood CD8-positive T-lymphocytes with HIV-1. Lancet 348:649.
599.Borrow, P. et al. 1994. Virus-specific CD8+ cytotoxic T-lymphocyte activity associated with control of viremia in primary human immunodeficiency virus type 1 infection. J. Virol. 68:6103.
600.Bouscarat, F. et al. 1996. Correlation of CD8 lymphocyte activation with cellular viremia and plasma HIV RNA levels in asymptomatic patients infected by human immunodeficiency virus type 1. AIDS Res. Hum. Retroviruses 12:17.
601.Yasutomi, Y. et al. 1993. Simian immunodeficiency virus-specific CD8+ lymphocyte response in

acutely infected rhesus monkeys. J. Virol. 67:1707.

602.Rabin, R.L. et al. 1995. Altered representation of naive and memory CD8 T cell subsets in HIV-infected children. J. Clin. Invest. 95:2054.

603.Utz, U. et al. 1996. Analysis of the T-cell receptor repertoire of human T-cell leukemia virus type 1 (HTLV-1) tax-specific CD8+ cytotoxic T lymphocytes from patients with HTLV-1-associated disease: evidence for oligoclonal expansion. J. Virol. 70:843.

604.Copeland, K.F.T. et al. 1996. Suppression of the human immunodeficiency virus long terminal repeat by CD8+ T cells is dependent on the NFAT-1 element. AIDS Res. Hum. Retroviruses 12:143.

605.Thompson, S.A. et al. 1996. Recombinant polyepitope vaccines for the delivery of multiple CD8 cytotoxic T cell epitopes. J. Immunol. 157:822.

606.Shen, L. et al. 1991. Recombinant virus vaccine-induced SIV-specific CD8+ cytotoxic T lymphocytes. Science 252:440.

607.Giorgi, J.V. et al. 1994. CD8+ lymphocyte activation at human immunodeficiency virus type 1 seroconversion: development of HLA-DR+ CD38+ CD8+ cells is associated with subsequent stable CD4+ cell levels. J. Infect. Dis. 170:775.

608.Prince, H. et al. 1989. Preferential loss of Leu 8-, CD45R-, HLA-DR+ CD8 cell subsets during in vitro culture of mononuclear cells from human immunodeficiency virus type I (HIV)-seropositive former blood donors. J. Clin. Immunol. 9:421.

609.Rubbert, A. et al. 1997. Multifactorial nature of noncytolytic CD8+ T cell-mediated suppression of HIV replication: b-chemokine-dependent and -independent effects. AIDS Res. Hum. Retroviruses 13:63.

610.Copeland, K.F.T. et al. 1997. CD8+ T cell supernatants of HIV type 1-infected individuals have opposite effects on long terminal repeat-mediated transcription in T cells and monocytes. AIDS Res. Hum. Retroviruses 13:71.

611.Franco, M.A. et al. 1997. Evidence for CD8+ T-cell immunity to murine rotavirus in the absence of perforin, Fas, and gamma interferone. J. Virol. 71:479.

612.Rosok, B. et al. 1997. CD8+ T cells from HIV type 1-infected seronegative individuals suppress virus replication in acutely infected cells. AIDS Res. Hum. Retroviruses 13:79.

613.Zhang, C. et al. 1996. Protective immunity to HIV-1 in SCID/beige mice reconstituted with peripheral blood lymphocytes of exposed but uninfected individuals. Proc. Natl. Acad. Sci. USA 93:14720.

614.Murphey-Corb, M. et al. 1989. A formalin-inactivated whole SIV vaccine confers protection in macaques. Science 246:1293.

615.Fult, P.N. et al. 1992. Vaccine protection of chimpanzees against challenge with HIV-1-infected peripheral blood mononuclear cells. Science 256:1687.

616.Miller, C.J. et al. 1997. Rhesus macaques previously infected with simian/human immunodeficiency virus are protected from vaginal challenge with pathogenic SIV_{239}. J. Virol. 71:1911.

617.Heeney, J.L. et al. 1994. Vaccine protection and reduced virus load from heterologous macaque-propagated SIV challenge. AIDS Res. Hum. Retroviruses (Suppl) 10:S117.

618.Wyand, M.S. et al. 1996. Vaccine protection by a triple deletion mutant of simian immunodeficiency virus. J. Virol. 70:3724.

619.Warren, J.T. et al. 1995. Fourth annual survey of worldwide HIV, SIV, and SHIV challenge studies in vaccinated nonhuman primates. J. Med. Primatol. 24:150.

620.Carlson, J.R. et al. 1990. Vaccine protection of rhesus macaques against simian immunodeficiency virus infection. AIDS Res. Hum. Retroviruses 6:1239.

621.Gardner, M.B. and S.L. Hu. 1991. SIV vaccines, 1991—A year in review. AIDS (Suppl.) 21:S115.

622.Gardner, M.B. and J. Stott. 1990. Progress in development of SIV vaccines: a review. AIDS (Suppl.) 11:S137.

623.Gardner, M. et al. 1992. SIV and FIV vaccine studies at UC Davis: 1991 update. AIDS Res. Hum. Retroviruses 8:1495.

624.Putkonen, P. et al. 1997. Protection of human immunodeficiency virus type 2-exposed seronegative macaques from mucosal simian immunodeficiency virus transmission. J. Virol. 71:4981.

625.Hartung, S. et al. 1992. Vaccine protection against SIVmac infection by high- but not low-dose whole inactivated virus immunogen. J. Acquir. Immune Defic. Syndr. 5:461.

626.Heeney, J.L. et al. 1991. Comparison of protection from homologous cell-free vs cell-associated SIV challenge afforded by inactivated whole SIV vaccines. J. Med. Primatol. 21:126.

627.Hilleman, M.R. 1992. Historical and contemporary perspectives in vaccine developments: from the vantage of cancer. Prog. Med. Virol. 39:1.

628.Haigwood, N.L. et al. 1992. Inactivated whole-virus vaccine derived from a proviral DNA clone of simian immunodeficiency virus induces high levels of neutralizing antibodies and confers protection against heterologous challenge. Proc. Natl. Acad. Sci. USA 89:2175.

629.Lewis, M.G. et al. 1993. Passively transferred antibodies directed against conserved regions of SIV envelope protect macaques from SIV infection. Vaccine 11:1347.
630.Luke, W. and G. Hunsmann. 1993. Protection of monkeys by a split vaccine against SIVmac depends upon biological properties of the challenge virus. AIDS 7:787.
631.Marx, P.A. et al. 1986. Prevention of simian acquired immune deficiency syndrome with a formalin-inactivated type D retrovirus vaccine. J. Virol. 60:431.
632.Marx, P.A. et al. 1993. Protection against vaginal SIV transmission with microencapsulated vaccine. Science 260:1323.
633.Murphey-Corb, M. et al. 1989. A formalin-inactivated whole SIV vaccine confers protection in macaques. Science 246:1293.
634.Murphey-Corb, M. et al. 1990. A formalin inactivated whole SIV vaccine and a glycoprotein-enriched subunit vaccine confers protection against experimental challenge with pathogenic live SIV in rhesus monkeys. Dev. Biol. Stand. 72:273.
635.Murphey-Corb, M. et al. 1992. A formalin-fixed whole SIV vaccine induces protective responses that are cross-protective and durable. AIDS Res. Hum. Retroviruses 8:1475.
636.Nishino, Y. et al. 1992. Major core proteins, p24s, of human, simian, and feline immunodeficiency viruses are partly expressed on the surface of the virus-infected cells. Vaccine 10:677.
637.Israel, Z.R. et al. 1993. Early pathogenesis of disease caused by SIVsmmPBj14 molecular clone 1.9 in macaques. AIDS Res. Hum.Retroviruses 9:277.
638.Redfield, R.R. and D.L. Birx. 1992. HIV-specific vaccine therapy: concepts, status, and future directions. AIDS Res. Hum. Retroviruses 8:1051.
639.Shafferman, A. et al. 1991. Protection of macaques with a simian immunodeficiency virus envelope peptide vaccine based on conserved human immunodeficiency virus type I sequences. Proc. Natl. Acad. Sci. USA 88:7126.
640.Shafferman, A. et al. 1993. Prevention of transmission of simian immunodeficiency virus from vaccinated macaques that developed transient virus infection following challenge. Vaccine 11:848.
641.Shen, L. et al. 1991. Recombinant virus vaccine-induced SIV-specific CD8+ cytotoxic T lymphocytes. Science 252:440.
642.Stott, E.J. et al. 1990. Preliminary report: protection of cynomolgus macaques against simian immunodeficiency virus by fixed infected-cell vaccine. Lancet 336:1538.
643.Mossman, S.P. et al. 1996. Protection against lethal simian immunodeficiency virus SIVsmmPBj14 disease by a recombinant Semliki Forest virus gp160vaccine and by a gp120 subunit vaccine. J. Virol. 70:1953.
644.Lu, X. et al. 1998. Targeted lymph-node immunization with whole inactivated simian immunodeficiency virus (SIV) or envelope and core subunit antigen vaccines does not reliably protect rhesus macaques from vaginal challenge with SIVmac251. AIDS 12:1
645.Thapar, M.A. et al. 1991. Secretory immune responses in the mouse vagina after parenteral or intravaginal immunization with an immunostimulating complex (SCOM). Vaccine 9:129.
646.Wyand, M.S. 1992. The use of SIV-infected rhesus monkeys for the preclinical evaluation of AIDS drugs and vaccines. AIDS Res. Hum. Retroviruses 8:349.
647.Clerici, M. et al. 1991. Immunization with subunit HIV vaccines generates stronger T helper cell immunity than natural infection. Eur. J. Immunol. 21:1345.
648.Le Grand, R. et al. 1992. Specific and non-specific immunity and protection of macaques against SIV infection. Vaccine 10:873.
649.Mestecky, J. 1987. The common mucosal immune system and current strategies for induction of immune responses in external secretions. J. Clin. Immunol. 7:265.
650.Lehner, T. et al. 1992. Induction of mucosal and systemic immunity to a recombinant simian immunodeficiency viral protein. Science 258:1365.
651.Miller, C.J. et al. 1993. Biology of disease: mucosal immunity, HIV transmission, and AIDS. Lab. Invest. 68:129.
652.Montefiori, D.C. et al. 1990. Complement-mediated, infection-enhancing antibodies in plasma from vaccinated macaques before and after inoculation with live simian immunodeficiency virus. J. Virol. 64:5223.
653.Cole, K.S. et al. 1997. Evolution of envelope-specific antibody responses in monkeys experimentally infected or immunized with simian immunodeficiency virus and its association with the development of protective immunity. J. Virol. 71:5069.
654.Shibata, R. et al. 1997. Live, attenuated simian immunodeficiency virus vaccines elicit resistance against a challenge with human immunodeficiency virus type1 chimeric virus. J. Virol. 71:8141.
655.Robinson, W.E., Jr. and W.M. Mitchell. 1990. Neutralization and enhancement of in vitro and in vivo HIV and simian immunodeficiency virus infections. AIDS Suppl. 11:S15.

656.Allan, I.S. et al. 1990. Enhancement of SIV infection with soluble receptor molecules. Science 247:1084.

657.Le Grand, R. et al. 1991. Antibody-dependent enhancement and neutralization pattern of sera from SIV-infected or HIV-2-vaccinated rhesus monkeys. J. Med. Primatol. 20:172.

658.Daar, E.S. et al. 1990. High concentrations of recombinant soluble CD4 are required to neutralize primary human immunodeficiency virus type 1 isolates. Proc. Natl. Acad. Sci. USA 87:6574.

659.Reimann, K.A. et al. 1993. In vivo administration to rhesus monkeys of a CD4-specific monoclonal antibody capable of blocking AIDS virus replication. AIDS Res. Hum. Retroviruses 9:199.

660.Salk, J. 1987. Prospects for the control of AIDS by immunizing seropositive individuals. Nature 327:473.

661.Clerici, M. et al. 1989. Interleukin-2 production used to detect antigenic peptide recognition by T-helper lymphocytes from asymptomatic HIV-seropositive individuals. Nature 339:383.

662.Clerici, M. et al. 1991. HIV-1 exposure indicated by HIV-specific T helper cell responses before detection of infection by polymerase chain reaction and serum antibodies. J. Infect. Dis. 164:178.

663.Clerici, M. et al. 1989. Detection of three distinct patterns of T helper cell dysfunction in asymptomatic, human immunodeficiency virus seropositive patients: independence of CD4+ cell numbers and clinical staging. J. Clin. Invest. 84:1892.

664.Clerici, M. et al. 1991. Detection of cytotoxic T lymphocytes specific for synthetic peptides of gp160 in HIV-seropositive individuals. J. Immunol. 146:2214.

665.Clerici, M. and G.M. Shearer. 1993. A TH1 to TH2 switch is a critical step in the etiology of HIV infection. Immunol. Today 14:107.

666.Clerici, M. et al. 1996. Chemokine production in HIV-seropositive long-term asymptomatic individuals [correspondence]. AIDS 10:1432.

667.Wahren, B. et al. 1987. Characteristics of the specific cell-mediated immune response in human immunodeficiency virus infection. J. Virol. 61:2017.

668.Joly, P. et al. 1989. Cell-mediated supression of HIV-specific cytotoxic T lymphocytes. J. Immunol. 143:2193.

669.Romagnani, S. et al. 1994. Role of TH1/TH2 cytokines in HIV infection. Immunol. Rev. 140:73.

670.Liu, S.-L. et al. 1997. Divergent patterns of progression to AIDS after infection from the same source: human immunodeficiency virus type 1 evolution and antiviral responses. J. Virol. 71:4284.

671.Lemaitre, F. 1997. No evidence for a shift from a Th1 to a Th2-type response in HIV infection: analysis of IL-2,IL-4 and IFN-g production at cellular level in peripheral blood lymphocytes [abstr 342]. 4th Conference on Retroviruses and Related Infections. January 22–26, Washington, DC.

672.Cardo, M. et al. 1997. A case control study of HIV-1 seroconversion in health care workers after percutaneous exposure. N. Engl. J. Med. 337:1485.

673.Koup, R.A. et al. 1994. Temporal association of cellular immune responses with the initial control of viremia in primary human immunodeficiency virus type 1 syndrome. J. Virol. 68:4650.

674.Luzuriaga, K. et al. 1993. Early viremia and immune responses in vertical human immunodeficiency virus type 1 infection. J. Infect. Dis. 167:1008.

675.Jurriaana, S. et al. 1994. The natural history of HIV-1 infection: virus load and virus phenotype independent determinants of clinical course. J. Clin. Invest. 204:223.

676.Spira, A. and D.D. Ho. 1995. Effect of different donor cells on human immunodeficiency virus type 1 replication and selection in vitro. J. Virol. 69:422.

677.Mattecucci, D. et al. 1996. Vaccination protects against in vivo-grown feline immunofecifiency virus even in the absence of detectable neutrilization antibodies. J. Virol. 70:617.

678.Lang, S.M. et al. 1997. Association of simian immunodeficiency virus Nef with cellular serine/ threonine kinases is dispensable for the development of AIDS in rhesus macaques. Nat. Med. 3:860.

679.Bryson, Y.J. et al. 1995. Clearance of HIV infection in a perinatally infected infant. N. Engl. J. Med. 332:833.

680.Rouges, P.A. et al. 1995. Clearance of HIV infection in 12 perinatally infected children: clinical, virological and immunological data. AIDS 9:19.

681.Baur, A. et al. 1989. Continuous clearance of HIV in a vertically infected child. Lancet 2:1045.

682.Kestler, H.W., III, et al. 1991. Importance of the nef gene for maintenance of high virus loads and/or development of AIDS. Cell 65:651.

683.Huang, Y. et al. 1995. Characterization of nef sequences in long term survivors of human immunodeficiency virus type 1 infection. J. Virol. 69:93.

684.Kirchhoff, F. et al. 1995. Brief report: absence of intact nef sequences in a long term survivor with non progressive HIV-1 infection. N. Engl. J. Med. 332:228.

685.Barker, E. et al. 1995. Effects of TH1 and TH2 cytokines on CD8+ cell response against human immunodeficiency virus: implications for long-term survival. Proc. Natl. Acad. Sci. USA 92:11135.

686.Lifson, A.R. et al. 1991. Long term human immunodeficiency virus infection in asymptomatic homosexual and virological characteristics. J. Infect. Dis. 163:959.
687.Buchbinder, S.P. et al. 1994. Long term HIV-1 infection without immunologic progression. AIDS 8:1123.
688.Bagnarelli, P. et al. 1992. Molecular profile of human immunodeficiency virus type 1 infection in symptomless patients and in patients with AIDS. J. Virol. 66:7328.
689.Ali, M. et al. 1996. No evidence of antibody to human foamy virus in widespread human populations. AIDS Res. Hum. Retroviruses 12:1473.
690.Gardner, M.B. 1996. Simian retrovirus vaccines: simian retrovirus and simian immunodeficiency lentivirus. AIDS Res. Hum. Retroviruses 12:399.
691.Fultz, P.N. et al. 1990. Prevalence of natural infection with simian immunodeficiency virus and simian T-cell leukemia virus type 1 in a breeding colony of sooty mangabey monkeys. AIDS 4:619.
692.Marx, P.A. et al. 1991. Isolation of a simian immunodeficiency virus related to human immunodeficiency virus type 2 from a west African pet sooty mangabey. J. Virol. 65:4480.
693.Legrand, E. et al. 1997. Course of specific T lymphocyte cytotoxicity, plasma and cellular viral loads, and neutralizing antibody titers in 17 recently seroconverted HIV type 1 infected patients. AIDS Res. Hum. Retroviruses 13:1383.
694.Franchini, G. et al. 1987. Genetic analysis of a new subgroup of human and simian T-lymphotropic retroviruses: HTLV-IV, LAV-2, SBL-6669, and STLV-lllagm. AIDS Res. Human Retroviruses 3:11.
695.Schnittman, S.M. et al. 1990. Increasing viral burden in CD4 and T cells from patients with HIV infection reflects rapidly progressive immunosuppression and clinical disease. Ann. Int. Med. 113:438.
696.Lewis, M.G. et al. 1992. Infection of rhesus and cynomolgus macaques with a rapidly fatal SIV (SIVsmmjPBj) isolate from sooty mangabeys. AIDS Res. Hum. Retroviruses 8:1631.
697.Binninger, D. et al. 1991. Mutational analysis of the simian immunodeficiency virus SIVmac nef gene. J. Virol. 65:5237.
698.Dewhurst, S. et al. 1992. Molecular clones from a non-acutely pathogenic derivative of SIVsmmPBjl4: Characterization and comparison to acutely pathogenic clones. AIDS Res. Hum. Retroviruses 8:1179.
699.Gardner, M.B. et al. 1993. Immune response of rhesus macaques to recombinant SIVgpl30 does not protect from challenge infection. J. Virol. 67:577.
700.Hirsch, V.M. et al. 1990. Molecular characterization of SIV in tissues from experimentally infected macaques. J. Med. Primatol. 19:287.
701.Thouless, M.E. and M.G. Katze. 1990. Inoculation of Macaca fascicularis with simian immunodeficiency virus, SIVmne immunologic, serologic, and pathologic changes. J. Med. Primatol. 19:367.
702.Mayne, A. et al. 1993. Quantitative differences in the levels of IL-2 and IFN-gamma produced by PBMC of naturally SIV infected sooty mangabeys and rhesus macaques experimentally infected with SIV [abstr]. 11th Annual Symposium on Nonhuman Primate Models for AIDS, Madison, WI.
703.Novembre, F. et al. 1993 Multiple viral determinants contribute to pathogenicity of the acutely lethal simian immunodeficiency virus SIVsmmPBj variant. J. Virol. 67:2466.
704.Rosenberg, Y.J. et al. 1991. Variation in T-lymphocyte activation and susceptibility to SIVPBj-14-induced acute death in macaques. J. Med. Primatol. 20:206.
705.Rosenberg, Y.J. et al. 1993. Decline in the CD4+ lymphocyte population in the blood of SIV-infected macaques is not reflected in lymph nodes. AIDS Res. Hum. Retroviruses 9:639.
706.Torres, J.V. et al. 1993. An epitope on the surface envelope glycoprotein (gp 130) of simian immunodeficiency virus (SIVmac) involved in viral neutralization and T cell activation. AIDS Res. Hum. Retroviruses 9:423.
707.Venet, A. et al. 1992. Cytotoxic T lymphocyte response against multiple simian immunodeficiency virus (SIV) proteins in SIV-infected macaques. J. Immunol. 148:2899.
708.Voss, G. and G. Hunsmann. 1993. Cellular immune response to SIVmac and HIV-2 in macaques: model for the human HIV- I infection. J. Acquir. Immune Defic. Syndr. 6:969.
709.Voss, G. et al. 1992. Potential significant of the cellular immune response against the macaque strain of simian immunodeficiency virus (SIVMAC) in immunized and infected rhesus macaques. Gen. Virol. 73:2273.
710.Veugelers, P.J. et al. 1994. Increasing age is associated with faster progression to neoplasms but not opportunistic infections in HIV-infected homosexual men. AIDS 8:1471.
711.Baskerville, A. et al. 1992. Pathological changes in the reproductive tract of male rhesus monkeys associated with age and simian AIDS. J. Comp. Pathol. 107:49.
712. Report of Consensus Workshop, Siena, Italy, Jan. 17-18, 1992. Maternal factors involved in mother to child transmission of HIV-1. J. Acquir. Immun. Defic. Syndr. 5:1019.
713.Yang, S.Y. et al. 1988. Differential in vitro activation of CD8-CD4+ and CD4-CD8+ T lymphocytes

by combinations of anti-CD2 and anti-CD3 antibodies. J. Immunol. 140:2115.

714.Miller, M.D. et al. 1992. Vaccination of rhesus monkeys with synthetic peptide in a fusogenic proteoliposome elicit simian immunodeficiency virus-specific CD8+ cytotoxic T lymphocytes. J. Exp. Med. 176:1739.

715.Knuchel, M. et al. 1994. Biphasic in vitro regulation of retroviral replication by CD8+ cells from non human primates. J. Acquir. Immune Defic. Syndr. 7:438.

716.Bouscarat, F. et al. 1996. Correlation of CD8 lymphocyte activation with cellular viremia and plasma HIV RNA levels in asymptomatic patients infected by human immunodeficiency virus type 1. AIDS Res. Hum. Retroviruses 12:17.

717.Sonza, S. et al. 1996. Human immunodeficiency virus type-1 replication is blocked prior to reverse transcription and integration in freshly isolated peripheral blood monocytes. J. Virol. 70:3863.

718.Zanussi, S. et al. 1996. Serum levels of RANTES and MIP-1α in HIV-positive long-term survivors and progressor patients [correspondence]. AIDS 10:1431.

719.Mackewicz, C.E. 1996. Role of β-chemokines in suppressing HIV replication. Science 274:1393.

720.Chen, Y. and P. Gupta. 1996. CD8+ T-cell-mediated suppression of HIV-1 infection may not be due to chemokines RANTES, MIP-1α and MIP-1β [correspondence]. AIDS 10:1434.

721.Blazevic, V. et al. 1996. RANTES, MIP and interleukin-16 in HIV infection [correspondence]. AIDS 10:1435.

722.Moriuchi, H. et al. 1996. CD8+ T-cell-derived soluble factor(s), but not β-chemokines RANTES, MIP-1α, and MIP-1β, suppress HIV-1 replication in monocyte/macrophages. Proc. Natl. Acad. Sci. USA 93:15341.

723.Biti, R. et al. 1997. HIV-1 infection in an individual homozygous for the CCR5 deletion allele. Nat. Med. 3:252.

724.Smith, O. 1997. HIV CCR5 resistance incomplete. Nat. Med. 3:372.

725.Mosoian, A. et al. 1997. Differential effects of recombinant RANTES, MIP 1\α and MIP 1\β compared to CD8+ supernatants on HIV-1 infection of primary macrophages [abstr 421]. 4th Conference on Retroviruses and Opportunistic Infection, Washington, DC.

726.Sachs, L. 1962. Transplantability of an X-ray-induced and a virus-induced leukemia in isologous mice inoculated with a leukemia virus. J. Natl. Cancer Res. 29:759.

727.Frucht, D.M. et al. 1991. Ultraviolet radiation increases HIV-long terminal repeat-directed expression in transgenic mice. AIDS Res. Hum. Retroviruses 7:729.

728.Klinman, D.M. et al. 1992. Effect of cyclophosphamide, total irradiation, and zidovudine on retrovirus proliferation and disease progression in murine AIDS. AIDS Res. Hum. Retroviruses 8:101.

729.Marx, P.A. et al. 1996. Progesterone implants enhance SIV vaginal transmission and early virus load. Nature Med. 2:1084.

730.Plourde, P.J. and F.A. Plummer. 1994. Oral contraceptives and the risk of HIV among hetrosexual women in Nairobi, p. 107. In A. Nicolosi (Ed.), HIV Epidemiology: Models and Methods. Raven Press, New York.

731.DiRienzo, A.M. et al. 1992. Modulation of cell growth and host protein synthesis during HIV infection in vitro. J. Acquir. Immune Defic. Syndr. 5:921.

732.Bagasra, O. and D. Tabor. 1986. Irradiation and cyclophosphamide induced alterations in Syrian hamsters T-cell population activity. J. Leukoc. Biol. 39:183.

733.Ho, W. et al. 1990. Reciprocal enhancement of gene expression and viral replication between human cytomegatovirus and human immunodeficiency virus type 1. J. Gen. Virol. 71:97.

734.McNally, T. et al. 1997. Interactions between HIV and hepatitis B virus in homosexual men: effects on the natural history of infection. AIDS 11:597.

735.Lathey, J.L. et al. 1994. Human cytomegalovirus-mediated enhancement of human immunodeficiency virus type 1 production in monocyte-derived macrophages. Virology 199:98.

736.Koval, V. et al. 1995. Differential effects of human cytomegalovirus on integrated and unintegrated human immunodeficiency virus sequences. J.Virol. 69:1645.

737.Tan, S.V. et al. 1993. Herpes simplex type 1 encephalitis in acquired immunodeficiency syndrome. Ann. Neurol. 34:619.

738.Liang, G.S. et al. 1993. An evaluation of oral ulcers in patients with AIDS and AIDS-related complex. J. Am. Acad. Dermatol. 29:563.

739.Choudhury, S.A. et al. 1994. Cutaneous herpes simplex virus infection in a child with acquired immunodeficiency syndrome. Clin. Pediatr. 33:698.

740.O'Brien, W.A. et al. 1995. HIV-1 replication can be increased in peripheral blood of seropositive patients following influenze vaccination. Blood 86:1082.

741.Smith, I.W. et al. 1980. Altered immunity in male patients with alcoholic liver disease: evidence for defective immune regulation. Alcoholism 4:199.

742.**Israelstam, S. and S. Lambert.** 1986. Homosexuality and alcohol: observations and research after the psychoanalytic era. Int. J. Addict. 21:509.
743.**Abrams, D.I.** 1986. Lymphadenopathy related to the acquired immunodeficiency syndrome in homosexual men. Med. Clin. North Am. 70:693.
744.**Bagasra, O. et al.** 1995. Do alcohol and other substance of abuse alter the natural evolution of and the susceptibility to human immunodeficiency virus type-1 infection? In R. Watson (Ed.), Alcohol, Drugs of Abuse, and Immune Function. CRC Press, New York.
745.**Avins, A.L. et al.** 1994. HIV infection and risk behaviors among heterosexuals in alcohol treatment programs. JAMA 7:515.
746.**Fong, I.W. et al.** 1994. Alcoholism and rapid progression to AIDS after seroconversion. Clin. Infect. Dis. 19:337.
747.**Mahler, J. et al.** 1994. Undetected HIV infection among patients admitted to an alcohol rehabilitation unit. Am. J. Psychiatry 151:439.
748.**Bagasra, O. et al.** 1987. Effects of alcohol ingestion on in vitro susceptibility of peripheral blood mononuclear cells to infection with HIV-1 and on selected T-cell functions. Alcohol. Clin. Exp. Res. 13:636.
749.**Bagasra, O. et al.** 1993. Alcohol intake increases human immunodeficiency virus type 1 replication in human peripheral blood mononuclear cells. J. Infect. Dis. 168:789.
750.**Bagasra, O. et al.** 1993. Increased HIV-1 replication in peripheral blood mononuclear cells in the presence of cocaine. J. Infect. Dis. 168:1157.
751.**Peterson, P.K. et al.** 1990. Morphine promotes the growth of HIV-1 in human peripheral blood mononuclear cell cocultures. AIDS 4:869.
752.**Bagasra, O. et al.** 1993. Increased HIV-1 replication in peripheral blood mononuclear cells in the presence of cocaine. J. Infect. Dis. 168:1157.
753.**Bagasra, O. et al.** 1993. Mechanisms of increased HIV-1 replication after exposure to cocaine and alcohol: prospect for molecular immunity, p. 683. In R.P. Watson (Ed.), Alcohol, Drugs and Immunomodulations in AIDS. Pergamon Press, New York.
754.**Des Jarlais, D.C. and S.R. Freidland.** 1988. Intravenous cocaine, crack and HIV-1 infection. JAMA 3259:1945.
755.**Bacchetti, P. et al.** 1989. Cocaine use and HIV-1 infection in intravenous drug users in San Francisco. JAMA 261:561.
756.**Sterk, C.** 1988. Cocaine and HIV-1 seropositivity. Lancet 1:1052.
757.**Peterson, P.K. et al.** 1991. Cocaine potentiates HIV-1 replication in human PBMC co-cultures. J. Immunol. 146:81.
758.**Zaretsky, M.D.** 1995. AZT toxicity and AIDS prophylaxis: is AZT beneficial for HIV+ asymptomatic persons with 500 or more T4 cells per cubic millimeter? Genetica 95:91.
759.**Mellors, J.W. et al.** 1996. Prognosis in HIV-1 infection predicted by the quantity of virus in plasma. Science 272:1167.
760.**Goedert, J.J.** 1997. Vertical transmission of human immunodeficiency virus type 1: insights from studies of multiple pregnancies. Acta Paediatr. Suppl. 421:56.
761.**Duliege, A.M. et al.** 1995. Birth order, delivery route, and concordance in the transmission of human immunodeficiency virus type 1 from mother infected twins with discordant disease courses. J. Pediatr. 126:625.
762.**Chang, J. et al.** 1996. Twin studies demonstrate a host cell genetic effect on productive human immunodeficiency virus infection of human monocytes and macrophages in vitro. J. Virol. 70:7792.
763.**Hutto, C. et al.** 1996. Longitudinal studies of viral sequence, viral phenotype, and immunologic parameters of human immunodeficiency virus type 1 infection in perinatally infected twins with discordant disease courses. J. Virol. 70:3589.
764.**Bex, F. et al.** 1994. Syngeneic adoptive transfer of anti-human immunodeficiency virus (HIV-1)-primed lymphocytes from a vaccinated HIV-seronegative individual to his HIV-1-infected identical twin. Blood 84:3317.
765.**Watson, A. et al.** 1997. Plasma viremia in macaques infected with simian immunodeficiency virus: plasma viral load early in infection predicts survival. J. Virol. 71:284.
766.**Siliciano, R.F. et al.** 1988. Analysis of host-virus interactions in AIDS with anti-gp120 T cell clones. Effect of HIV-1 sequence variation and a mechanism for CD4+ cell depletion. Cell 54:561.
767.**Chun, T.W. et al.** 1997. Presence of an inducible HIV-1 latent reservoir during highly active antiretrovial therapy. Proc. Nat. Acad. Sci. USA 94:13193.
768.**Fowke, K.R. et al.** 1997. Immunologic and virologic evaluation after influenza vaccination of HIV-1-infected patients. AIDS 11:1013.
769.**Tseng, C.K. et al.** 1991. Syphilis superinfection activates expression of human immunodeficiency

virus I in latently infected rabbits. Am. J. Pathol. 138:1149.

770.**Hibbs, J.R. et al.** 1997. Prevalence of human immunodeficiency virus infection, mortality rate, and serogroup distribution among patients with pneumococcal bacteremia at Denver General Hospital. Clin. Infect. Dis. 25:195.

771.**Best, S. et al.** 1996. Positional cloning of the mouse retrovirus restriction gene Fv1. Nature 382:826.

772.**Lilly, F. and T. Pincus.** 1973. Mouse leukemia: a model of a multiple-gene disease. Adv. Cancer Res. 17:231.

773.**Benit, L.** 1997. Cloning of a new murine endogenous retrovirus, MuERV-L, with strong similarity to the human HERV-L element and with a gag coding sequence closely related to the Fv1 restriction gene. J. Virol. 71:5652.

774. **Kozak, C.A. and A. Chakraborti.** 1996. Single amino acid changes in the murine leukemia virus capsid protein gene define the target of Fv1 resistance. Virology 225:300.

775.**Jolicoeur, P. and D. Baltimore.** 1975. Effect of the Fv-1 locus on the titration of murine leukemia viruses. J. Virol. 16:153.

776.**Goff, S.P.** 1996. Operating under a Gag order: a block against incoming virus by the Fv-1 gene. Cell 86:691.

777.**Wong, J.K. et al.** 1997. Recovery of replication-competent HIV despite prolonged suppression of plasma viremia. Science 278:1291.

778.**Bagasra, O. et al.** 1992. Detection of human immunodeficiency virus type 1 in mononuclear cells by in situ polymerase chain reaction. N. Engl. J. Med. 326:1385.

779.**Bouziane, M. et al.** 1996. Alternate strand DNA triple helix-mediated inhibition of HIV-1 U5 long terminal repeat integration in vitro. J. Biol. Chem. 271:10359.

780.**Bagasra, O. and M. Amjad.** 1997. Natural immunity against HIV-1: Prospect for AIDS vaccine. Front. Biosci. 2:387-402.

781.**Tsukahara, S. et al.** 1996. Inhibition of HIV-1 replication by triple-helix-forming phosphorothioate oligonucleotides targeted to the polypurine tract. J. Biomol. Struct. Dyn. 13:835.

782.**Putkonen, P. et al.** 1989. Experimental infection of cynomolgus monkeys (Macaca fascicularis) with HIV-2. J. Acquir. Immune Defic. Syndr. 2:359.

783.**Putkonen, P. et al.** 1992. Clinical features and predictive markers of disease progression in cynomolgus monkeys experimentally infected with simian immunodeficiency virus. AIDS 6:257.

784.**Gulizia, J.M.P. et al.** 1994. Reduced nuclear import of human immunodeficiency virus type 1 preintegration complexes in the presence of a prototypic nuclear targeting signal. J. Virol. 68:2021.

785.**Prakash, K. et al.** 1992. Generation of deletion mutants of simian immunodeficiency virus incapable of proviral integration. J. Virol. 66:167.

786.**Reyes, R.A. and G.L. Cockerell.** 1996. Unintegrated bovine leukemia virus DNA: association with viral expression and diseases. J. Virol. 70:4961.

787.**Donahue, R.E. et al.** 1992. Helper virus induced T-cell lymphomas in nonhuman primates after retroviral mediated gene transfer. J. Exp. Med. 176:1125.

788.**Pauza, C.D. et al.** 1994. 2-LTR circular viral DNA as a marker for human immunodeficiency virus type 1 infection in vivo. Virology 205:470.

789.**Kukolj, G. et al.** 1997. Subcellular localization of avian sarcoma virus and human immunodeficiency virus type 1 integrases. J. Virol. 71:843.

790.**Purcell, D.F.J. et al.** 1996. An array of murine leukemia virus-related elements is transmitted and expressed in a primate receipient of retroviral gene transfer. J. Virol. 70:887.

791.**Rey-Cullie, M-A. et al.** 1998. Simian immunodeficiency virus replication to high levels in sooty mangabeys without inducing disease. J. Virol. 72:3872.

792.**Feichtinger, H. et al.** 1990. Malignant lymphomas in cynomolgus monkeys infected with simian immunodeficiency virus. Am. J. Pathol. 137:1311.

793.**Rademakers, L.H.P.M. and H.-J. Schuurman.** 1992. Simian immunodeficiency virus (SIVsm) infection of cynomolgus monkeys: effects on follicular dendritic cells in lymphoid tissue. AIDS Res. Hum. Retroviruses 8:2021.

794.**Kaaya, E. et al.** 1993. Accessory cells and macrophages in the histopathology of SIVsm-infected cynomolgus monkeys. Res. Virol. 144:81.

795.**Dittmer, M.T. et al.** 1997. Biological charaterization of human immunodeficiency virus type 1 clones derived from different organs of an AIDS patient by long-range PCR. J. Virol. 71:5140.

796.**Cann, A.J. and I.S.Y. Chen.** 1996. Human T-cell leukemia virus type I and II, p. 1849. In B. Fields et al. (Eds.), Fields Virology, Vol. 2. Lippincott-Raven, Philadelphia.

797.**Chen, I.S.Y. et al.** 1983. Molecular characterization of the genome of a novel human T-cell leukemia virus. Nature 305:502.

798.**Hjelle, B. et al.** 1991. Incidence of hairy cell leukemia, mycosis fungoides, and chronic lymphocytic

leukemia in first known HTLV-II endemic population. J. Infect. Dis. 163:435.
799.Beilke, M.A. et al. 1994. Laboratory study of HIV-1 and HTLV-I/II coinfection. J. Med. Virol 44:132..
800.Beilke, M.A. et al. 1992. Detection of HTLV-1 in clinical speciments. J. Virol. Methods. 40:133.
801.Sarr, A.D. et al. 1998. HIV-1 and HIV-2 dual infection: lack of HIV-2 provirus correlates with low CD4+ lymphocyte counts. AIDS 12:131.
802.Bottiger, D. et al. 1992. Prevention of HIV-2 and SIV infections in cynomolgus macaques by prophylactic treatment with 3′-fluorothymidine. AIDS Res. Hum. Retroviruses 8:1235.
803.Durand, J.P. et al. 1995. Increased risk for a second retroviral infection (SIV or STLV type 1) for wild African green monkeys already infected by one retrovirus in Senegal (West Africa). AIDS Res. Hum. Retroviruses 11:985.
804.Mariani, R. et al. 1996. High frequency of defective nef alleles in a long-term survivor with nonprogressive human immunodeficiency virus type 1 infection. J. Virol. 70:7752.
805.Baba, T.W. et al. 1995. Attenuated retrovirus vaccines and AIDS. Science 270:1218.
806.Kanki, P. et al. 1992. Prevalence and risk determinants of human immunodeficiency virus type 2 (HIV-2) and human immunodeficiency virus type 1 (HIV-1) in West African female prostitutes. Am. J. Epidemiol. 136:895.
807.Cavaco-Silva, P. et al. 1998. Virological and molecular demonstration of human immunodeficiency virus type 2 vertical transmission. J. Virol. 72:3418.
808.Bagasra, O. et al. 1993. Frequency of cells positive for HIV-1 sequences assessed by IS-PCR. AIDS Suppl. 7:S7.
809.Wolthers, K.C. et al. 1998. Rapid CD4+ T-cell turnover in HIV-1 infection: a paradigm revisited. Immunol. Today 19:44.
810.Nowak, M.A. et al. 1997. Anti-viral drug treatment: dynamics of resistance in free virus and infected cell populations. J. Theor. Biol. 184:203.
811.Pakker, N.G. et al. 1997. Patterns of T-cell repopulation, virus load reduction, and restoration of T-cell function in HIV-infected persons during therapy with different antiretroviral agents. J. Acquir. Immune Defic. Syndr. Hum. Retrovirol. 16:318.
812.Kootstra, N.A. et al. 1997. Analysis of CD8+ T lymphocyte-mediated nonlytic suppression of autologous and hetrologous primary human immunodeficiency virus type 1 isolates. AIDS Res. Hum. Retroviruses 13:685.
813.Pollack, H. et al. 1997. CD8+ T-cell-mediated suppression of HIV replication in the first year of life: association with lower viral load and favorable early survival. AIDS 11:9.
814.Mellors, J.W. 1997. Plasma viral load and CD4+ lymphocytes as prognostic markers of HIV-1 infection. Ann. Intern. Med. 126:946.
815.Sepkowitz, K.A. 1998. Effect of HAART on natural history of AIDS-related opportunistic disorders. Lancet 35:228.
816.Williams, A.B. 1997. New horizons: antiretroviral therapy in 1997. J. Assoc. Nurses AIDS Care 8:26.
817.Coffin, J.M. 1996. HIV viral dynamics. AIDS (Suppl 10) 3:75.
818.Finzi, D. et al. 1997. Identification of a reservoir for HIV-1 in patients on highly active antiretroviral therapy. Science 278:1295.
819.Perrin, L. and A. Telenti. 1998. HIV treatment failure: testing for HIV resistance in clinical practice. Science 280:1871.
820.Kaufmann, D. et al. 1998. CD4-cell count in HIV 1 infected individuals remaining viraemic with highly active antiretroviral therapy (HAART). Swiss HIV Cohort Study. Lancet 351:723.
821.Bloom, F.E. 1996. Breakthrough of the year. Science 274:1987.
822.Fiala, A.M. et al. 1996. Divergent effects of cocaine on cytokine production by lymphocytes and monocyte/macrophages: HIV-1 enhancement by cocaine within the blood-brain barrier. Adv. Exp. Med. Biol. 402:145.
823.Drew, P.A. et al. 1984. Polyclonal B cell activation in alcoholic patients with no evidence of liver dysfunction. Alcoholism 57:479.
824.Adams, H.G. and C. Jordon. 1989. Infection in the alcoholics. Med. Clin. North. Am. 68:179.
825.Bailey, R.J. et al. 1979. Histocompatibility antigens, autoantibodies and immunoglobulins in alcoholic liver disease. Br. Med. J. 2:727.
826.Kilby, J.M. et al. 1997. Effects of tapering doses of oral prednisone on viral load among HIV-infected patients with unexplained weight loss. AIDS Res. Hum. Retroviruses 13:1533.
827.Balla, A.K. et al. 1994. Human studies on alcohol and susceptibility to HIV infection. Alcohol 11:99.
828.Cole, S.W. and M.E. Kemeny. 1997. Psychobiology of HIV infection. Crit. Rev. Neurobiol. 11:289.
829.Yang, Y. and R.R. Watson. 1994. Chronic ethanol consumption before retrovirus infection is a cofactor in the development of immune dysfunction during murine AIDS. Alcohol Clin. Exp. Res.

18:976.
830.Margolick, J.B. et al. 1989. Development of antibodies to HIV-1 is associated with an increase in circulating CD3+ CD4- CD8-lymphocytes. Clin. Immunol. Immunopathol. 51:348.
831.Kaslow, R.A. et al. 1989. No evidence for a role of alcohol or other psychoactive drugs in accelerating immunodeficiency in HIV-1-positive individuals. JAMA 261:3424.
832.Eyster, M.E. et al. 1987. Natural history of human immunodeficiency virus infections in hemophiliacs: effects of T-cell subsets, platelet counts and age. Ann. Intern. Med. 107:1.
833.Bagasra, O. et al. 1996. Increased HIV-1 replication in human peripheral blood mononuclear cells induced by ethanol: potential immuno-pathologic mechanisms. J. Infect. Dis. 173:550.
834.Bagasra, O. et al. 1987. Functional analysis of T-cell subsets in chronic alcoholism. Immunology 61:63.
835.Williams, L.M. et al. 1992. Polymorphic human gene determines differential susceptibility of CD4 lymphocytes to infection by certain HIV-1 isolates. Virology 184:723.
836.Saksela, K. et al. 1994. Human immunodeficiency virus type 1 mRNA expression in peripheral blood cells predicts disease progression independently of the numbers of CD4+ lymphocytes. Proc. Natl. Acad. Sci. USA 91:1104.
837.Donahoe, R.M. et al. 1986. Coordinate and independent effects of heroin, cocaine and alcohol abuse on T-cell E-rosette formation and antigenic marker expression. Clin. Immunol. Immunopathol. 41:254.
838.Ginzburg, H.M. et al. 1985. HTLV-III exposure among drug users. Cancer Res. (Suppl.) 45:4605.
839.Marmor, M. et al. 1985. Risk factors for Kaposi's sarcoma in homosexual men. Lancet 1:1082.
840.Bigger, R.J. et al. 1984. Low T-lymphocyte ratios in homosexual men. JAMA 251:1441.
841.Havas, H.F. et al. 1987. Effect of cocaine on the immune response and host resistance in Balb/c mice. Int. Arch. Allergy Appl. Immunol. 83:377.
842.Van Dyke, C. et al. 1986. Cocaine increases natural killer cell activity. J. Clin. Invest. 77:1387.
843.Ou, D.W. et al. 1989. Effects of cocaine on the immune system of Balb/c mice. Clin. Immunol. Immunopathol. 52:305.
844.Peterson, P.K. et al. 1987. Opioid-mediated suppression of interferon-gamma production by cultured peripheral blood mononuclear cells. J. Clin. Invest. 80:824.
845.Shapshak, et al. 1997. Cocaine and cocaethelene accelerate HIV progression in African American women [abstr 488]. 4th Conference on Retroviruses and Opportunistic Infection, location?.
846.Bagasra, O. and L.J. Forman. 1989. Functional analysis of lymphocyte subpopulations in experimental cocaine abuse. I. Dose dependent activation of lymphocyte subsets. Clin. Exp. Immunol. 77:289.
847.Burns, D.N. et al. 1997. Influence of other maternal variables on the relationship between maternal virus load and mother-to-infant transmission of human immunodeficiency virus type 1. J. Infect. Dis. 175:1206.
848.Nair, M.P. et al. 1994. Selective effect of alcohol on cellular immune responses of lymphocytes from AIDS patients. Alcohol 11:85.
849.Caiaffa, W.T. et al. 1994. Drug smoking, Pneumocystis carinii pneumonia, and immunosuppression increase risk of bacterial pneumonia in human immunodeficiency virus-seropositive injection drug users. Am. J. Respir. Crit. Care Med. 150:1493.
850.Seage, G.R., III et al. 1992. The relation between nitrite inhalants, unprotected receptive anal intercourse, and the risk of human immunodeficiency virus infection. Am. J. Epidemiol. 135:1.
851.Shibata, R. et al. 1990. Generation and characterization of infectious chimeric clones between human immunodeficiency virus type 1 and simian immunodeficiency virus from an African Green Monkey. J. Virol. 64:5861.
852.Shibata, R. et al. 1992. SIV/HIV recombinants and their use in studying biological properties. AIDS Res. Hum. Retroviruses 8:403.
853.Li, J. et al. 1992. Infection of cynomolgus monkeys with a chimeric HIV-1/SIVmac virus that expresses the HIV-1 envelope glycoproteins. J. Acquir. Immune Defic. Syndr. 5:639.
854.Levy, J. et al. The Retroviridae, Vol 3. Plenum Press New York, NY 1994.
855.Robertson, D.L. et al. 1995. Recombination in HIV-1. Nature 374:124.

Index

Q

R

S

T

V

Y

Z

Omar Bagasra was born in India in 1948, the son of Muslim refugees who eventually settled in Pakistan. When war broke out between India and Pakistan in 1965, he volunteered for the Pakistani Army, and his interest in medical studies led him to be trained as a medical corpsman. At the end of the war he turned his attention to the study of Buddhism in a monastery in Tibet. After two years of Lamaistic study, he chose to pursue a more scientific understanding of nature.

He earned a bachelor's and a master's degree in biochemistry at the University of Karachi; by 1979, he earned his PhD in microbiology and immunology and completed his post-doctoral training in infectious diseases at the University of Louisville, KY.

Dr. Bagasra studied medicine for two years at the Universidad Autónoma in Ciudad Juarez, Mexico, and completed his clinical medical education at Temple University. He held an Associate Professorship at Hahnemann University and served as Professor and the Director of Molecular Retrovirology Laboratories and the Section Chief of Molecular Diagnostics and the AIDS Clinical Trial Group Immunology Laboratory at the Center for the Study of Human Viruses at Thomas Jefferson University.

Dr. Bagasra is recognized internationally for his invention of the in situ PCR technique, by which a single copy of a gene can be amplified inside a single intact cell. This technique has become uniquely important in the investigation of a large number of infectious and pathologic conditions in situ. He was recently awarded two separate international patents for this technique.

Dr. Bagasra has long been interested in the study of human retroviral pathogenesis. Utilizing the in situ PCR technique and other approaches, he has published on the levels of HIV-1 infection in various cell types. These studies have been critical in the development of our understanding of in vivo pathogenesis of this retrovirus, and his papers are cited widely. In addition, his work on cofactors that affect HIV-1 expression, including molecular effects of cocaine and alcohol on CD8 T-lymphocytic function, has demonstrated the unique effects of environmental agents on the natural history of HIV-1 and its variable course in certain patients.

Dr. Bagasra's dedication to his work has resulted in over 150 scientific articles, books, and book chapters, and he is invited to speak at scientific conferences throughout the world.

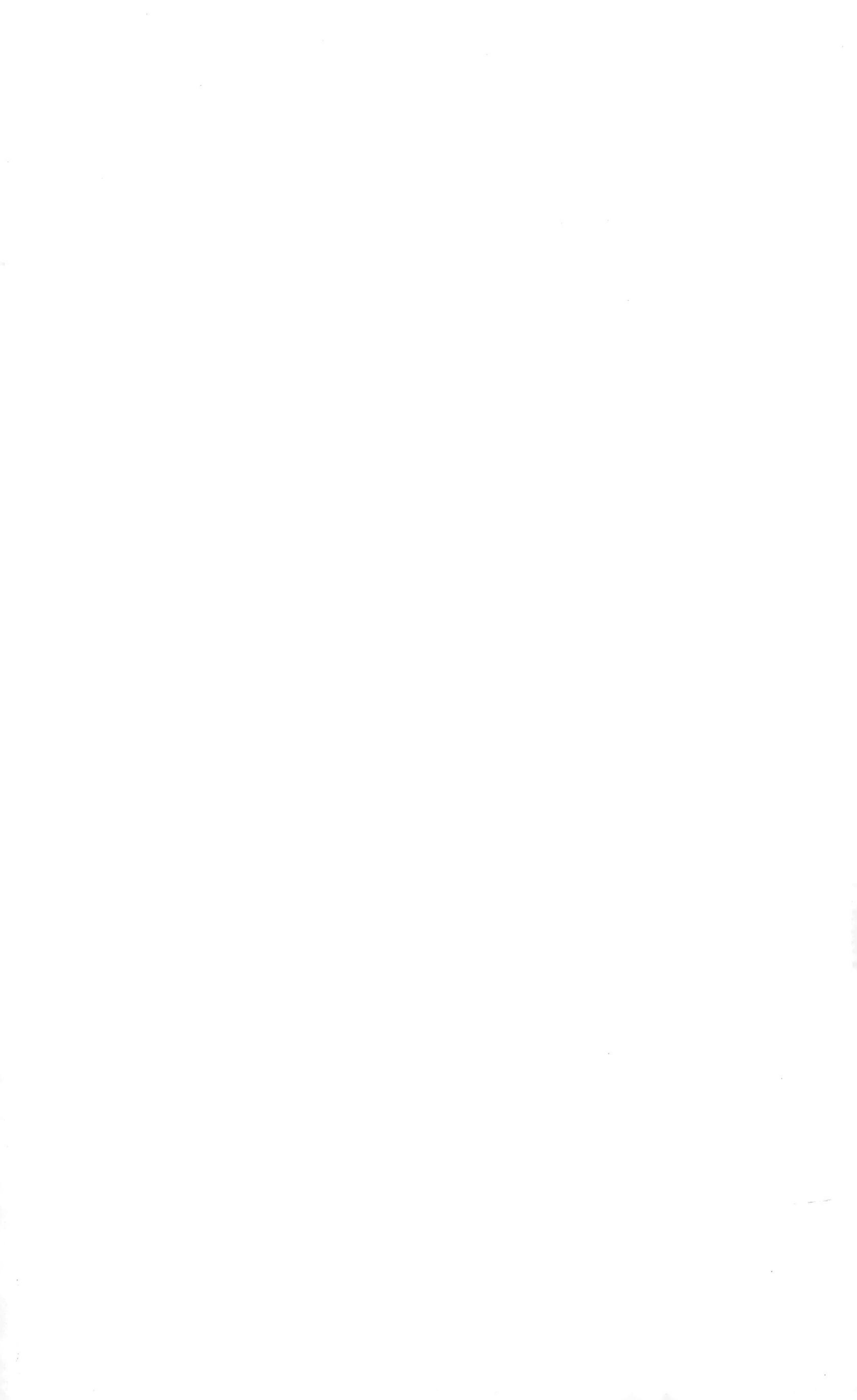